HEART TO HEART
Care for Your Heart Naturally

BY LETHA HADADY, D.AC.,
AND MICHAEL FOSTER

Heart to Heart: Care for Your Heart Naturally
Copyright© 2017 by Letha Hadady.
All rights reserved.

Above all else, guard your heart for it is the wellspring of life.

Proverbs 4:23

In the present is the past, in the present is the future.

Sogyal Rinpoche

WHY THIS BOOK NOW?

by Michael Foster

Your heart is a miracle. Its beating, which it does some 35 million times in a year, defines your being alive. Through a complex network of blood vessels that, if laid end to end, would extend 60,000 miles, your heart carries life giving nutrients to all your organs, muscles, limbs, and brain. Yet like most of us, myself included, you probably take your heart for granted—until it suffers an attack, failure, or just stops. Then you're gone. A few years ago I almost went over that hill.

During several precarious days and nights the medical staff at Dartmouth Hospital helped me pull through, though frankly not as deeply as the author of this book, Letha Hadady, who stayed by my side, sharing, worrying, reassuring each twenty-four hours. Once my struggling heart reached an equilibrium and I felt stronger, and a cardiac catheterization procedure was done to locate the blockage in my arteries, I was faced with vital decisions. My heart failure, which felt more like an attack, could be treated with a cocktail of advanced medical drugs, with the implant of stents, with arterial bypass surgery (recommended by one cardiologist), or even by a heart transplant (there is a waiting list). Still somewhat groggy and more learned in medieval history than human anatomy, how was I to decide? Fortunately, I had Letha by my side, and she has long studied, practiced, taught, and written about several healing traditions, and between us we made the right choice for me. These days I write books, exercise, and play the market as keenly as ever.

Heart To Heart is just that—an offering from Letha to the reader. It is a means to "Prevent and Care For Heart Illness Naturally" as the subtitle says. The book is packed with information about how to stay healthy, to favor instead of wearing out your heart. It offers the reader his/her choices of remedies from Traditional Chinese Medicine (TCM), Ayurvedic (Indian), homeopathic and Western holistic and complementary medicine. It is especially addressed to the sixty million caregivers in this country, who whether trained or just family are mainly women. There are numerous good books written by cardiologists, but they often seem to write to one another. Here, the caregiver is the audience—and the patient. Indeed, this is the first time the patient (namely me) is heard from in Realtime updates.

Reader, keep your heart happy. Listen to Letha and avoid becoming a cardio patient. But if it happens, keep *Heart To Heart* nearby. It won't kiss you like a partner, or purr and lick your hand like our two pet cats, but it's the next best thing for your heart ease.

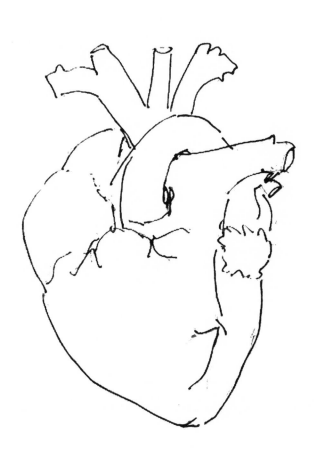

CONTENTS

Part Four: Looking at You

Part Five: Your Loving Heart

PREFACE

MY HEART AND YOURS

This book celebrates the long, productive lives of my love, Michael Foster, and my dear mother Letha Helen Hadady. They were both of great heart--generous and noble. Michael wrote brilliant biographies and novels for over sixty years. Many times we shared a look, a kiss and knew each others' thoughts. Michael took me to my first yoga class, encouraged me to study Asian medicine, and to write books.

Mother lived for her children. Self-sacrifice was her gift and pride; her home a gallery of her paintings of flowers and cherished family. Her generosity and sweetness were matched by a tenacity of spirit that kept her strong. Michael and Mother both had heart disease and refused heavy medication and surgery. Mother died quietly at home in her bed at age 93. Michael would have lived longer in the Vermont woods that he loved. But New York is home. He worked every day writing important books and at night trading stocks with the ebb and flow, and occasional crash, of the market, caring for us and his elderly wife. Natural remedies kept him comfortable and able to live a courageous, heroic lifestyle and a romantic sexual life until age 80.

American health insurance coverage is being hotly debated in Congress, and the elderly, poor and sick may expect cruel slashes in health protection. It is vitally important to realize that *prevention* is our best protection against illness. Wellness can and must be supported at home every day with love, patience and Nature's tools. This book will help you, your family and heart patient to work toward improved wellness. Michael wrote brief, delightful "Real Time" heart health updates for this book. He began this preface years ago:

"We'll have to admit you," said the nurse on the phone. "It's an emergency. They'll bring you in by helicopter." I'm Michael, and my partner Letha had just explained to the assistant of Dr. Alan Kono, senior cardiologist at Dartmouth Medical Center, that I had been unable to sleep for three days and nights and had difficulty breathing. I felt like I had been socked in the stomach. Previously, I'd had symptoms of minor heart trouble, and I did a yearly check-up at Dartmouth that included the usual blood tests, an EKG, even an echocardiogram. The latter, using Doppler ultrasound something like a submarine, shows your heart muscle working on a screen, pumping blood through the chambers and valves. It's a wonderful diagnostic tool but it makes me uneasy to watch the old ticker at work.

Until this summer my heart health checked out stable to improving. My blood pressure was under control, cholesterol nothing special, no chest pains. I particularly watched the "ejection fraction" from the echocardiogram, which told how well the heart was pumping blood to the body. I was approaching the normal range. Except for a vicious sweet tooth, my habits weren't harmful. I hadn't smoked in decades, drank a whiff of Bourbon before dinner. My success in avoiding heart failure was largely owing to Letha Hadady, an acclaimed writer and practitioner of natural health, who had me on a regimen of a heart-healthy diet and natural remedies. That and love had worked increasingly well until this financially disastrous year.

Letha, who had been urging me to speed-up my appointment at Dartmouth, made the call to Dr. Kono's office, and I was on the extension. It was close to the Fourth of July and the doctor was on vacation, but my symptoms were those of severe heart failure. Still I resisted the nurse's suggestion, thinking I was a pretty tough guy. My grandfather on my mother's side was the village blacksmith back in Russia and built like one. My mother's nickname on New York's lower East Side was "Little Stone," and my Dad was a Golden Gloves boxer. But I'd become soft and round, corrupted by a life of reading and writing books at a desk. As an AARP magazine headline declared: "Sitting Is the New Smoking." I gave in and agreed to get to the hospital early next day.

We were in our condo on Killington Mountain, Vermont, almost two hours drive east to Dartmouth Hospital near Hanover, New Hampshire. The usual procedure is for an ambulance to transport the patient to nearby Rutland Hospital and from there, if the case is serious enough, a helicopter flies him/her to Dartmouth. I hate to fly. So next morning, under hovering rain clouds, we drove through a thin mist, and at my insistence, I was at the wheel. The road was typical of Vermont, narrow and winding past woods and meadows with cows lowing in deep greenery among rolling hills. A couple of crows squawked and flew overhead as a farmer on a tractor pulled to the side, waiting for us to pass. I was wary of a sheriff whose car lurks behind a turn past Bridgewater Corners. He pounces on tourists for speeding, which means anything over 25 mph, and the fines keep the village going.

We passed a local brewery of whose Long Trail Ale I had fond memories. I wasn't paying attention, and the sheriff, parked ahead of his usual spot, nabbed me doing 35 mph. Looking at him standing by my windshield--overweight, face lined, paying the price of an unpleasant, sedentary job--I wasn't inclined to argue. Letha explained where and why we were headed, and the man's face lit up. "Why didn't you say so?" he exclaimed. No ticket, instead a sheriff's escort through the larger village of Bridgewater, after which we waved goodbye. Woodstock was next, and though the tourist Mecca could be busy at this season, I knew a short cut back of town. It was strange making this trip, which I usually drove toward the stately Dartmouth College library, but now tense, sick, I was concerned more about Letha, obviously worried, than myself. Edgar Allen Poe wrote, "There is no dying without a dying of the will." I believe that.

At Dartmouth Hospital we were fortunate to be installed in a single room with a view over the parking lot and out toward the woods. The helicopters came buzzing in every so often, reminding me there were others who, like me, hadn't expected to spend the Fourth of July in a hospital bed. My arm was soon hooked up to an IV tube descending from a stand, to which I would be wedded for the next few days. The doctor on call had listened to my heart through a stethoscope, remarking to a nurse, "His heart is galloping." I soon had sensors attached to my chest, and at a central station down the hall my heart beats were being monitored. A cart was wheeled in to check my blood pressure, breathing, and I knew not what else, and the day and night round of tests, taking of blood samples, being attached to gizmos, and swallowing unpleasant things had begun.

You will hear from me again, for the first time a patient tells how it feels in a book on heart health. I believe especially the tens of millions of home caregivers, whether relatives, friends, or employees, will appreciate this. Now, I turn the telling of the story over to the author, Letha. The threat of premature illness occurs too frequently, since heart attack/failure is America's number one killer for men and women. But it can also be a tale of hope and rejuvenation. Letha witnessed every moment. She slept at my side on an adjustable but uncomfortable couch, and she observed with a professional eye. While I remained conscious, the hospital stay and the excellent doctors and nurses came across as a surreal blur. After one difficult procedure I experienced temporary amnesia, not knowing who or where I was. Naturally impatient, as Letha managed me, I began on an inner dialogue: talking to my heart. Try it, get to know your heart. Learn what your most vital organ desires and needs and can't tolerate. Or you may find yourself in an ambulance or helicopter hospital bound, your life hanging on a wing and a prayer. . .

***

A few days earlier, while I was in New Mexico visiting my mother, who was past ninety and in fragile health, Michael had consulted a sports medicine doctor at a nearby clinic because pain and swelling in his foot made exercise difficult. Michael thought it was gout. But when I cut short my visit and flew back to Vermont, I saw that his spirits were low, both feet swollen, and breathing difficult. I realized the problem was his heart. The clinic doctor, without consulting Michael's cardiologist, had changed his blood pressure prescription, the only prescribed medicine he took, by *omitting* the diuretic drug that helped prevent heart failure. The result was almost final.

A major problem with modern medicine, though wonderfully exact and in many ways highly effective, is that it does not routinely take into consideration the entire patient but breaks up our body into medical specialties. To date, there isn't a viable universal computer data base of patient information from one clinic to another. Nowadays Facebook and Google may know more about us than do our doctors. Another problem is that the heart patient is typically hit with a barrage of highly technical tests often with little or no explanation of what they mean, how the results impact health, and how the prescribed heart drugs work. For practical reasons, such as a doctor's lack of time or staff, the patient is forced to accept medical advice on face value without taking part in the decisions concerning treatment or understanding what is involved. About half the patients stop taking their cardio medications, either because of troubling side effects, the expense, or the bother. Many harm their health and vitality by continuing a damaging lifestyle that led to their heart problems in the first place. Another issue is the marginal attention given to the day-to-day caregiver, whether spouse, relative, or nurse, usually female, sometimes unprepared to be a caregiver.

Michael had not been sleeping because he had difficulty breathing. The omitted diuretic drug would have helped prevent his lungs from filling with fluid, and the result was a crisis when Michael's overworked heart could not pump out the excess. When walking on the streets of New York, in which we spend most of the year, we had attributed his occasional shortness of breath to the ozone-polluted air. It's part of life in always interesting, densely packed Manhattan. Michael slept with several pillows and occasionally woke up with sleep apnea, common among older men with hypertension who are even slightly overweight. A carefully considered regimen of remedies, taken from my study of both Traditional Chinese and Ayurvedic medicines, had kept Michael's health improving despite age and overweight. However, during the Spring, when the price of gold suddenly plunged on the market, Michael lost a million dollars, at least on paper. This sort of thing had happened before, and his holdings had recovered, but such shocks came too often. I was alarmed, though Michael had no typical heart symptoms, neither chest pain, arm pain, or sudden rise in blood pressure. But I knew this was serious. For the lion-hearted, the heart is most at risk.

In polluted New York streets, Michael took a tiny Chinese herbal pill to help open his air passages, ease circulation and send more oxygen-rich blood through the heart. Driving to the hospital that morning I saw him reach for the tiny bottle of Suxiao Jiuxin Wan pills in his pocket. It smells fresh and invigorating because medical grade camphor, a main ingredient, dilates clogged blood vessels and cools the throat as it melts. Another Chinese herb, ligusticum, encourages heart action. The pill quickly eases discomfort when used in a small dose. Taken in a larger dose it can relieve chest pain during a heart attack. While driving to the hospital, Michael melted three tiny pills in his mouth and smiled at me.

I loved him during my entire adult life. We were together lovers forty years along with our cats, spending time in New York, midwinter in Miami and summers in Vermont, chasing fair weather. I knew his every mood, every tone of voice, every curve and wrinkle of his body. We were united by love and even by painful separations. We worked together on writing projects and critiqued one another's work. His heart was in my keeping a long time and I treasure our love.

That summer we drove from Killington to Dartmouth Hospital for checkups with one of the best cardiac teams in the nation. My many years of experience with herbal medicines and acupuncture, the five previous health books I have written, and a natural health practice that made it through the AIDS epidemic helped mount our defense. Natural remedies had helped prevent his heart disease for a long time, but chronic stress, sitting long hours at the computer, weight gain, age, and the ups and downs of a writer's life had temporarily won out. I urged Michael to stay on his blood pressure medicine but added herbal tonics to facilitate healing. According to "Diagnosis: Heart Failure," a special report from Harvard Medical School patients have a life expectancy of fewer than five years after onset of the disease. But heart disease begins years earlier. We build or harm health daily, too often ignoring warning signs, expecting emergency medicine to save us. I listen to my heart and respect its yearning: I send prayers to Michael every day and, when necessary, take Tibetan Precious Pills for my blood pressure. But you do not have to follow Buddhist teachings to benefit from herbal advice.

Stay well, stay strong. This book offers practical, natural alternatives, including diet, easily available natural remedies, and enjoyable lifestyle advice for prevention and complementary and alternative treatment of common heart ailments. However, a careful working explanation of the standard medical approach given here is also necessary to help heart patients and caregivers to understand and participate in healing. I appreciate the caring, professional work of cardiologists and related physicians and their willingness to share information that helps clarify the patient's point of view and responsibilities of the caregiver.

The biggest challenge of this book is neither the new material nor the natural methods to achieve wellness. The herbal medicines described here are researched by an international community and available from health food outlets and online. The biggest challenge of this book, and of your heart wellness, is to learn how to effectively pay attention to your body and with that observation to preserve wellness. Many of us seem to live our lives out in space caught up in thoughts, emotions, and our cell phones literally transmitting into space. Coming back to your body and to Nature will help you to feel real, will give you a solid basis upon which to heal.

The medical community does not entirely agree on the optimum practices for preserving the wellbeing of your heart. Many cardiologists believe that the main causes of heart disease are genetic disposition, overweight and/or diabetes, and an excessive buildup of cholesterol in the coronary arteries (especially LDL or "bad" cholesterol) that leads to fragile blood vessels and an eventual heart attack. Excess intake of salt and/or sugar is sometimes fingered. Our addictions to sugar, processed foods and stress, our obesity epidemic are large topics. The diet advice and herbal medicines described here will help you to gain vitality and heart health. You can find additional natural ways to maintain a healthy weight with my previous book *Feed Your Tiger*.

Several cardiologists featured in this book believe that cholesterol, which is produced by the body, is essential for general health and longevity and is an *indicator* of heart disease rather than a *cause* of its malfunction. Clearly, the heart is challenged by inflammation, an empty, high-caloric diet, and lack of nutrition at the cellular level. However, the many tests for heart health, and the resulting prescribed medicines, are complex, difficult to understand and come with risks and side-effects. Then there are the supposedly decisive cures of inserting stents and/or open heart surgery. It is not likely that you, patient or caregiver, presently have the grasp of information to choose your treatment modalities. But choose you must, or simply be led. Find out how your heart works and fine distinctions among various heart ailments in Chapter 4. More than this, observe your own heart health.

Heart To Heart uniquely offers you personalized guideposts at the end of each chapter called "Heart Health Checkups" to help you judge how you feel, how your heart is doing, and your best options for health and wellbeing. The Resource Guide at the back of the book and my website www.asianhealthsecrets.com offer links to many of the health products described in the book, in my writing and Net and live radio broadcasts. Ultimately, patients must decide on their correct health maintenance program. Aging Baby Boomers need special attention, as do the Millennials (sons, daughters) who often serve as caregivers. Many of us Boomers continue to lead a life full of experience, including travel, love, new work and new families. We live longer, have more free time, and chronic health concerns than previous generations.

Anyone, including children, can develop high blood pressure, which greatly increases the risk for heart disease and stroke, the first and third leading causes of death in the United States. A 2013 study in the *JAMA* (*Journal of American Medical Association*) magazine, reports hypertension and obesity are major instances where Boomer health falls short of our goals. Smoking, drinking, a diet high in animal fats, salt and sugar, and lack of exercise harm health and appearance. There is a better way.

While taking selected medicines, finding natural substitutes for others, Michael added heart supportive supplements and herbal remedies. That allowed him to increase his exercise and enjoy our deeply enriching sex life. Although health improvements are a changing process as new natural supplements become available, I knew that Michael could neither give up writing difficult, groundbreaking books based on years of laborious research nor his daily dealing with the ebb and flow of the stock market. Neither a fad diet nor a miracle herb of the week can fix a heart burdened with tiring work and worries. I, though younger, more fit, and food conscious, follow the same lifestyle as Michael and most of you reading this book. We need to care for our heart. Most people have no idea how their heart works or what personally threatens it. That is why we have written this book, a love story about health and happiness and a practical guide to realistic life choices to heal and protect your heart and loved ones.

INTRODUCTION

YOUR HEART IS YOU

Heart disease, our nation's number one killer for men and women, is found everywhere regardless of advanced age, sex, income and social status. According to recent data from Harvard Medical School, over 70 million Americans have high blood pressure, often the first warning of heart trouble, more than 7 million have suffered a heart attack, and another 11 million have other types of cardiovascular disease. But statistics, clinical studies, and global medical or dietary data cannot ultimately prevent heart disease: You have to become personally involved in supporting your healthy lifestyle.

Heart to Heart is both a comprehensive and intimate look at the personal causes of heart disease and what we can do to prevent illness, end suffering and stay well at home. It's our lifestyle and habits more than anything else that give us heart disease. We often make a typical disconnect: Heart attack happens over time when inflamed blood vessels clogged with cholesterol and toxins become blocked. Narrowed blood vessels starve the heart of blood and heart tissue can rapidly die. Our adrenal vitality can become challenged or there may be a hormonal or thyroid imbalance that provokes an irregular heart rhythm. Our experience or fear of heart attack is so dramatic and painful that we fail to make any connection between the incident and our everyday life.

Health troubles often come in bunches. A study reported in 2015 at the American College of Cardiology's annual scientific session exposed a causal link between heart disease and cancer. It's known among cardiologists that cancer treatments, including chemotherapy and radiation therapy, may lead to future heart damage, including weakened heart tissue or heart rhythm irregularities. New evidence shows that patients who survive their first heart attack are at higher risk for cancer overall, and lung and bladder cancer in particular. (1.) [The particulars of scientific studies, lists of select product ingredients and other such information are listed numerically and can be found at the back of the book in "Notes."]

Heart attack is sudden and can be fatal in minutes. Heart failure is often chronic, but one often leads to the other. Heart failure happens when blood backs up in a heart weakened by illness, chronic overwork, a rich diet combined with a sedentary lifestyle, severe blood loss, and physical or emotional trauma. Heart failure can occur when we least expect it. My aunt died suddenly the day following knee surgery. No doubt her heart had been checked prior to the operation. It's typical these days for doctors, if unwillingly, to send patients home the day following surgery. Hospitals may be crowded and understaffed. Patients are happy to go home, but for some it may be too soon so that complications set in. One young surgeon at a top American hospital told me, "Like it or not we doctors take orders from insurance companies."

It is better to prevent heart problems to avoid stents and surgery, but if surgery is necessary, we need to carefully prepare and recover. For one thing, chronic anemia, preventable with herbal remedies, dangerously weakens the heart and threatens survival. This book contains many valuable tonics that have been respected for generations as well as new concentrated extracts. Survival now more than ever requires planning, coordinated action of medical and natural healing professionals and lifestyle improvements. In 2017 I was pleased to attend a conference offered by my acupuncture alma mater and Sloan Kettering, a leading cancer hospital in New York, to learn they are using acupuncture for cancer patients to help prevent side-effects from chemo-therapy, depression, weight loss and other treatment-related trauma. One day, I hope the broader medical community will follow.

Heart disease is not what we're prepared for. Women dutifully check their breasts while in the shower and perhaps drink green tea. While we fear breast cancer, the numbers tell a different story. Yearly 40,000 women die from breast cancer and 300,000 women from heart disease. Relying too heavily on regular cholesterol testing, the modus operandi for many cardiologists, is controversial. I treat the issue in a several chapters, including "The Cholesterol Wars." If cholesterol is indeed a causal factor in heart disease, it is only one of the warning aspects of trouble. Most subtle signs of heart disease such as shoulder pain, swollen ankles, disturbed digestion, circulation-related jaw pain, and emotional imbalance often go unexplained.

Natural holistic medicine gives us a special window through which we can view disease. For example, Chinese acupuncture meridians for the heart run up the inside of the arm to the heart but are energetically paired with meridians located on the outside arm, shoulder, jaw and sides of the head. It is as though the outer energy of the heart is in our upper back. A relaxing shoulder massage can sometimes ease a tense heart by improving circulation in the upper chest, ease tensions, not to mention win approval from your heart-throb. A natural approach to everyday heart health stresses wholesome foods, exercise, appropriate curative herbs and relaxing revitalizing treatments. Fear and chronic anxiety, often underlying causes of heart trouble, are capable of leading to frozen circulation, emotional imbalance, relationship problems and worse.

I have met heart patients who, following a heart attack, are using the standard regimen of prescribed drugs. Their heart works more effectively, but traumatized by the experience, sedated by drugs that rule the heart's action, lacking vitality, they give up their revivifying activities--arts, sports, sex--nervously fearing another heart attack. Their heart has become a machine that works smoothly but feels no joy. Traditional Chinese medicine TCM doctors believe the heart to be the master organ that controls life and is the giver of joy. When the spirit in our heart (our *shen*) loses its bearings, our understanding of self and others, our emotional health and comfortable sense of well-being fall away. Everyday uncertainties, chronic stress, poor habits and pollution have created our heart disease. Overuse of antibiotics have created superbugs and genetically modified foods weaken immunity. We have lost heart—the courage necessary to live our life to the fullest.

This is my six natural health book featuring practical tips and expert advice from medical and alternative health sources. It takes a wider aim than most heart books because our wellness and joy reach for fulfillment and achievement. Speaking of ourselves or loved ones, we may touch our chest. Our heart's work is who we are. I am often asked about the effectiveness of a particular supplement or herb for various problems. However, for your heart there is no one simple answer. Modern medicine regulates the heart with drugs that stimulate its actions and prevent blood vessels from narrowing, drugs to eliminate sludge, stents to replace clogged parts, and electro-shock devices to keep its rhythm steady. But our heart, more than a pump, requires nourishment, rejuvenation and stress-relief derived from our healing lifestyle, a comprehensive individualized program of highly effective ongoing home treatments that comfort and protect you and those closest to your heart. We need to heal our heart at home.

Not everyone has the time, energy, or patience to absorb the complex aspects of heart illness and healing. For that reason I have created levels of information in this book. Many of you will enjoy reading the book's detailed information, including the referenced studies found in the Notes and Resource Guide. You, heart patient or caregiver, are strongly encouraged with a "Heart Health Checkup," located at the end of most chapters, to observe your heart daily in order to become sensitive to your wellness. If you want a quick answer to a pressing question along with a link to a helpful natural health supplement, that can be found at the end of most chapters in the sections called "Q & A." You might use that quick information guide on your cell phone or android anywhere.

As in all my books I describe many wonderful foods, herbal tonics, and rejuvenating techniques appropriate to your symptoms. The herbal medicines are easily available from health shops, pharmacies, and online from trusted manufacturers and huge distributors such as Puritan Pride, Vitamin Shoppe, Wal-mart and amazon.com. Do not be distracted by the wide array of easily available natural products described in this book. You cannot and should not use them all because your needs are individual. Keep it simple. Make small changes at first. Great benefits can occur from only one healing food or herbal if you give yourself fifteen minutes daily to sit quietly, breathe calmly, and visualize your wellness with a remedy that you make your own.

While writing this book I realized important differences not only in the medical approach to heart health, but in natural treatments. A Western naturopathic approach features supplements such as D-ribose, a sugar naturally occurring in the body, L-carnitine, a supplement used for weight loss, and Co-enzyme Q10. These are helpful, easily available energy supplements that work on a cellular level allowing the heart to better pump blood and relax. In addition, traditional Asian herbal medicines aim to rejuvenate the heart and improve digestion, reducing the effects of stress and inflammation that affect heart muscle and blood vessel tissue. An approach as ancient as the Vedic texts and the Chinese discovery of tea aims to guide the heart in ways that prevent illness and aging. There are many benefits derived from heart-oriented herbs for the entire body. For example, the Ayurvedic herb, guggul, a relative of myrrh, reduces harmful dietary fats, toxins, and phlegm creating the sludge that clogs blood vessels while it reduces body fat and fibroids.

Another thing to consider is that Asians traditionally use medicinal herbs in everyday foods without knowledge of scientific studies. Herbal teas, soups, even desserts have healing herbs easily found in Asian communities and online. One example is Guilinggao, a refreshing south China dessert, an herbal jelly and cooling/detoxifying medicine. This powder, made like Jello, contains anti-inflammatory herbs such as dandelion, honeysuckle, smilax, and sophora and is recommended to cure acne and itchy skin and urinary inflammation. Often served with honey or coconut milk after its jelled. Sinophiles love it especially in humid hot weather. There is laboratory research evidence that Guilinggao reduces heart cell death. (2.)

I am sometimes asked how to use certain high quality tonics that are hard to swallow, such as moringa bark powder from a tree that grows in Africa and is used medicinally throughout the Middle East and India as well. Friends have told me, "It tastes so bitter I can't use it." My own morning superfood pudding recipe is made adding moringa powder to nutritional yeast, chia seeds, bee pollen, olive oil steeped with fresh garlic and rosemary, a hint of raw honey, and water. In ten minutes the flavors blend and chia seed become soft. The high protein snack beautifies skin and hair, strengthens nails and nourishes internal organs. Another answer is to add moringa powder to warm water and soak your feet to absorb the vitamins, minerals and antioxidants and benefit from the anti-inflammatory, anti-cholesterol treatment. Or add the powder to ghee, clarified butter, and massage it into the bottom of your feet or use it as a skin moisturizer. We absorb herbals through our skin as well as from ingesting them. The same goes for the strong chemicals and preservatives used in skin creams, shampoo, and cosmetics.

I take my own advice when writing books. Using a dual approach by blending natural health treatments East and West we can achieve optimal heart health documented with modern heart testing. This approach of improving lifestyle is the basis of my final chapter, which covers your individualized heart health protocol. It relies on your guided self-observations done throughout the book. Whether you are a heart patient or caregiver, you can use simplified Asian diagnosis adapted for this book to choose positive lifestyle changes that insure wellness. The "Heart Health Check-up" at the end of most chapters is a simplified form of traditional Chinese medical diagnosis that helps us to gather information about the heart and allied organs. By participating in healing we develop courage and independence.

The Center for Disease Control and Prevention in Atlanta, in discussing our national heart problem, says "early action is key." For the CDC that means tests and treatments. But well known warning signs such as chest pains may come too late or not at all. Can you recognize that aching shoulders, shortness of breath, a grayish or reddish facial hue, or an unusually breathy vocal quality signals low vitality that affects your heart? Noticing such subtle changes in appearance and behavior gives us a great opportunity for improving heart health. A heart-healthy lifestyle rewards us with overall wellbeing. Many people live alone. We live longer and strive to remain active. Make your heart's work your life work, confident to accomplish your heart's desire.

A growing problem is a subtle killer called "broken heart syndrome." It resembles a heart attack but is actually an enlarged heart leading to heart failure. Brought on by chronic stress or grief, ninety percent of "broken heart" cases are women. Traditionally most caregivers are women. According to AARP a growing number, over 25% of caregivers, are millennials, most of whom have little experience in natural non-medical alternatives. This book may helps us to observe important symptoms, organize a health routine, and maintain heart wellness. Our heart likes regularity with calm, gradual lifestyle improvements that lead to a predictable positive outcome.

According to a Harvard Medical study some 65 million Americans are presently caregivers for their kids, a spouse, partner, or aging relatives. Researching heart remedies it became clear to me how our heartaches, like a subtle melody playing in the background of daily life, affect mood and actions. Together mind and body express the love in our heart as well as our vulnerability and frustration. I have rediscovered delightful natural treatments, including flower essences for long-standing emotional distress, that alleviate caregiver frustration and anxiety.

This book helps avoid herbal/drug interactions by describing when curative herbal remedies and rejuvenating tonics may either compromise your heart medicines or in some cases may replace them. Although not heart herbs per se, rejuvenating herbal medicines raise our level of wellness, resilience and courage. Nature's tonics also affect the emotional contents of our heart not just its structure and function.

Traditional Chinese culture has much to offer our health and wellbeing. Qigong and tai chi movement meditations, with highly developed styles, is practiced daily not only in China but many North American gyms, in parks, and community senior centers. I have adapted its simple, graceful movements so that you can enjoy this healing method in the comfort and privacy of your home. Opening our heart to universal energy known as qi is a source of inspiration and long life. Qi energy in the environment comes from air we breathe and foods we consume. Qi inside our acupuncture meridians keeps our heart beating and protects all aspects of health and wellness. We cannot live without the breath of life.

Illness may seem inevitable given our fast food, lack of exercise lifestyle, but heart disease and a broken heart can be avoided or managed by developing a greater love with care, patience, and the right natural remedies. One of my friends had a heart attack some years ago. She tried a few medicines but mainly recovered by having a practitioner give her healing touch. My friend was so impressed with the results that she became a Reiki master herself. She involved her husband in her healing practices and confided to me that otherwise they could not have stayed together. Many heart troubles are aggravated by anxiety, a feeling of hopelessness or isolation. The patient/caregiver relationship is an intimate bond, as important as our inner dialogue.

Are you listening to troubled mental chatter? Are you worried, depressed, frustrated with your life? Together we will protect our heart and capacity to love and live with confidence, creativity, and compassion. You may notice with your heart ease while using supportive remedies that you no longer feel so vulnerable or obsess over painful problems. You have better energy for work and pleasures.

That is because our mind and heart play in tune to our emotions and life issues. Heal your heart and change your life. Start by imagining your wellness. Give yourself the opportunity of radiant health, and we will take the road to heart wellness together.

Most of us take for granted that our stamina, courage, patience and mental clarity will serve us. But we need to take better care of our heart as we age and are challenged by illness, chronic pain, and stress. A low fat diet and exercise are not enough to insure health and happiness. The heart's energy system is a messenger that sends nourishment to every cell, maintaining the ebb and flow of fluids underlying life force. Our complementary medical approach to heart health stresses up-to-date medical testing and select natural treatments to speed healing. Some of you will add natural treatments from this book to your medical protocol, or you might drop certain medicines, with your doctor's approval, after discovering natural substitutes. I have a chapter that details natural drug alternatives and targeted information throughout concerning drug/herb interactions. Aside from lifestyle issues, unforeseen events can set off heart troubles. Even younger people or those who follow a healthy lifestyle can suffer illness, infections, and blood loss following an accident or surgery and other environmental factors.

How easy is it to add natural heart tonics to your life? Very simple. I enjoy eating seasonal heart healthy red and purple foods like watermelon in summer and pomegranate in the fall, fats from nuts and select omega 3 seafood. I drink tasty, slimming oolong tea. One of the best-known Chinese herbs for maintaining heart health without medical drugs is Salvia milt. also called Chinese red sage root or danshen. It comes in pills or powder but I like to soak a handful of the sliced dried roots steeped in a jar of spring water on my windowsill. I might add other tonics that are foods to the water such as goji berries and black cumin seeds (Nigella sativa) for enhanced energy and immunity. The sun makes a mild tea that gradually improves circulation and increases fluid to quench thirst. Another windowsill tea I love is made adding a handful of select Maine seaweeds to water overnight. It fills my bones with sunshine and mermaid songs, sea minerals that enhance vitality in every cell. Using herbs to benefit our heart increases courage and clarity.

It is good to know that we may feel protected despite life's shocks. Improve heart health and you enhance your capacity to love and live a fulfilled life. I may already know you from social media, my website, from my writings or Net radio interviews. Many of you live on the other side of the globe in Asia, Europe or Africa. We everyone share a common desire for wellness and wholeness. This book is a gift from my heart to yours.

Special Alert: What doctors don't take time to tell you

1. A pacemaker placed in your chest or abdomen can be thrown off kilter by someone near you using a cell phone or computer. Electromagnetic interference (EMI) a type of low-frequency electromagnetic radiation is emitted from virtually everything electrical and electronic in our modern world. (3)

2. Commonly prescribed heart drugs have resulted in memory loss, sexual dysfunction, kidney and liver damage. For statin drug users there is an increased risk of developing type 2 diabetes. (4)

3. Medical professionals are themselves at high risk of infections. It is estimated that over 60 percent of doctors and nurses have been exposed and may be carriers of drug-resistant super-germs.

4. Doctors, hospital administrators and insurance companies provide for treatments that are acceptable to Medicare (the government) and drug companies (big business.) Patient treatments may vary due to fear of non-payment or lawsuits. From a November, 2014 article in the *New York Times*: "Contracts for medical care that incorporate 'pay for performance' direct physicians to meet strict metrics for testing and treatment. . . that do not take into account the individual characteristics and preferences of the patient or differing expert opinions on optimal practice."

5. Doctor-speak based on research and test results and doctors who have no time to explain tests or test results make it difficult to communicate your degree of sickness and reason for treatment. When a doctor recommends an invasive treatment we assume the decision is based upon our test results but in fact the doctor may be simply following hospital policy regardless of your needs.

The bottom line

Although numerous treatments for heart disease, including heart attack, heart failure and other heart irregularities are effective and may be necessary to save your life, the final burden for prevention and health maintenance falls upon you the patient or caregiver. A serious illness is a wakeup call: You need to change your lifestyle by improving your diet, exercise, the way you handle stress, your emotional involvements, and your tools for enhancing immunity. This book provides trusted methods to maintain heart health, guided personal observations to chart your progress, and encouragement along the way. It offers a Patient- and Caregiver-Centered Approach to natural heart health.

PART ONE

BE A FRIEND TO YOUR HEART

Would you starve, exhaust or ignore your friend?
Age, Emotions, and Weather

ONE

EVERYDAY HEART CARE

They used to keep a caged canary in coal mines because as long as the bird sang the miners knew there was enough oxygen and no deadly methane gas in the mine. If the song bird died the miners had to run. A canary in the coal mine has become a popular financial and political idiom meaning a harbinger of the future. Our heart is like that canary because it signals our overall health and it can suddenly stop beating. The world would be a sad place without sunshine and bird song. We would be sad without friends. But most people do not know their best friend, their heart, neither how it works nor how to keep it well. We need clear directives for preserving the smooth flow of vitality and emotions, simple ways to enliven our day. Let us begin.

You may not be able to add all these heart healthy suggestions at once, but this is our aim: Start the day with an invigorating splash and heart massage. Enjoy a heart-wakeup breakfast. Spend at least 15 minutes during the day walking, and improve sleep and cushion your nerves with my simple breathing, stretching and heart-mind-centering exercises at bedtime.

1. A Power Splash and Heart Massage

Our lymph system collects toxins, cancer cells, and infection to be eliminated from our body. A lymphatic drainage massage reduces pain, swelling and water retention while it reduces impurities from the body. That allows your heart to work with more ease. There are lots of lymph glands located at the sides of the neck, upper chest and underarm. Swollen lymph glands and fever are a signal that immune cells are multiplying to fight off invaders, including bacteria, fungi, viruses or parasites that can harm the heart.

Before your morning shower, do a 5 minute lymphatic-drainage massage either with or without oil. Use oil during winter's cold, dry weather or if you have very dry skin. Olive and coconut oils are fragrant and cooling. Sesame oil is warming and relaxing. Add a few drops of Ayurvedic organic neem oil if you need to eliminate skin infections or rashes. Spread a little oil on your palms and lightly apply it with very gentle strokes from the face downward towards the heart and from the feet upward towards the kidneys and your lower back in order to stimulate lymph-cleansing. Spread the oil on your face lightly with your fingertips from the hairline to your mouth, from your face to your neck and top of your shoulders. Gently smooth the oil from your hands up the arms to your underarms, making circles on the breasts and stomach, and upward from the feet to the groin and hips. Light feathery strokes encourage the skin cells to eliminate excess fluid retention.

Massage these acupuncture points to improve circulation

Two acupuncture meridians on the inner side of each arm are located closest to your trunk and help to regulate heart action. Massage firmly on each inner arm for up to one minute while having relaxed, deep breathing. Start by rubbing together the palms of your hands. With the thumb of one hand massage the center of the palm of the other hand. Then reverse. That encourages stuck circulation away from your heart and out through your fingertips. Move the thumb up halfway to the inside elbow and massage a point between the wrist and the crook of the elbow. It may be painful so be gentle. Then firmly tap with your palm along the inner arm from the wrist to the underarm and firmly massage the underarm make circles as though creating a crevice in each underarm. The light stroking and tapping encourages lymph fluid to flow toward and into that crevice. Now take a warm bath or shower.

Do the King Kong

Remember the King of Apes? He was pretty tough and climbed to the top of the Empire State building. You too can have a big strong heart. During your morning shower, turn the water temperature to cold and let it run on your chest for a few seconds to awaken circulation.

Drum your thymus, an important gland located below the collar bone in front of the heart and behind the sternum or breast bone in your upper middle chest. It runs out of steam as we age which reduces our energy and immunity. The thymus is lymphoid tissue, tightly packed white blood cells and fat, and its function is to transform lymphocytes (white blood cells developed in the bone marrow) into T cells that protect immunity. T cells are transported to lymph glands where they fight infections and disease. But our T cell production is reduced by stress, illness and depression.

King Kong beat his chest to show his strength. Tap your chest just below the center of your collar bone daily to stay strong, awaken your sleeping thymus, end your shower and start the day. You might also run cold water for no more than 15 seconds on your feet. Cold water on the feet stimulates blood circulation in the head and chest. Later when we discuss energizing, detoxifying foot soaks, we will apply the traditional Chinese adage: "The feet are the second heart." After your bath or shower, towel dry your body and apply a few drops of an essential oil such as lavender to relax tension and balance heart action. Lavender both stimulates and relaxes heart circulation that can liberate sluggish vitality and what TCM doctors call "stuck" emotions. Think of it as obsession.

2. The Heart-Wake-up Breakfast

Don't skip breakfast. According to a July, 2013 report published in the medical journal *Circulation*, men who skip breakfast have a 27 percent higher risk of suffering a heart attack or developing heart disease than those who start the day with something in their stomach. "Men who skip breakfast are more likely to gain weight, to develop diabetes, to have hypertension and to have high bad cholesterol." (5) If you skip a healthy breakfast you are more likely to snack on junk or binge later in the day or evening. Our culture supports a gulp and go breakfast. Not a good idea. Chewing food sends a message to our brain to prepare our digestive enzymes to reinforce smooth digestion for our meals and for the entire day. You might chew some nuts with your smoothie or chew raw carrots and celery before eating a protein in order to prime your digestive enzymes.

Protein for breakfast

Eat a simple protein for breakfast or brunch in order to reduce muscle-wasting during morning hours. Avoid a heavy, hard to digest (meat) protein in order to reduce digestive and heart stress. What food offers high quality protein with slimming heart health benefits? Seaweeds. Nori is one third protein plus iodine that tones the thyroid to speed metabolism and enhance healthy weight loss. Nori is also a great source of micronutrients, containing more vitamins and minerals than most vegetables and fruits. It's a particularly full of vitamins B12 and more vitamin C than a comparable amount in an orange! It contains iron, calcium and zinc more omega-3 fatty acids than a cup of chopped avocado. Many people eat sheets of roasted nori with sushi, but that is a processed food. I prefer eating the real thing ordering my seasonal dried seaweeds from a pristine environment in Maine from theseaweedman.com.

What makes a tasty, slimming breakfast? Fresh fruit, tea and an organic boiled egg, chia seed pudding, or low fat, thick Greek yogurt spiced with curry powder or a dash of turmeric. To tone your digestion try a little dried dulse seaweed or pickled vegetables or a green apple. These health foods are sources of fiber, antioxidants and essential nutrients. I have several entire chapters that describe heart foods and herbs including recipes. In general, a heart-awakening meal includes stimulating bitter and sour flavors such as fresh dark leafy greens or dried tart cherries to eliminate harmful cholesterol and regulate water retention and heart rhythm. Chief among heart healthy foods is real tea (Latin: Camellia Sinensis.) Tea reduces absorption of dietary fat and harmful cholesterol in the digestive tract which makes it a perfect slimming food. You will enjoy discovering various types of teas, including my recipes for cooking with tea.

Before breakfast enjoy a liver-cleansing beverage such as warm water or tea and lemon juice. It helps to rid undigested foods and obsessive thoughts from the day before. Eat a ripe persimmon in season, fresh berries or grapes or mix a tall glass of pomegranate juice, 1 teaspoon of unsweetened cranberry concentrate, adding water to cut the sugar content, and a tablespoon of fresh organic lemon juice for liver cleansing. A persimmon has more fiber and valuable nutrients than an apple. Cranberry is diuretic (increases urination and is useful for urinary infections) and lemon is a source of vitamin C. Both reduce water retention to help normalize blood pressure.

You might have a whole grain cracker with your favorite oat breakfast cereal and non-dairy milk. Or enjoy a carefully chosen old favorite the egg. There are health benefits from eggs that may surprise you. An egg a day adds vitality and may improve memory. A chicken egg has protein, fat and carbohydrate a near perfect food with 70 calories. (Duck eggs have higher fat/cholesterol content and are nourishing for a dry, aging complexion.) Protein makes up our hair, skin and nails. Research from North Carolina State University shows that despite cholesterol warnings of the 1990s, the good old egg is still our friend. Eggs contain vitamin A, potassium and many B vitamins like folic acid, choline and biotin. Eating organic free-range eggs daily may reduce macular degeneration, blood clots, and breast cancers. (6)

There are caveats. Chickens regularly given antibiotics to prevent infections or bulk their weight potentially lead to drug allergies and stronger resistant bacteria in the chickens, eggs, the egg farmer and consumer. Free-range eggs actually show greater resistance to salmonella, but egg safety depends upon the clean environment and handling practices in which the chickens are raised. Please see my Resource Guide section at the back of the book for suggestions of safe farm-fresh foods that have been raised in a humane and sustainable manner.

Oils aid absorption

Absorption is another important health issue. As we mature, we require more dietary oil to improve absorption in the colon. An Asian cook might suggest starting the day with a teaspoon of sesame oil. I prefer taking my oils in capsules such as vitamin D3, hemp or flaxseed oil capsules and evening primrose oil, an anti-inflammatory supplement, together with breakfast. Or I might have a breakfast boiled egg garnishing with a pickled vegetable made with turmeric, salt, and pepper or a bit of Dijon mustard and a healthy oil such as grapeseed, pumpkin seed, or black cumin seed oil (Nigella sativa). Avoid oils such as corn oil and canola which quickly spoil. If you have a sodium restricted diet, add a dash of cayenne or curry powder or cooling spices turmeric and cumin and avoid table salt.

Chia power

If you don't cook, a high protein, energy-packed, super-healthy, slimming breakfast dish you might try is chia seed pudding. Chia seeds are found in your supermarket, health food store and online. To make the pudding just add water, tea, or milk substitute in a glass bowl to 1 tablespoon of chia seeds. It is only 70 calories. It bulks up with fiber to make you feel more full. Stir it once with a plastic spoon and again in 15 minutes and when the seeds absorb the liquid you have a pudding. Flavor it with spices, a fresh fruit, stevia, vanilla extract, your favorite juice or cocoa extract. Chia has two times more protein than most grains and five times more calcium than milk. Plus, it has high levels of omega fatty acids which are healthy oils, soluble fiber, potassium and anti-oxidants. You will enjoy the slimming benefits and easy, fast digestion. Foods are everyday protection against stress, illness, and aging. Part Two of this book will help you to find your best dietary heart remedies.

3. Walk, Walk, Walk

Whether we were meant to swing from trees or spend a lifetime in prayer our fragile hips and knees were not designed to sit at a computer day and night. Walk, walk, walk with a steady, easy rhythm to deepen your breath, bring oxygen to your muscles, and ease your mind. A slim volume called *Walking* was written by Henry David Thoreau (1817 –1862) the naturalist philosopher poet who spent entire days walking in the Massachusetts woods. He wrote, "I enter a swamp as a sacred place, --a *sanctum sanctorum*. There is the strength, the marrow of Nature. . . A township where one primitive forest waves above, while another primitive forest rots below,--such a town is fitted to raise not only corn and potatoes, but poets and philosophers for the coming ages."

Nature refreshes what is highest and most human in us. I have sat at the pine wood school desk Thoreau kept in his rustic cabin at Walden Pond while he translated the ancient Greeks. Grooves left by student's pencil marks are still there as well as the philosophy Thoreau practiced--simplicity.

Clear your mind of everyday chatter his way. In nice weather, get outside in the city and walk to the supermarket or post office. In the country walk around your garden or a local pond. If homebound, watch a DVD of ocean, mountains or other pleasant landscape while walking inside your home. Stand tall, swing your arms, and breathe the air of the great outdoors. If you use a stationary bike don't read or your blood will flow to your brain not your joints. You might hum your favorite music to steady your breath.

You can burn tummy fat after walking 30 minutes daily. Start by walking 15 – 20 minutes three times a week. Then increase to 30 minutes up to five times a week. The nineteen century Christian mystic and health expert Edgar Cayce advised: After breakfast to read a while, after lunch rest a while, after dinner walk a mile. In later chapters you will find out why it is so important to ground yourself, detoxifying your body and mind from harmful electromagnetic rays. So if possible, walk barefoot on grass, sand, wood floors or leather shoes. Let your heel strike the ground first, then roll from the heel to the ball of your foot. Push off with the ball of your foot for better momentum taking long, smooth strides. Brisk walking with natural, deep breathing improves circulation to protect your heart and memory.

4. Breathing for Life

Our muscles that support bones and enable us to sit, stand, and walk contain water and oxygen. Heart muscles send blood and oxygen wherever needed in the body. City dwellers, smokers, and people who breathe from the chest-up don't get enough oxygen. Asian health traditions such as yoga, tai chi and qigong have long recognized the vital connection between stretching the body along with deep, rhythmic breathing to achieve mental and emotional balance and muscle strength. In Part Four we will deepen our commitment to healthful breathing with natural treatments used to improve asthma and reduce chronic cough in order to protect the heart and enhance vitality and mood.

For now, try this simple exercise. Stand relaxed with both feet pointing forward spread slightly apart. Your jaw should be relaxed with shoulders soft, your back is relaxed and knees slightly bent. Allow your head to float above your shoulders. Place your palms together in front of your chest as though in prayer. This position aligns internal organs so that circulation is eased.

Now without making a sound breathe gently, slowly and deeply into the lower abdomen allowing the breath to warm your lower body. When you reach nearly full capacity, exhale with a quiet, long hiss. Exhale as though sending the air like honey melting down through your legs. Repeat this several times and imagine how your breath, a column of air, connects your head with the sky and feet with the earth. If you feel dizzy, sit down, relax and, if comfortable, try the exercise sitting in a chair. You may also want to try this breathing exercise while lying in bed. Reduce back pain by placing a round pillow under the arch of your neck and behind the knees in order to support a healthy spinal curve. Do not force your breath.

The point is to gain an even, steady relaxed breathing rhythm that eases tension. You may feel that your back and neck find a new comfortable position. Don't allow your jaw, shoulders or legs to stiffen. If troubling thoughts arise during the exercise let them dissolve. With this simple qigong breathing practice, we are not trying to exercise or solve problems but only to relax and deepen the breath so that oxygen is available to nourish every cell.

5. Stretch for Comfort

Your shoulders and neck are connected through acupuncture meridians to your heart so anything you can do to relax them, ease tension, and deepen breath will help remove stress from the heart. One of my favorite stretches is done while standing to avoid interference from our large white cat Fluffy who likes to jump on my chest. You might do this stretch standing next to your desk. Put your arms behind your back and interlock your fingers to open the chest. Relax the shoulders and neck and comfortably bend forward inhaling then backwards while exhaling slightly through the mouth. Breathe comfortably. My favorite stretch is passive. I lie on top of a soft rubber ball with a diameter of about 7 inches placed between my shoulder blades in order to open chest circulation and reverse computer crunched shoulders.

Try not to make a big deal about exercising. If you live in a city you can often see someone doing a Chinese qigong exercise such as walking in a park, standing on a porch or in a city street with his arms open wide allowing qi energy to penetrate his heart. He may be walking along smiling, seated or standing. It's perfectly natural and enjoyable to welcome a garden or a lovely friend into your open arms. Welcome a healing breath.

6. Comfortable Sleep or Rest

Sleep is so important for healing that I am putting it up front so you can't miss it. There is a section covering heart-safe herbals for insomnia in Chapter 5, however it is best to achieve adequate sleep without drug- or herbal-dependence. Over time they might weaken the heart. Most experts agree that seven hours is an optimum night's sleep. If you can't sleep, experts recommend lying in bed quietly resting. That would drive some of us crazy. But relaxing in bed is still better than taking a sedative. Try deep breathing, listening to music or reading to relax. You might also use a heart-rhythm normalizing herbal pill such as danshen wan made from Salvia miltiorrhiza which you will read about later.

Here is how the mind/body creates insomnia. First you feel a discomfort. The bed is lumpy, the room temperature is too cold or hot, or your stomach is upset after eating so that you are tired but awake. There are a million reasons why you might have a dream or turn in your sleep and wake up. The discomfort provokes a memory. You awaken more thinking about the memory. The interruption of sleep increases discomfort in the chest, jaw or shoulder pain or indigestion for example. You are awake, uncomfortable and thinking. The worst thing you could do is take a sedative because that supports a pattern of imbalance that weakens vitality and heart health. A big part of insomnia is our overactive mind. How can we stop mental chatter without sedating the heart?

A homeopathic remedy to correct insomnia

Homeopathic coffee (Coffea cruda 6x to 30C strength) is recommended to reduce the effects of caffeine-like stress including hypersensitivity to noise, pain, weather and nervous insomnia. There may be neuralgia and overactive mind from sudden emotions and nervous heart palpitation. Many coffee and tea drinkers can benefit from this remedy that takes caffeine out of the body. Always use homeopathic remedies as directed, separated from food, drink and toothpaste by two hours.

Acupressure for insomnia

Two acupuncture points may be stimulated with massage and essential oils in order to slow mental chatter that keeps us awake. Do not worry about finding the exact point because pressing and holding the area is often sufficient. Acupressure helps you to observe your energy. Use this natural method to feel comfortably relaxed.

One area to press is on the inner crease of the wrist, where the hand bends inward, and below the little finger. Points located at the inner side of hand and wrist affect heart rhythm and can moderate an anxious heart. With the thumb of one hand press and hold the inner crease of the wrist of the opposite hand. Hold to the count of ten. Breathe slowly, calmly and let your mind go blank. Imagine your mind emptying from your head downward through your fingers as you breathe.

The other point is on top of each foot near the space between the second and third toes. That area corresponds to a meridian that begins in the face and moves downward to the second toe. Pressing that area of the foot tends to moderate an over-active energy and hyper emotions. Pressing there may feel calming and help to deepen breath. Let your troubles leave through your toes.

The Heart Mudra

Here is another ancient method still used today by people who practice yoga and meditation. A mudra is a hand position often used before or during meditation and prayers. It helps us focus our breath and thoughts. A mudra also engages our deep meridian energies in ways to achieve mental, physical and emotional harmony. Each fingertip is the end of an acupuncture meridian. By holding a mudra we engage those meridians, allowing vitality to circulate freely and encourage relaxed mental focus. Try it while breathing deeply, softly and listening to the sounds of a waterfall, a singing bowl, chimes, or soft music. Don't expect to empty your mind completely. That takes practice. You may remember things to do while holding the mudra, but note them for later. Allow your schedule to empty. Mental house-cleaning encourages clarity as troubling emotions become pale and distant–washed away with breath.

See the illustration of the Heart Mudra. It looks like a flower bud opening.

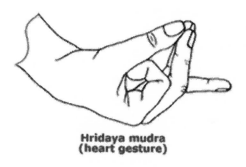

**Hridaya mudra
(heart gesture)**

Imagine yourself in the middle of the soft, fragrant flower. Sitting comfortably or lying on your back, breathe into your lower abdomen. With each hand, place the tips of your thumb, third and fourth fingers together as shown. Curl the pointer finger and place it to rest on the thumb. It is the green sprout inside the opening bud. The little finger is free, pointing away from the palm. That is where heart tension escapes from the body. Continue to breathe softly and allow the lovely opening flower to create peace.

In Chinese medicine, the tips of the thumb and pointer finger correspond to acupuncture meridians of the lungs and large intestine our pathways to breath and detoxification. Bringing together the thumb with the middle fingers joins earth and spirit to the air that fills us and surrounds us. You are made of earth and spirit blended in air.

The mudra reminds us of our choice of health and high intensions, the opening flower. Enjoy it.

You will notice that my daily approach to heart health is simple, just a cold splash and light massage, a healthy meal, walking, and some relaxing breathing practices. Simplicity is key to enduring good health. Take one new step at a time, develop the habit that becomes a part of your daily routine. A week of crash dieting or occasional aerobic exercise soon becomes a chore that has little effect.

Heart Health Checkup

Here is your first self observation on your path to improved heart health. It concerns your breathing impacted by lifestyle and pollution.

- Do you smoke or live and/or work in a polluted environment?
- Do you have dry or chronic cough or chronic thirst? Is your tongue red and dry indicating internal inflammation and dehydration?
- Do you have chronic fevers, menopausal hot flashes, or night sweats? These may be increased by diabetes, feverish illness or spicy or inflammatory foods and alcohol. Lung dryness and irritation increase stress, anxiety, arterial inflammation and atherosclerosis also called hardening of arteries.

Quitting smoking, avoiding smokers and as much as possible limiting your exposure to pollution can save your life. After Michael had several days of medical testing at Dartmouth Hospital, he and I slowly walked down the corridor of the cardiology department for exercise. A sickly looking man with a grayish complexion huffed along to catch up with us. This was his second heart attack he said, "I have smoked for thirty years." I could not help but think, "Strike three and you're out."

I asked a cardiologist on duty whether there were more men or women hospitalized with heart trouble on the cardiology floor at the time. He hesitated saying it varied, one week more men another week more women. When asked the number one reason they were there he didn't hesitate a moment and replied, "Smoking."

Cooling, moistening foods nourish lung tissue and help reduce cigarette craving. Eat more asparagus, cooked oatmeal, and greens. Chew a carrot, celery stalk or a cinnamon stick instead of a cigarette. Cinnamon is spicy sweet and helps support blood sugar balance for diabetes. Get acupuncture to stop smoking and ease nervous tension. Don't try to quit all at once. Take a yoga class or get massage to help you relax. Cut your smokes in half. Heat and dryness from smoking a pipe, cigarettes or marijuana are inflammatory to endanger blood vessels and increase dry cough, thirst and parched skin.

Whether or not you currently smoke, here is a lung-soothing detoxification plan to get you on a path to overall physical and mental health.

1. Try to build a rhythm of wellness. If possible, get up and go to sleep at regular times so your body and mind get used to rest. Listen to relaxing music and breathe.

2. Eat real food. Chapters in Part Two describe cooling foods.

3. Try a new beverage, a juice or tea or other non-soda drink, not your usual beverage after which you are more likely to crave a cigarette. In other words break old habits of association like smoking a cigarette along with a meal, while reading the paper or the TV news.

4. Wash your clothes, linens, drapes, furniture covering, rugs as much as possible to remove the smoke stink or else you will crave what you smell.

5. Move the furniture around so that you get a new view of things. That helps break old habits like reading the paper with a cigarette and coffee.

6. There are lots of stop-smoking aids such as patches, pills and smoking substitutes. You will need something to help with withdrawal, to quiet your nerves as you detoxify body and mind from your habit and your polluted environment. This can also make all your lifestyle improvements easier. Ease Plus pills

are made by Health Concerns, a California company that uses traditional Chinese herbal formulas made under strictly controlled safety conditions. Ease Plus, a vegetarian formula, has been proven effective for improving insomnia, nervousness, headaches and mood swings and withdrawal from tobacco, drugs, medicines, and other addictive substances. It treats gastric acidity, ulcers, hiccupping and belching. It is wise to start slowly with two pills with or without meals and increase to the recommend dose when comfortable. If you are pregnant, avoid this as well as any laxative such as rhubarb or act according to the guidance of your health advisor.

Q & A: Addictions and Substitutes

I want a healthy substitute and a natural treatment for my addictions:

Sugar and sweets – *stevia reduces harmful cholesterol and replaces sugar*

Salt – *dried dulse seaweed, powdered cumin, coriander and turmeric*

Alcoholic drinks – *Party Night capsules, a combination of liver-saving supplements:* http://www.absorbyourhealth.com/product/party-night/?ref=4041

TWO

HEART HEALTH WARNINGS

Some people can smell rain and feel the barometric pressure drop as their muscles stiffen and joints ache from an approaching storm. That's the time to grab your rain gear. By paying attention to details, we avoid getting drenched. However, by the time we experience the typical signs of heart trouble it is already late in the game. Doctors warn us to pay attention to chest discomfort, arm pain, and shortness of breath because they are dramatic signs of heart disease. Because blood flow may be greatly reduced these are signs of an attack on the heart itself. Much of modern medicine is based on warlike tactics. We explode harmful cholesterol with drugs, prop-open blood vessels with stents, and using emergency measures prevent heart tissue death that happens within minutes of a heart attack. This saves lives when prevention is too late. In addition to this chapter, to learn the difference between angina, which is chest pain, and heart attack, to understand how blood pressure readings measure heart health, see Chapter 4. "Heart Works."

Heart attack symptoms must be taken seriously. Call 911 as soon as possible. A matter of minutes in delaying treatment can cause death when a fragment of cholesterol breaks away from inside a blood vessel to choke off circulation. That problem most likely took years to develop and there were warnings that the patient, his family and doctors failed to recognize or adequately treat.

Presidential Stress Imbalance

Photos of former President Bill Clinton taken before his heart attack and stents show an overweight, tired looking man who enjoyed eating hamburgers. He lost 25 pounds after changing to a vegan diet in order to recover and prevent future heart episodes. Bill, prior to diagnosed heart trouble, had excess fat at the waistline, had a puffy face with bags under the eyes from chronic water retention. Former President George W. Bush, in 2012 before his heart episode and stents, had a flushed complexion and looked tight-lipped and tense. Since retiring, G.W. again has his handsome, relaxed smile and he exhibits his paintings. Some have linked President Donald Trump's rotund shape to his diet of burgers and fries. Our digestion processes our food as well as mental clarity and emotional balance. No one expects presidents to look healthy: Their job requires the utmost in personal energy and sacrifice. Anyone with a demanding life should take special care of their heart. My motto is: The larger the waistline the shorter the lifeline.

This chapter describes important warning signs typically unrecognized by modern Western medicine. There was a time when people regularly took time to observe how well their body looked and felt. They avoided extremes in diet and fatigue, they examined the contents of their mind and the reach of their spirit. You will be given that opportunity throughout this book.

Let's face it: we spend more time looking at a computer or caring for our car than observing our health. Most of us living a busy life do not consult a doctor unless we feel urgent discomfort. We ignore a backache or blame the weather or arthritis. Life-threatening heart symptoms, such as sudden, severe long-lasting sharp pain in the center of the chest, gasping for breath and swollen ankles, are cause to call 911. Those are not everyday little discomforts, indicating heart issues. We will pay attention to heart symptoms that can be prevented, the discomforts we most often ignore.

From a holistic view our heart is subject to our digestion, adrenal vitality, hormones, and emotional balance. For example, the heart needs hormones and enzymes regulated by the adrenal glands and liver to help maintain healthy water balance in the body. Diuretic and other drugs prescribed for hypertension, because they affect the liver, need to be monitored for liver and kidney damage. Over time, these organ malfunctions become as important an indicator as chest pains. More than likely your doctor will give you a barrage of tests. They may be required because of age, infection or injury affecting the heart.

Warning Signs of Heart Troubles (Traditional Asian Medicine)

At home, before medical testing, there are a lot of signs we may observe for ourselves and our family that indicate our heart health. That is a great strength of Asian medicine. At the end of most chapters you are given guidelines for self-observations. As you get to know your energy, the imbalances you find will make sense. You will be better able to predict your vitality level and adjust habits accordingly. I have a shorthand version of these observations in this chapter. Call it a ten minute "heart selfie." or what to notice daily. To help recognize health issues that indirectly affect the heart I have included a couple of examples along with a simple flash remedy to improve the symptoms. The main points to notice are:

- Waistline and "love handle" fat
- Adrenal weakness: severe back and leg pain, shortness of breath, poor hearing, poor memory, disturbed sleep
- Troubled digestion: burping, bloating, constipation/diarrhea
- Fluid imbalance: swollen face, belly, hands or feet
- Physical and emotional vulnerability: depression, anxiety, oversensitivity to weather

Belly Fat

Age and a sedentary lifestyle cause an increase in fat around the waist and an increase in harmful triglycerides, the dense fat that is hard to lose and clogs circulation. Experts advise that women and men who are overweight should monitor their waistline as a potential danger to heart health. An acceptable measure for women is a waistline 35 inches or less and 40 inches or less for men. You can measure your BMI ratio of fat to body weight later in the book. For now notice where you collect fat and start to take steps to lose pounds as necessary. For example, cut back on sugar, extra salt, sodas, alcohol, processed foods, and sweets and increase exercise.

Adrenal Energy

Your adrenal glands float on top of the kidneys near the level of your waist in your lower back. Adrenal vitality is necessary to energize the heart, supply needed hormones, and insure proper circulation. If adrenal energy is weak, heart muscle becomes weak, blood backs up in the heart and fluid in the body. In extreme cases of weakness or blockage, blood flow supply is reduced for the brain and could lead to muddled thinking or stroke. Healthy people can usually rebuild their strength after illness or exhaustion by resting and eating nourishing foods. Most of us experience discomforts from jet lag, overwork, or when taking certain medications for blood pressure or diabetes. However chronic adrenal weakness can eventually aggravate circulation problems. Here is an example.

Terry is overweight especially from the waist down. Her face and hands are puffy from excess water. During the day she is lethargic. She cannot sleep at night because she has leg cramps, has to urinate and often stays awake doing crossword puzzles or playing computer games. She feels weak much of the time with a backache and sore legs. She is short of breath when climbing stairs or walking her dog. She has developed hypertension and can't always remember if she took her medicines. When tired she is weepy and withdraws from everyone. Generally we feel stronger, less vulnerable, and more capable of dealing with life when adrenal energy is adequate.

A flash remedy for adrenal wipeout is an adaptogen, a general tonic that supports internal organs and vital processes and reduces the effects of fatigue and stress. For example, ashwagandha a great Ayurvedic tonic herb used to rejuvenate muscles, nerves, and reduce mental and physical exhaustion. Terry could take capsules available from health food stores or she could add ¼ of powdered ashwagandha root to warm water and (optional) a little raw honey.

A tonic may not be enough to correct long term water retention. Another important consideration is that despite having no urinary discomforts a heart patient may have cardiac edema which is fluid backed up in the heart. Chinese Wu Ling San capsules address this sort of edema very well. That classic vegetarian formula made from digestive and diuretic herbs is recommended for general edema (body swollen with water retention), cardiac edema, heart failure, dizziness, swollen waistline from liver disease. It reduces bloating while improving energy. Consult an herbalist trained in traditional Chinese medicine before adding any such herbal supplement.

Our heart and circulation impact our appearance and personality in many ways. Hormone imbalance or excess plaque buildup may look red, inflamed and feel hot. Here is an example. Natalie was a go-getter. She lead workshops, traveled to give lectures, and promoted her slogan: "My hot flashes are power surges!" Her tongue was red and dry with a grayish coating, signs of chronic inflammation affecting internal organs including the heart. Her voice was strident and manner brusque. Her complexion was oily and ruddy and her hair was becoming thin. She had arthritis. Acidity, plaque, and inflammation were jamming her circulation, digestion and elimination. She had an odor of burnt paper and projected high enthusiasm bordering on chronic hype. Eventually she had a stroke.

A flash remedy for chronic inflammation, dehydration and hormone imbalance might contain berberine an anti-inflammatory chemical for example coptis sinensis. But that herb is very bitter and not a common household herb. An easier everyday remedy is aloe vera from the health food store. Drinking up to ¼ cup of aloe juice is soothing and alkaline for the digestive tract, which improves constipation, body odors and complexion blemishes. It cools by reducing excess acidity. Evening primrose oil capsules, recommended for acne and arthritis, also reduce inflammation markers affecting blood vessels.

PAD

A special case is PAD, peripheral artery disease, corresponding to a build-up of plaque impairing circulation in the legs. If you sit at a desk all day and eat animal fats for protein, check out your legs for signs of this illness right now. The main symptoms are leg discoloration and leg pain following exercise. Other common symptoms include cramping in thighs or calf after walking or climbing stairs. Also leg numbness, shiny reddish skin on legs, leg or foot sores that don't heal, a weak pulse in legs or feet, and erectile dysfunction in men. If peripheral artery disease progresses, leg pain may occur when lying down and it disrupts sleep. Walking around the room may temporarily relieve pain but that is not enough. PAD is not considered heart trouble by Western medicine, but excess plaque collected in leg veins known as PAD indicates a risk of stroke.

You can see that heart and circulation troubles usually take a long time to develop and many signs go unnoticed so it is a good idea to stress prevention no matter whether you are officially considered at risk of heart trouble or not.

Who is considered most at risk of heart attack?

Allopathic Western and Holistic medicine more or less agree on these factors:
- Men over 45 and women over 55
- A Family history. Having a father, brother or grandfather who had a heart attack before age 55 and/or a mother, sister, or grandmother who had a heart attack before age 65. But family histories are impacted by diet, attitude and habits.
- Race. African-Americans typically have higher rates of heart disease and stroke but racial profiling may be related to poverty, depression, abuse, poor dietary habits, and other social factors.
- Lifestyle health factors such as high blood pressure, high cholesterol, diabetes, smoking, unhealthy diet, extra weight, and physical inactivity are key factors.

Heart troubles around the world

The more you acquaint yourself with medical traditions stemming from other countries, the more you find that illness is, at least in part, defined culturally. In Latin America being plump is desirable, attractive, a sign of wealth. In modern India you will find kids wearing jeans carrying cell phones. However traditional Indian medicine, Ayurveda, suggests that the cause of heart disease comes from our emphasis on personal achievement, competition, financial survival and material wealth which leads to broken hearts or spiritual starvation. Heart diseases reflect deeper issues of identity, feeling and consciousness. In other words, hearts fail from stress and spiritual neglect as well as from a diet of sweet and salty food, animal fats and fried food. Ayurveda recommends lifestyle changes aimed to connect us with our feelings and enhance deep-relaxation, including yoga and meditation, also cleansing and rejuvenating health practices, as well as highly effective herbs, we will study later, that regulate cholesterol and support blood vessel health.

Traditional Chinese medicine TCM teaches us to protect our qi or vital energy and immunity. Eating unwisely, ignoring inclement weather and germs and exhausting our sexual vitality weaken qi energy that activates our organs, moves our blood, and keeps us alive. Qigong exercise aims to build vitality and longevity.

Emotional problems play a role in heart disease and should also be considered in acupuncture and herbal treatments. Herbs are chosen to relieve chest oppression, enhance circulation, reduce cholesterol, reinforce the elasticity of blood vessels, correct anemia, increase adrenal vitality, and reduce inflammation as needed. One main difference between a Western and Eastern medical approach is that herbs, like foods, do not take over the work of the heart, as drugs do, but support the heart's actions, stimulate metabolism and eliminate toxins that cause congestion pain. Chinese herbal doctors may diagnose by observing chest pain along with other conditions. For example, they will look at the tongue and observe various pulses at the wrist for what they call phlegm and/or blood stasis symptoms. You are not normally expected to notice such problems. It takes years to become a good doctor or any alternative health practitioner because it requires sensitivity and experience. Here is what they are looking at.

"Phlegm" and "Blood Stasis"

Phlegm (roughly translated as dampness or in Chinese *she* pronounced back in the throat like grrr) is a complex concept in TCM. For a picture of phlegm imagine your difficulty slogging through a knee-deep swamp while wearing heavy weights on your legs. Phlegm feels like heaviness of limbs, water retention, and thick mucus congestion resulting from slow metabolism, excess dietary fat and sweets, lethargy or damp weather. A large waistline indicates we have trouble processing fats, sweets, and sedating foods. In other words, our digestion cannot adequately handle foods that increase phlegm, dampness, water retention etc. If you have chest pain along with a thick tongue coating then what the Chinese call dampness or phlegm is impairing circulation and digestion. This flash remedy is slimming dietary advice for reducing tummy fat and harmful cholesterol: sliced raw or lightly steamed zucchini squash and chopped chives. Notice they are bitter and pungent foods, not sweet and rich.

Blood stasis presents another picture that suggests blood is not moving freely through blood vessels. Imagine squeezing a tube of toothpaste so that toothpaste can't move through the tube. If blood stasis is caused by weakness (qi deficiency) symptoms will include fatigue, a wan or sallow appearance, shortness of breath, palpitations and chest pain, a purplish tongue may have a coating or a thin or no coating, and an uneven pulse. To correct underlying weakness and get blood moving again, stimulating tonic herbs that affect the heart such as tienchi ginseng (AKA tianqi, sanqi, notoginseng) are used. The single or combination herbal formula used should reflect your individual needs observed by your herbal doctor.

A typical herbal formula used to correct poor circulation stirs up toxins and eliminates them. It may include a vitality tonic such as astragalus root (huang qi) which supports immunity. Other ingredients will include blood tonics such as tangkuei (dang gui) and semi-sweet flavored ligusticum. Red peony root (chi shao), herbs that clear inflammation in lungs and liver, laxative peach kernel (tao ren) and diuretic herbs are used to eliminate fluid. Carthamus flower (hong hua) a medicinal form of safflower enhances circulation. Visits to your herbal doctor can keep you on track for your heart herbs. The ingredients and dosage should vary as your condition improves. You can see that holistic medicine comes in the side door to treat heart troubles by improving vitality, digestion, circulation, and water balance.

Heart Health Warnings: Your Tongue

Your tongue is an internal organ you can easily observe and adjust your diet accordingly.

If your tongue is large or scalloped around the edges indicating water retention and if it is coated indicating phlegm, cut back on salt, friend foods, unhealthy fats including meat, cheese, and sweets because they slow digestion and increase phlegm. Continue an anti-phlegm low fat, high fiber diet until there is less coating on the tongue and your energy improves.

If your tongue looks mauve or red purple you have stuck circulation (what Chinese doctors call "blood stasis") that needs to be addressed most likely with medical as well as holistic health checkups. To help nourish the body as you lose excess weight, you might take 2 – 3 alfalfa pills or capsules with meals until your tongue becomes a pink color. Alfalfa supplies minerals and is an alkalizing green food.

What not to do

When using herbal remedies for prevention or treatment of heart health, don't medicate yourself without consulting an herbal expert who can advise you and follow-up with regular visits in order to maintain optimal energy and immunity. In *Heart to Heart* many useful traditional foods and easily available herbal tonics and cooking herbs are explained. You can use them with confidence, but the best medical herbal formula for you should be individualized and changed according to your symptoms, age, health conditions and seasonal climate changes.

Can you increase your chances of developing heart discomfort by making wrong natural health choices or using remedies at the wrong time? Yes. It seems obvious but sometimes we forget that any supplement taken at the same time–herbs, vitamins, minerals, foods, drugs, etc.,--becomes a *combination* remedy. Here is an example of how things can go wrong.

Arthur, a seventy year old overweight heart failure patient takes diuretic medication and herbs to control high blood pressure. He has no symptoms that indicate heart trouble and his yearly echocardiogram test shows improvement. He gets little exercise and eats sweets and salty cheese daily. It is winter and he feels weakened by cold weather and fatigued from his desk job. People sneezing in the office near Arthur make him feel anxious about catching a cold so that he takes an over-the-counter cold pill containing echinacea and elderberry, herbs which increase sweating. But, to save time, he takes the diaphoretic (sweat-inducing) cold pill at the *same time* that he takes his heart medication and heart health herbs.

The heart does not and should not sweat. Mixing remedies for such unrelated problems as colds and flu and heart action is a bad *combination* that confuses the body. (The sweat-increasing supplement is taking energy away from the heart at a time it is vulnerable.) Arthur quickly becomes nauseous and feels a lump in his throat as his chest circulation becomes stuck. He can't swallow and has difficulty breathing. He has cold sweat and feels weak. His legs feel numb. He panics and tries to vomit but can't. Is he giving himself temporary heart trouble?

It is possible to stress the heart especially of a weak, elderly patient so that an arrhythmia problem can result. Luckily I was able to help Arthur by rubbing acupuncture points in the legs around the knees and on the feet to encourage the chest circulation stuckness to move downward which helped ease nausea and deepened his breathing so he could relax and regain balance. But this problem could have been avoided. Here is my simple golden rule about using curative herbs.

If the problem is poor digestion or absorption, take digestive herbs with meals. If the problem is not digestive, for example treating pain or injury, colds/flu, or skin problems, take appropriate herbs between meals and at least 2 - 5 hours separate from medicines.

The same general rule applies to heart herbs. Take heart medicines as directed by your physician and take recommended heart health herbs between meals, for example at 10AM, separate from medicines so that the body does not become confused and overloaded with treatment. Now you have lots of indicators to notice about your heart's energy--your tongue color and shape, circulation comfort, and emotions. Let's continue to heal the heart by opening our awareness to higher consciousness.

Heart Health Checkup

1. Observe your tongue first thing in the morning before brushing your teeth. Your tongue is a map of your vital energy and heart health that you can observe directly. Try to relax, opening the mouth gently without forcing the tongue so that you can observe the natural shape and color. What are the shape, color and texture? They may temporarily change with dietary changes but we want to get an overall sense about your vitality, circulation, digestion, and immunity. Their indications are slow to change and therefore will look the same overtime.

Your tongue may look:

- Large and puffy – indicating water retention or weak metabolism. You will be helped by upcoming chapters covering herbal tonics for kidney/adrenal health and digestive strength. Also see my article "Low Sodium Alternatives" for further information and low sodium recipes at www. asianhealthsecrets.com. It's important to reduce excess water retention when preventing heart failure symptoms such as swollen ankles and shortness of breath when walking or sleeping.
- Narrow, dry or cracked – indicating dehydration, chronic thirst or inflammation. This may result from smoking, stomach ulcers or a pre-diabetic condition. If the condition is chronic you may benefit from nourishing, moisten foods that help balance blood sugar. If you have a fever or you recently ate drying, spicy foods your tongue may be temporarily appear red and dry. Another way to check whether you are temporarily dehydrated is to pinch the skin on top of your hand. If the skin pops up quickly to regain normal elasticity, you are hydrated. If the pinched skin remains a raised ridge it is a dehydration symptom.

2. Do you tend to easily catch colds? Do you feel run-down, often tired? Your immunity may be low from stress or chronic weakness. Dietary changes may also bring on cold-like symptoms. For

example if you consume lots of raw or cold foods, salads, ice drinks and cooling, moistening herbs your fluids will increase. In extreme cases cooling or raw foods or herbs can give you diarrhea, excess urination, cramps, a runny nose, nausea or other signs of excess fluids. Later chapters explain many health foods and tonics. Most people can use them but your best most appropriate use of foods and herbs will come with your daily self observations. After all if you had stomach cramps after eating raw or iced foods, and runny diarrhea and runny nose, would you drink ice water or salad or ice cream? They would make the runny symptoms worse. You might also notice chills, lower back weakness, leg cramps and low motivation for daily work.

Herbal energy tonics we will learn about such as astragalus (huang qi) and anti-oxidant-high foods such as tart cherry help keep our immunity in good shape. Finding the right dietary pleasures and herbal remedies for your needs are part of the adventure. The remedies may change as your health improves and with seasonal climate changes. An important part of healing is being able to recognize your discomforts using the ongoing self-observations from this book.

Q & A: Energy and Immunity
  I have low energy – *High dose, highly absorbable vitamin C has been shown to reduce colds, flu, fatigue, heart trouble and stroke. Liposomal Vitamin C absorbs into the body more than 10x efficiently than traditional oral Vitamin C. Liposomal Vitamin C is broken down into nano-sized particles.*
  http://www.absorbyourhealth.com/product/liposomal-vitamin-c-best-price-net-1-gram-vit-c-every-teaspoon/?ref=4041

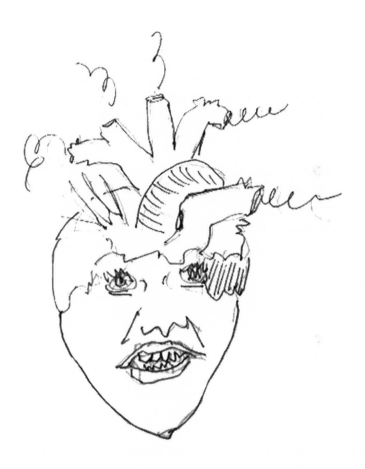

Stop Smoking!!

THREE

CLEAN UP YOUR ACT

Arianna Huffington says, "Fearlessness is like a muscle. I know that the more I exercise it the more natural it becomes." I agree that dealing with anxiety requires a sort of Emotional Calisthenics. Fear, worry, frustration and depression threaten heart health. Calisthenics are simple movements refined with practice. Likewise a positive attitude requires our working toward and expecting something better. It takes skill and practice. Normally we do not experience gripping fear that jams our vital forces. More likely, we have day to day worries about financial survival, health issues or relationship troubles. Caregivers get a big dose. Doctors suggest reducing stress by taking walks, petting your dog or calling a friend. But they do not provide a lasting cure.

Anxiety is a physical response to a real or imagined threat. We are wired to get out of the way of on-coming danger. Our heart pounds, we sweat and breathe with difficulty as our energy and blood circulation shift into high gear. The problem is that most of us get used to a milder form of these discomforts until they trouble our sleep and make life difficult. We should enhance health not simply sedate our heart, mind, and adrenal energy. Fear has its place. It can save your life, but it should fit the situation. Fight or flight reactions are made worse from irritating or stimulating foods such as caffeine or alcohol, hormonal shifts, fatigue. With chronic anxiety we may feel chilled. Our hands may sweat or shake. A warm soothing bath, a foot rub with a massage oil, and a good night's sleep work wonders to ease fatigue, pain and stress. Anxiety can feel hot, quick, painful, abrupt. Try slow deep breathing, a cool shower – seek the opposite in the treatment.

Unfulfilled Desires

Have you watched a television program or an artistic performance that moved you to anger or tears? Something about it touched your sense of identity, your feelings about being you. Have you dreamt of someone you miss? Our desires echo in dreams. Sleep is a time when our brain heals itself by incorporating and organizing new and old information. Our unresolved feelings, the shadow part of who we are, make up our old information that can be revealed naturally. For example you may dream of someone after using calming, blood-enhancing rejuvenating herbs because their memory remains deeply hidden from ordinary life. The herbs reach a part of you that is younger, fresher. Respect your feelings as they evolve and continue using the rejuvenating treatments in this book to feel light and free. Accepting our hidden self we feel whole, but that is only the beginning. Emotions demand expression.

I know a cardiologist who after suffering a heart attack took up water color painting. He told his colleagues that his hobby was stress-management, but he told me confidentially that painting expressed the "unfulfilled female" part of himself. He is happy to feel whole. Unfortunately, there are people who have an artistic, creative, even a courageous temperament with no outlet for their emotions except injury and illness. Time, space and society set limits to self-expression. So do outdated ideas. Have you avoided trying something different, taking time for yourself because it seemed selfish or silly? Self expression is the voice of your emotions, your heart. By developing a different part of our brain/body connection our learning expands and memory improves. Old habits of brain-boring repetition and set ideas cause our senses, intelligence and memory, literally our brain, to shrink. Unfortunately we too often fail to listen to our heart until we become sick. One of my friends, a former financial executive, described her heart attack at age forty and recovery this way:

> I had my coronary when I was in a high pressure job that did not suit me at all. A friend and healing touch practitioner came to the hospital and did a treatment for a whole hour. The recovery weeks were some of the most relaxed times I'd had in a long time and so really gave me a message that something in my life needed to change. I got regular natural treatments,

61

including energy healing modalities with caring practitioners, herbal remedies, and I made a real commitment to enjoy life and not push myself past comfort zones in my life, no matter what others told me to do. I learned to detoxify on all levels, both internal, external and who I spend my time with.

Whether you use herbal remedies, meditation, exercise or a form of energy balancing, it's important to respect your heart's needs and in so doing respect your life force.

Let's pretend we can clear the air of troubling emotions like cleaning a cluttered room. The aim is not to sweep feelings under a rug but to create an approach whereby we feel safe, able to forgive our self and others, and reduce useless blame, guilt, and worry. The steps seem simple but require practice: Eat well, clear mental clutter, and use protection against harm. Actress Betty Davis had good advice on that. She said, "Your enemy is someone who keeps you from doing your work." We can expand that to include someone who intrudes into your space and tries to prevent or harm your health and positive, creative self-expression.

Inside your Home and Heart

Our appearance and living space are extensions of our body/mind. Depressed people, some with damaging habits and poor self-esteem, need constant reminders—like wearing heavy scents, soiled clothing, or dirty skin--to verify their reality. Stifled anxiety means living in clutter, overcome by our messy surroundings as though unable to control excretions. Confused thinking and panic easily take hold when we feel helpless, sick, alone in a hostile, unpredictable world.

In panic, the heart pounds and blood leaves vital organs to energize muscles and escape danger. Within three seconds our adrenal glands shoot out stress hormones adrenaline and cortisol that prompt sweating, rapid breathing and heartbeat to pump oxygen to muscles used for running and fighting. The eye pupils dilate. It's a lousy way to live. But caregivers, as well as depressed people, may be faced with this sort of panic mode either in themselves or their patient. A nightmarish mental landscape challenges the heart.

To defeat a sick mindset, increase habits that support kindness to yourself and others. Start fresh with good nutrition and internal "housekeeping." Take a deep, relaxing breath. Do you use baking soda to remove stains inside your teapot? How wonderful it feels to take a warm twenty minute soak in a bath tub adding 1 cup of baking soda. It leaves your skin clean and smooth because baking soda makes the water more alkaline. We feel like a sparkling diamond. Some people add apple cider vinegar to balance the alkaline base (baking soda) with an acid. The combination dries the skin if used too often. At the end of Chapter Sixteen we cover Borax added to bathwater to reduce heavy metals.

If you feel weak and vulnerable, reconnect with the healing powers of Mother Earth. You may enjoy adding ¼ cup of powdered bentonite clay to your bath. It leaches out harmful heavy metals and adds needed minerals such as calcium and potassium. Your bath feels grounding yet energizing. Redmond's clay from Utah is sodium- and calcium-based bentonite clay that can be used internally, one teaspoon mixed in a glass of water, to ease indigestion and constipation. Clay water can be used as a gargle, a facial pack for acne or as an anti-inflammatory, detoxifying poultice for arthritic joints, bug bites, or bruises.

A Rhythm of Wellness

We forget that adults as well as kids need to regularly wake up, eat meals, use the bathroom, and fall asleep at about the same time each day to create a comfortable rhythm of wellness. Mind and emotions need to be nourished as much as the body. I met an artist I will call Steve who never ate regular meals, only worked and smoked, and occasionally ate candy bars. His thin hair was sickly and limp and his wrinkled skin looked much older than his years. He had lost his sense of taste and told me he could eat nails. His doctor warned him about lung cancer, but he still smoked. Overwork was his identity.

If you are going to snack instead of eat meals, at least, snack healthy. For Steve I suggested nourishing, rejuvenating black sesame Tahini paste. He loved the taste. Sesame is a good source of protein and calcium. Beans and lentils in any form—hummus, bean soup, etc—are also a source of protein, starch and fiber that help to keep blood sugar in balance. Steve lived on takeout junk food so I advised easy things to grab while on the job such as low fat yogurt, dried fruit, nuts and real unsweetened cocoa powder in his coffee instead of candy bars. Eating habits are under your control. It is easy to add one healthy food at a time. Eventually you can enjoy a better diet. Avoiding meals and ignoring good nutrition makes blood sugar balance and nervous tension go whacko which overworks your heart.

Detoxify properly

The basics are to drink enough water, some say one liter a day, so that internal organs work properly. It is more important to listen to your body than to follow hard set rules. Few people drink enough water. I enjoy warm tea all day which is cleansing and stimulating to mind and body. For weight loss black coffee is recommended. If you add water to juices you can reduce calories and sugar content. Observe yourself. Your daytime urine should be abundant, with a clear pale yellow color not oily, thick, flakey, dark or odorous. Urine with a greenish tint indicates the liver is not working well enough and you need to eat bitter green foods like chicory and dandelion greens in order have more laxative bile.

For example, add 1 teaspoon of Angostura aromatic bitters or other herbal digestive bitters containing gentian [Gentianae Radix] to a wine glass of water before dinner. Gentian is used for digestion problems such as loss of appetite, fullness, intestinal gas, diarrhea, gastritis, and heartburn. It has also been used for fever, hysteria, muscle spasms, and high blood pressure. Avoid excess use during pregnancy.

You can make your own digestive bitters by steeping dried sliced dandelion root, gentian root, orange peel, and raw ginger for two weeks or more in a liter of gin or vodka. Take capsules of dandelion, alfalfa, or eat fresh greens or cooked or toasted seaweed with meals to supplement needed minerals. Seaweeds such as dried dulse work well if you crave salt but are on a salt-restricted diet.

You should have one or more fast, easy bowel movements daily with a stool shaped like a brown banana, neither formless nor hard balls. It should not be black or red from blood or contain undigested food or parasites. Here is a highly effective internal cleansing method promoted by health food researcher Prof. Dr. İbrahim Saraçoğlu.

The Cabbage Cure

Boil 4 leaves of green cabbage in 2 cups of water for 15 minutes and drink the liquid when cooled either one hour before breakfast or during the afternoon separated from meals by two hours. Cabbage, an alkaline, anti-cancer food, reduces dietary fats and poisons that can choke circulation. Your urine may appear oily for a few days as toxins leave your body. Dr. Saracoglu recommends drinking the cabbage cooking liquid for five days, rest for three days and resume the treatment until you have cleansed for five consecutive days three or four times as needed. Eventually your urine will be clear and light, cellulite will be reduced, and your energy and mood will have improved. Proper internal cleansing assures a clear complexion, freedom from body odor and bad breath, and a healthy heart because harmful cholesterol does not clog blood vessels when the body is working properly.

Two homeopathic remedies for emotional relief

A homeopathic remedy is made from a mere trace of a substance, often an irritant, because it engages the body's healing response against it. It is energy medicine, a highly refined and studied art. One important thing to know about homeopathic remedies is that they work quickly on the cellular level and, after they have done their job, no trace of the remedy remains in your body. In most cases you can cancel a remedy with a cup of coffee. With an ineffective remedy choice, you won't notice improvement of symptoms. There are quite a number of homeopathic remedies that directly affect heart action and chest comfort, but their use is beyond the scope of this book and require a great deal of knowledge about homeopathy and the patient's condition. However, here are two flash remedies that improve mood and may overcome underlying problems affecting energy. Choose one to change your rhythm of wellness. Also see the chapter Caregiver's

Survival Kit. Do not mix homeopathic remedies with foods or beverages, toothpaste or medicines:

> **Do you frequently cry a lot, obsess or complain? Homeopathic Pulsatilla**
> **Do you feel overcome by anxiety and exhaustion? Homeopathic Gelsemium**
> **Do you feel overcome with grief, loss, ambivalent feelings? Homeopathic Ignatia amara**

Shortness of Breath, Weeping and Whining – Homeopathic Pulsatilla

Excess weeping or complaining can be related to a hormone imbalance or stress. Of course crying is perfectly normal and beneficial at times, but homeopathic pulsatilla treats a long standing physical and emotional imbalance. Chronic shortness of breath with thick white phlegm, water retention that collects in the abdominal area and legs, a feeling of constrained breathing as though being shut in a room without air, heartburn and chest-tightness after eating–these all improve by using homeopathic pulsatilla.

Pulsatilla, the wind flower, is used in Chinese herbal medicine to help dry the digestive tract and reduce parasites. Homeopathic pulsatilla on the other hand works for the mind as well as body. Pulsatilla 30C is a constitutional treatment for someone who moans, complains and constantly asks for help. Their sticky, heavy nature matches their phlegm. They may fear being alone. They may appreciate massage to calm painful colic. The pulsatilla heart patient or caregiver will feel sad or moody much of the time and unable to cope with crowds of people or tiring work. They will have slow difficult digestion and shallow breathing.

Homeopathic pulsatilla may help heart failure patients and caregivers who are addicted to sugar, soda drinks, or fattening foods. They will have difficulty breathing, require more than one pillow in bed, get out of breath walking up stairs and have water retention that looks like puffiness or fat in the middle, a swollen face, hands, and legs. Swelling [AKA edema], cough and shortness of breath are also common side-effects of certain heart drugs, for example, calcium channel blockers. (7) Consider the emotional aspects when using pulsatilla. The pulsatilla patient who requires emotional support, who over-worries, whines and obsesses over unhappy past events may improve with better breathing. For them homeopathic pulsatilla may clear the air, support vitality, and feel calming like a yoga session.

Exhaustion, Anxiety – Homeopathic Gelsemium

A lot of people today are anxious about the future. They fear illness or situations that place them in jeopardy like flying, public speaking or being with new people. Homeopathic gelsemium, made from yellow jasmine, though not a sedative, bolsters courage by calming free-floating anxiety and easing discomforts of nervous exhaustion. It has been recommended to reduce aches, pains and fever during early stages of the common cold. Do you overwork to the point of dizziness and trembling? A slow pulse, muscular weakness, mental apathy, headache with a sore scalp, stiff neck and shoulders are common discomforts for the Gelsemium patient. The heart will frequently have palpitations with a slow, weak pulse that becomes accelerated when moving around. This useful remedy bolsters confidence in the patient and fortitude in the caregiver whose heart is oversensitive to anxiety and fatigue.

Grief, Shock, Loss, Ambivalence – Homeopathic Ignatia amara

Ignatia, amara made from a trace of the Saint Ignatius bean, which is, if taken as the bean, is deadly. It quickly kills so that the homeopathic remedy, made from only a trace of the original substance, retains the ability to counter collapse. It awaken our immunity and frees life force. It has been recommended for grief. It takes the sharp edge off loss. It helps settle anxiety and indecision due to panic. I have recommended it for unhappy people in the midst of divorce, bankruptcy, separation from family and it works by shifting our energy. One girl who couldn't stop crying after breaking up with her boyfriend. She had heartbreak and indecision whether to attack or ignore him. She took a dose of homeopathic ignatia amara, developed cold symptoms for a day or two, and then felt fine, relieved as though her body and mind had been detoxified from the grief.

When using a homeopathic medicine for enhanced emotional support or to brace up your courage, take the appropriate remedy as directed under the guidance of a homeopathic expert. You may find that relief feels like taking a deep breath and stepping away from a difficult situation.

A refreshing mind trip

Whenever possible take a break from your worry and work routine. We often see caregivers smoking or talking on a cell phone outside hospitals. It would be better if they did qigong movements or took a walk. I like to use calming visualizations that involve nature but you can make up your own escape from stress. Here are a few ideas to get you started.

1. Imagine you are with your loving pet in a garden at mid-day. You both are drowsy and happy. Birds are singing and the sunshine feels wonderful. There is nothing to do so you decide to take a nap with your pet nearby. A soft light surrounds you and you sense that the garden flowers expand and relax with each breath you take. The garden protects you and you enjoy its perfume.

2. While in your bathtub imagine you are a frog or fish in a shallow pond. You are happy not moving while a quiet breeze stirs the air. Let cool water cover your body as your head floats. Your legs and arms float like lily pads and your cares melt away in the water.

3. This is a walk through the desert at sunset with your best friend. You are the only two people for miles and no sound can be heard except a bird circling high above in the sky. Pale colors of mountains, sand and sky are exquisite and the scent of pine and sage crackle in the dry air. This unforgettable moment gives you courage when you remember how much you love your friend.

Placing your arm on your friend's shoulder you share this moment of contentment.

Outside Forces

We cannot assume that our emotional troubles all stem from our own heart. There are troubling forces at work in the world. Let us consider demons and vampires, who they are and how to foil them.

Demons

Do you know someone who smiles when you stub your toe? The demon enjoys others' suffering. In extreme cases a mute, staring expression reveals their need to feel or inflict pain in order for them to feel emotion. An everyday demon stands fascinated at traffic accidents, smiles when hearing bad news or watching a quarrel. It may be a nervous reaction, but still a smile. Their unsettling presence makes you feel uncomfortable and they enjoy that.

A skillful demon may play the clumsy child who repeatedly makes dumb mistakes, breaking things, generally causing an uproar in order to get attention. They thrive on chaos and confusion, their twisted world view. Depression, hopelessness, a sour outlook may become lifelong for the demon. Their imbalance usually has physical symptoms such as an unhealthy grey cast on oily, troubled skin and strong body odor like rotten fish which are signs of adrenal exhaustion, liver toxins, and dehydration. Other inflammatory symptoms may include a red tongue, fast pulse, shrieking laughter and a determined, mean-sounding, shrill voice. Their tense body is ready to spring.

The best defense against a demon is to leave quickly although they love an audience and will try to stop you. If you offer help they will inevitably foul it and blame you for the horrendous outcome or, true to their stubborn nature, they will refuse your help believing that they know better. Their stubbornness resembles the slurping tenacity of the vampire, although demons are meaner and more dangerous. They want you to fail in order to prove they are right, better, prettier, smarter or whatever they want to prove.

What if you are caregiver to a demon? If you are healthy, strong and emotionally centered you might let a demon know that you are on to their game, but don't expect to win. They will simply move on to another victim. They often cycle through numerous caregivers, doctors, friends, and spouses so be ready for a ride. Demons hate light and fresh air. Try to get out into the sun for at least fifteen minutes daily, avoiding sun glasses. We absorb healing rays of the sun through our eyes as well as skin. Do not stare at the sun but look at a distance and that will help you relax. If you want to avoid the sun for health reasons or live in a dark climate, take at least 1,000 iu of natural vitamin D3 daily to protect your bones and immunity. Take D3 along with an oil such as flaxseed oil capsules for better absorption.

Demons are full of acidic toxins. They may also be troubled by an inflammatory hormone imbalance such as menopausal hot flashes no matter what their age. You can suggest or let them discover for themselves the healing benefits of liver cleansing greens and cooling foods such as tart cherries detailed in Part Two. That way they will have fewer headaches, skin rashes, arthritic problems and temper tantrums. Their tendency for hypertension and insomnia may also improve.

Vampires

Vampires are a common problem among intrusive friends, in-laws, bothersome ex-spouses, emotionally draining co-workers, and dinner guests who stay too long or call you at midnight for a recipe. In extreme cases they are the houseguest from Hell, but they can be anyone, a stranger, who loves to suck your energy. Your blood supplies their vitality. Unlike the demon who seeks to defeat you, the vampire toys with you, keeping you at bay and interested in order to protect their blood supply. In a word, they always want MORE. Vampire patients are a pain for caregivers. While you patiently explain how that if they pour hot sauce on to a wound it will hurt, they are already planning the next attack with their mind rambling and mouth babbling at top speed. Sit them quietly and start again at zero. The vampire loves to prove you are dumb and they are dumber. Their aim is to enslave you.

After a few tries, they get destructive. They have to work on a project broken into little steps. That may help calm their anxiety and yours.

Bela Lugosi (born Béla Ferenc Dezső Blaskó, 1882 –1956) played the most famous vampire, Dracula, in American films. Before he arrived in the States he was a suave leading man on the Budapest stage. The vampire has great appeal because he needs you so very much. How attractive is someone who cannot live without you? Do you need to be needed? After all, your blood must be quite valuable if the vampire desires it so very badly. A coy vampire calls you over to change a light bulb, clean a messy house, or fix a computer they have unplugged. They are more annoying than deadly. Free yourself from vampires by building a healthy defense so that you can stand alone without teeth marks in your neck.

One traditional way to ward off vampires in Transylvania was wearing a necklace of garlic. These days you might eat it in your salad dressing. Garlic, an antimicrobial food, reduces cholesterol and acts as a blood thinner. The pungent odor coming through your pores after eating garlic is enough to kill small flying insects. However another old cure works better to enhance energy and ease your guilt over not allowing the vampire to consume you whole.

Vampire-wort

St. Johnswort (Hypericum perforatum) like other herbs ending in "wort" is recommended for magical protection against evil. This herb gives us a clue how to deal with threats to our peace and wellbeing, including vampires. St. Johnswort works against depression on an energetic level by enhancing our breathing. It has been recommended by John Lust, an early herbalist, for asthma and wheezing. If we stand firm and breathe freely, our vitality is a natural defense. The vampire is slurpish because of their real or imagined vulnerability. They need you after all. If you become stronger, building a defense with enhanced oxygen, you will need them less and humor them less. You might share a pot of tea, adding ten drops of St. Johnswort extract, with your vampiric friend or patient so that you both feel more emotionally resilient and independent. Let them know that you have boundries.

Oxygen kills germs, fortifies all our cells and protects against invaders. Because St. Johnswort corrects depression and shortness of breath, it improves those typical signs of heart weakness. In later chapters we will cover specific heart tonics such as artic root [AKA rhodiola] which fortifies circulation as it improves mental clarity and memory. The best defense against demons and vampires is your physical vitality and peace of mind.

Heart Health Checkup

1.   Observe your urine first thing in the morning. See the amount, color, quality, odor, and frequency of urination. Also if you urinate frequently at night, it is a sign of adrenal weakness or too much caffeine consumed at night. Healthy urine as described by Asian traditional doctors is clear, light yellow, without an oily, gritty, flakey, cloudy or reddish appearance, unpleasant smell or burning sensation. These can be broken down into Hot and Cold Symptoms:

Your tongue and urine diagnosis may correspond. If your are weak, chilled and rundown, your tongue and urine are more likely to look pale—TCM calls it internal cold symptoms not confused with colds and flu but a chronic state of weakness and chills. You may have too much saliva. If everything is a normal color and flowing well--saliva, urine, sinus drainage, and stools, and if there is no effort necessary, no sign of weakness, blood, or shortness of breath–elimination is going well. If, on the other hand, you are weakened for some reason, indicated by excess urine and diarrhea, chills, pallor etc. you are more likely to be drained by emotional vampires. See the chapters on herbal tonics and use digestive and adrenal tonics as you watch your tongue color and shape to observe improvements in energy and mood.

If you are a smoker or dehydrated, not drinking enough water daily, or for some reason overheated, your urine will more likely appear thick, sparse, dark yellow to orange and odorous. It may be from temporary or long term internal heat--a fever illness, or hormone changes. If that continues and especially if there is pain upon urination, have it checked for possible infection or prostate issues. You may also have other signs of inflammation such as joint pains, headaches, and night sweats. Inflammation that can eventually damage blood vessels will be addressed with cooling herbs including aloe, nopales cactus useful for diabetes, and numerous heart health tonics we will cover later.

2.   It is difficult to change negative mental chatter because it is an old habit. Observing our mind and emotions is one aim of meditation. For our purposes we will begin by simply noticing our thoughts especially when and under what circumstances we feel troubled. Our mental chatter is barely audible as we go about our business. However a pattern of trouble begins. Do you feel unhappy, angry, or frustrated while doing something particular or thinking about a particular person? Something simple, out of the ordinary, may provoke a memory. Or do you feel that way at predictable times of day such as bedtime or in the morning? Our thoughts may actually correspond to physical discomforts and health issues. Thoughts come to the surface when we finally relax in bed. It is hard to say which comes first the thought/memory or the physical pain or muscle tension. Acidity aggravates inflammatory joint and muscle pain and mental upset. We may feel pain after lying in bed throughout the night and feel stiff and emotionally drained upon waking. Heart burn and indigestion affect heart rhythm. Anxiety and anger increase when we are sexually frustrated or insomniac.

Try to determine the *quality* of your emotional pain. Is it cold and stiff like fear or anxiety, hot and sharp like hatred and distain, or soggy like despair? And why do you feel it? Listen to your heart's dialogue. Sometimes simply asking your heart what it feels is enough to reach an epiphany.

Do certain images repeat? What is the tone of the chatter? That is your heart speaking. It may be a health warning. Do angry thoughts occur late at night or first thing in the morning? Do you have pain in the right ribs—a sign of inflammation or stuck circulation affecting the liver? According to TCM the liver, our major detoxification organ is, like the heart, key for emotional balance. Do your lower back or joints hurt? That may be muscle strain or a pinched nerve. If anti-inflammatory herbs such as aloe and liver cleansing foods and herbs covered in this book do not help, you may need treatment for a structural problem.

Weak adrenal energy may cause daytime sleepiness and night time difficulty falling asleep and staying asleep. Do you have cold hands and feet? You may have early morning diarrhea, sexual dysfunction and feel chilled and weak if vital energy [AKA kidney qi; adrenal energy] is low. After reading the chapters covering energy tonics come back to this **Heart Health Checkup** to observe at what times and under what circumstances you feel uncomfortable. That will help you to determine your best health plans for short and long term. Improving vitality creates a defense against challenging situations and people. Your vitality, what Chinese herbalists call qi, gives you quick energy for work and play and it also supports immunity, sexuality and emotional balance over time.

Improve your qi this way: First reduce physical and mental poisons. A clean diet, herbs to enhance elimination and deep breathing will help. Then build strength and calm resolve with appropriate tonics that reinforce resilience, immunity and courage. You will learn to observe your vitality and discover natural treatments throughout this book.

Q & A: Anxiety
I am afraid of having heart trouble or a stroke -- *Reduce nervous anxiety and stress, improve mood and reduce addictive behavior*:: If not using medication for depression, some people prefer using lithium with guidance from a health expert. http://www.absorbyourhealth.com/product/lithium-orotate/?ref=4041

FOUR

HEART WORKS

I am listening to an excellent performance of Vivaldi's Concerto for Four Violins. Four violins in nine minutes create bliss, flowing as smoothly as the movement of blood through the heart's four chambers and four valves.

Heart Diagram

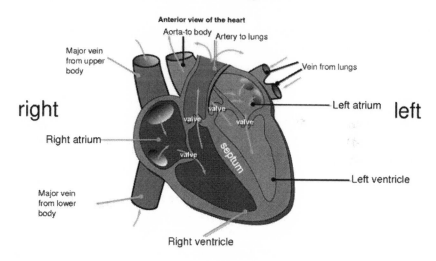

This is how our heart works: Oxygen-poor blood comes from veins into the right atrium for a brief second then down to the right ventricle and out through a large artery into the lungs. Refreshed by oxygen blood flows back from the lungs into the left atrium and ventricle, and out the aorta, our largest blood vessel, to every part of the body. The entire squeeze and release, lasting a few seconds, moves one cup of blood through a ten ounce heart, the size of a fist, sending blood through 60,000 miles of blood vessels to energize body, mind, and spirit. The Vivaldi concerto and the heart are each a masterpiece of brilliant, economic construction. How does this marvel of Nature get into trouble? We need to clarify several medical terms before we can discover natural alternatives. What do we mean by hardening of the arteries, heart attack and heart failure?

Atherosclerosis

Atherosclerosis, hardening of the arteries, is the usual cause of heart attacks, strokes, and peripheral vascular disease which are together called "cardiovascular disease." Do all you can to keep your blood free-flowing. We learned how blood flows through the body and the heart. Arteries that carry blood from the heart throughout the body are lined by a thin layer of cells, the endothelium, which keeps the inside of arteries toned and smooth, and that keeps blood flowing. According to the accepted view expressed by Richard Stein, MD, spokesperson for the American Heart Association, "Atherosclerosis starts when high blood pressure, smoking, or high cholesterol damage the endothelium. At that point, cholesterol plaque formation begins."

Bad cholesterol (LDL) crosses damaged endothelium and enters the wall of the artery. Plaque is formed over time. Your white blood cells stream in to digest the LDL cholesterol. Over years, "a jumble of lipids, or cholesterol, cells, and debris. . . creates a bump on the artery wall," explains Stein. As the process of atherosclerosis continues the bump gets bigger. A big enough bump creates a blockage from plaque in your heart or throughout the body increasing the risk of stroke.

The bad news is we cannot feel the clogging mess in our blood vessels, there are no symptoms until middle or older age. Once hardening of arteries become severe, the blockage chokes off blood flow and causes pain. Pain on exertion (in the chest or legs) is the usual symptom.

Blockages can also suddenly rupture, causing blood to clot inside an artery at the site of the rupture. Stable plaques in the heart's arteries may cause angina which is chest pain upon exertion. In that case the chest hurts because the heart lacks blood and oxygen, which is going out to tired muscles. Angina pain is usually temporary as normal circulation returns with rest. But sudden plaque rupture in blood vessels and clotting that blocks blood flow to the heart causes heart muscle to die. This is a heart attack, or myocardial infarction. In Chapter two we learned about PAD, narrowing in the arteries of the legs caused by plaque also called peripheral artery disease. This causes leg pain after walking, discolored purplish legs, and poor wound healing. Severe PAD disease may lead to amputations.

Experts say a large number of asymptomatic young people have evidence of atherosclerosis. A 2001 study of 262 apparently healthy people's hearts atherosclerosis was present in 85% of people over age 50 and 17% of teenagers had atherosclerosis. Not one of them had noticeable symptoms! That's pretty shocking. And very few had severe narrowing of the arteries detectable by special tests. If you are 40 and generally healthy, experts say you have about a 50% chance of developing serious atherosclerosis in your lifetime. Atherosclerosis is progressive, but preventable. For example, nine risk factors are to blame for upwards of 90% of all heart attacks:

- Smoking
- High cholesterol
- High blood pressure
- Diabetes
- Abdominal spare tire
- Stress
- Not eating fruits and vegetables
- Daily more than 1 alcoholic drink for women, more than 1 – 2 for men
- Not exercising regularly

This book covers foods such as tree ear mushrooms, garlic, cayenne pepper, garlic and tea which are blood thinners as well as cholesterol-reducing, blood pressure-regulating treatments that are safer then taking low dose aspirin which irritates digestion and can cause bleeding stomach ulcers. It is a wonder we don't all have PAD if we sit at a computer all day with our knees bent and back crunched forward to stare at a screen. Getting up to stretch and walking around the room may help, but lifestyle changes are necessary.

Medical intervention including stents, angioplasty, and bypass surgery come with risks and are usually saved for people with significant symptoms or limitations caused by atherosclerosis. Such intervention is the end game of heart troubles, after there is no other effective treatment. Let's look closer at heart attack and heart failure symptoms which are usually the reasons why we consult a cardiologist.

Heart Attack

If you tune a string instrument too tightly the strings break. If we create excess tension in fragile artery walls, they crack. A wound on the skin is normally healed when the body sends "glue" to seal the crack, a cut or burn, with a scab. Eventually it forms a scar. But inside blood vessels this healing glue made of fat, calcium, and wastes, is *plaque* that can quickly blocks blood flow, cutting off oxygen to heart muscles, in effect, quickly killing heart muscle.

A heart attack can kill a person within twenty minutes. After years of poison from dietary mistakes, junk foods, harmful chemicals, and inflammation from stress, smoking, environmental pollution among others, blood vessel walls thicken, harden and become brittle, eventually leading to congestion and cracks. What comes first and is most damaging to blood vessels– harmful cholesterol or inflammation-- is a point argued by present day cardiologists. For our purposes we shall address both issues because they are real problems that affect us all.

Blood Pressure

I guess most people begin to pay attention to heart health when their blood pressure becomes elevated. Someone with so called normal blood pressure can still have a stroke so it is only one measure of heart health that we can easily monitor. Blood pressure measures the strength or pressure of blood flow against arterial walls. In other words how hard your heart is working and how much blood is being pumped through blood vessels. Your cardiologist will likely place his fingers on your neck and ankles to measure the strength of the pulse. But you can measure your blood pressure at home using an inexpensive device. Measure if possible during the same time of day and same arm to get a more accurate reading.

The systolic or top number measures tension when the heart contracts and the bottom number, the diastolic, measures arterial tension when the heart relaxes between heartbeats. With arteries constricted by cholesterol or edema (water retention) from heart weakness, the heart works harder to push blood forcefully through arteries and there is your higher blood pressure measurement (higher than 120/70.) If a crack or rupture develops in an artery made brittle by inflammation and is healed with glue, it shuts off blood flow like stepping on a garden hose.

Breathing and Walking

The four heart valves and many little valves in the veins prevent blood from flowing backwards the wrong way. There is no tension, no blood pressure, in veins those large bluish blood vessels that carry blood to the heart. So how does blood get from your feet and your head to your heart? Breathing and walking move your blood. The heart is resting on the diaphragm. Every time you inhale your abdomen pushes up the diaphragm which makes the heart pump.

When you move, your muscles push against the walls of blood vessels moving blood as muscles undergo contraction and relaxation cycles that propel blood within the veins. Gravity also moves blood from the head to the heart. So blood in the veins is squished by muscles toward the heart and cannot fall backward because the tiny valves in the blood vessels prevent blood from collecting in our feet.

Walking is for most of us the easiest and best daily exercise. Watch to see if you develop swollen feet, painful, hot feet or leg pain and muscle fatigue after walking. They are signs of heart weakness or blood vessel congestion that you should not ignore. Here is another sort of gentle exercise/meditation for your pleasure and comfort.

Gently flows the stream

Try this free-flowing exercise to move the current of ocean waves filled with light and life reaching every pore of your body. Wear loose-fitting comfortable clothing and bare feet in a quiet room. Lie on your side with your knees up toward your chest in a fetal position. Support your hips and lower back by placing a pillow between your bent knees. Extend the arm you are lying on from your shoulder so that it does not constrict your breathing and with the other bent arm support yourself. Breathe smoothly without pause throughout this exercise. Focus on your breath and allow tensions to relax.

Using a slow, steady movement, and without moving your legs, flex and extend your feet as though you are walking, without stopping the rhythmic flow of your breathing. You might inhale as you stretch your feet up toward your head and, as you exhale, let the feet relax downward. You are a gentle jelly fish. Open and close your hand to the slow rhythm set by your breath and feet. You might be a slowly opening lotus as long as you continue breathing smoothly, opening, closing, opening, closing with your delicate feet and hands.

Congestive Heart Failure

When the heart contracts it sends blood through the aorta, our largest blood vessel, out to the body. When the heart relaxes it fills with oxygenated blood from the lungs. Blood flows in the right side of the heart and out the left side of the heart to the tissues. When the heart muscle is weak from age, stress, medications, illness, grief, shock, anemia, then it can leak from behind the left atrium into the lungs. The fluid build-up causes congestive heart failure. The dietary and herbal approach necessary to reduce heart stress in this case would reduce excess fluid retention (edema) and strengthen the heart muscle and tissue. Most often weight loss especially reducing belly fat can improve heart function. The heart can stay strong if it has to work less hard to pump excess backed-up fluids.

Signs of congestive heart failure include labored breathing. Do you need several pillows to improve breathing as you sleep? Do you huff and puff when climbing stairs or walking more than a few blocks? Are your ankles, face or hands bloated with excess fluid? Sometimes dietary changes as simple as reducing salt and canned and processed foods, often high in sodium, and taking diuretic herbs such as parsley tea are adequate to reduce excess water retention and heart stress. We will cover many such cleansing health foods and slimming herbs in later chapters.

Broken Heart Syndrome

"Broken heart syndrome" has been described as a condition prompted by emotional upset, grief and loss that leads to heart failure even though other signs such as cholesterol are normal. It happens when the left ventricle, the part of the heart that has to pump blood out to the lungs, swells with fluid and takes on the appearance of a Japanese pot used to catch octopus. Illustrations of this condition show the swollen left side of the heart and leads us to wonder how emotions can be seen and felt.

TCM traditional Chinese medicine teaches that grief damages the lungs and heart, especially the lung's aspect of promoting vitality and our *desire* to preserve our health. The heart has been called the master organ, the giver of joy. Modern heart medicines and surgical procedures aim to preserve life, the steady rhythm measured in heartbeats. Can this be done while ignoring the joy we may feel with a healthy heart? Do our heart drugs sedate joy, while avoiding pain and plaque? A Chinese herbalist may advise a treatment that enhances circulation for someone with a broken heart—pain in the chest resulting from intense emotions that impair blood flow. For example holly (Mao Dong Ching capsules) or Salvia (danshen.) The correct choice and dosage of herbs is best left to experts.

We have come a long way since the time when medicine aimed to kill disease with no thought of preserving wellness. We have come a long way in women's health, in accepting the vulnerable side of emotions and the ebb and flow of hormones, our internal ocean. The real work of protecting wellness begins and ends at home and with us. We have come a long way in our appreciation of Asian herbs. Years ago searching for heart remedies in a health food store we might have found fish oil, a source of healthy fat, hawthorn berry to strengthen the heart muscle, or co-enzyme Q-10 to help reduce heart stress, but little else. Today at Asian food markets, online, and in national chain stores such as Vitamin Shoppe we find arjuna, a tree bark Ayurveda's primary herb to prevent heart troubles. It protects a weak heart, reduces excess cholesterol, and helps correct arrhythmia.

During the British colonization of India, British writers documented the use of arjuna as an effective treatment for heart disease. In the 1990s, medical doctors used arjuna tree bark as a clinical treatment for heart conditions. If we had an ideal diet and exercise program, if we walked an hour daily and added more fruits, vegetables, nuts, seeds, teas, and healthy protein to keep a sensible weight then perhaps we could avoid heart trouble. However we cannot avoid grief and loss: they are part of life. Herbs give us an advantage in that they allow us to experiment with foods, audaciously travel and abuse vitality when necessary. They allow us to recover naturally from jet lag. A tree when well rooted can bend in the wind without breaking. I like adding a pinch of arjuna powder to my tea when I need courage.

Angina and Arjuna

You will read in later chapters about the Ayurvedic herb arjuna's action as a natural cardio-tonic and cardiac restorative. Arjuna, a tree bark, has also shown promising success in decreasing the persistence of angina attacks. Angina is experienced as a pain or tightness in the chest that is caused by reduced blood flow and oxygen to the heart. Angina attacks normally occur in times of intense emotional stress or during physical activity. Arjuna reduces angina in much the same way as prescription drugs such as nitroglycerin do—but without the side effects and complications (such as headaches, nausea, light headedness, allergic reactions and breathing difficulty.) Nitroglycerin may mask symptoms, but arjuna improves the heart, regenerating the heart muscle and stimulating healthy heart function. Heart rhythms are normalized, blood clots reduced, and hardening of the blood vessels reversed.

A double-blind placebo-controlled study published in the International Journal of Cardiology reported that volunteers treated with 500 mg. of arjuna four times a day experienced a 50% reduction in angina attacks. Results also included an overall improvement in cardiac function, lower blood pressure levels, and LDL cholesterol levels, as well as weight loss. According to Ayurveda, arjuna is astringent. By strengthening the heart muscle arjuna, which has been used for thousands of years, helps the heart to push blood out to the lungs. East has met West, heart to heart, to help ease suffering and cure illness.

The loves songs we know express the heart's longing, the joy of love and our grief at losing it. In dreams we may relive our feelings, however our unexpressed, barely noticeable discomforts also express the depth of the heart's dialogue as though our heart is speaking to us. We cannot bring back the past but we may with the help of natural remedies enhance physical comfort that enables resolution of feelings and eventual peace of mind.

A Woman's Heart

Are women particularly at risk of heart disease by simply being women? Does our capacity for feeling, communication, and expression open us to vulnerability and illness? We share the same risk factors as men except for one. Both sexes are susceptible to hypertension, unhealthy cholesterol, and high levels of homocysteine an amino acid. According to PeaceHealth, the official website of Oregon's Sacred Heart Medical Center, excessive amounts of that amino acid can damage the lining of arteries and promote plaque. However, that imbalance may be regulated by increasing our intake of vitamins B6 and B12 and folic acid. Both men and women are more susceptible to heart disease if they have diabetes, but in many cases that may be controlled with diet. (Also see chapters in Parts Four and Five for women and caregivers and the article "The Villain Sugar" at my website www.asianhealthsecrets.com)

Your heart and hormone replacement

One major factor of heart disease we do not share with men is also under our control. Some women opt for synthetic hormone replacement therapy after menopause a practice that has been linked to increased incidence of cancers and heart troubles. After the body gradually stops producing estrogen the risk of developing heart disease steadily climbs. Our natural estrogen aids in the absorption of calcium for strong bones and is soothing for nerves. However, if you are risk of breast and/or uterine cancers and if, like most of us, you live with stress, consider using natural hormone replacement with estrogenic foods and herbs instead of drugs. Herbs such as coptis (huang lien) which is very bitter and anti-inflammatory reduces hot flashes and hypertension discomforts. It comes in pills and has been studied for its estrogen-balancing, anti-inflammatory effects. Yucca, an estrogenic food and herbal capsule, reduces arthritic swelling and pain. Estrogenic herbs are safe for women who do not have active estrogen-sensitive cancers. Our body accepts herbs as it does foods so that they become part of our energy system. Nature's plan is for us to live long and well, learn from our heartaches, and enjoy the riches of health and happiness. Our human heart embodies a perfectly simple design for love which is to give and take.

Heart Health Checkup

Listen to your heart beat.

Traditional doctors from the Asian healing arts still take your pulse without using an instrument other than their fingertips and sensitive training in pulse diagnosis. They listen to the speed, strength and quality of the heartbeat but also to meridians—lines of energy that course through the body to bring blood and qi (energy circulation) to organs. Chinese doctors find twelve superficial and deep pulses on the radial artery, six on each hand, corresponding to the nervous system, circulation, breathing, digestion, and elimination. Ayurvedic doctors feel the quality of the pulse to identify humors that may be translated *wind, bile* and *phlegm* – nervous energy; digestion, also aggressive or feverish conditions; and phlegm conditions and metabolism. We will apply this diagnostic specialty to our needs in a very simple, easy to use way.

Speed, strength and quality

Many heart patients are advised to take their blood pressure at the same time daily and record it along with any sudden weight gain or swollen ankles which indicates water retention or heart weakness. That offers a method to listen to your heart. You need an old fashioned blood pressure arm cuff and stethoscope so you can listen to the heartbeats. Notice the speed of the beats.

Your healthy heartbeat speed is about 5 beats per inhalation/exhalation. Inhale and exhale slowly and count the beats. A faster heartbeat may indicate inflammation or stress and a much slower beat may indicate weakness or congestion when heart muscles cannot adequately empty the heart of blood.

If the beat is fast, heavy, sharp and you have other signs of inflammation such as fever, dizziness, intense thirst, skin rash or night sweats inform your doctor and you may need to adjust medicines and your diet away from inflammatory substances. You may be headed for diabetes. Or hormonal shifts during peri-menopause may be playing tag with your heart. For Heaven's sake stop smoking. See my chapter on cooling heart foods like sour cherries and grapes.

If the beat is slow, sluggish or halting and you have water retention in your face, hands, belly or ankles and feet, fluids are backing up and can damage the heart. Cut back on salt and other sodium often hidden in canned and processed foods. See the article "Low Sodium Alternatives" at www.asianhealthsecrets.com

Finally listen to how your heart feels as though listening to a friend talking to you. If the heart beat is irregular, liver or digestive circulation may feel stuck. Are your ribs and sides sensitive to touch? Is life frustrating you? Anyone with circulation issues, no matter what the cause, affecting the abdomen, the liver located under the ribs on the right side, or chest may develop an irregular heart beat. Fatigue plays a big part in that problem as well. But many people hold in emotions.

When the pulse or in this case the heart beat is irregular and indicates stuck circulation, for example, if there is a jaundiced (yellowish) complexion, frustration or anger, a good herbal supplement that works for many people is one that addresses digestion as well as circulation. For example the Chinese patent remedy Xiao Yao Wan recommended for "stuck liver qi." Other options might include a tea made with ginger, mint, and lemongrass. It improves digestion and eases digestive spasms. Another thing that can work wonders for many people is quiet, deep breathing. Take your pulse or blood pressure again after sitting quietly for 20 minutes and breathing as though alone in a pastoral setting. You can sense a difference.

Q & A: Heart Regularity
I have a nervous heartbeat -- *Support heart muscle energy with D-Ribose powder, a healthy sugar substitute.* Add it to teas as needed to ensure heart health. http://www.absorby-ourhealth.com/product/d-ribose-powder-100g-increase-ener-gy-endurance-enhance-atp-production-sweet-tasting-easily-soluble/?ref=4041

FIVE

A HEART FOR ALL SEASONS

Many birds fly south in winter to hatch their chicks where they first saw light. Not everyone is as lucky. Weather affects our heart and blood pressure more than we suspect. Did you know that cold temperatures tend to raise blood pressure by narrowing blood vessels? Cold weather tightens muscles increasing stiffness and aches which weakens immunity. It challenges circulation and breathing. Be sure to protect your neck with a scarf, your head, hands and feet to avoid a stiff neck and sore throat, often the first signs of a cold.

Inhaled air penetrates deep inside the body and through meridians affects not only the skin surface and muscles but the lungs, large intestine, adrenal glands, and kidneys. That's why we feel chilled and urination is increased after being in cold weather. Is your tongue usually pale and complexion wan? Do you feel weak during cold weather? To enhance your qi consume warming herbs and cooked foods instead of salads and iced drinks.

Great Regulator

Your temporary chill due to cold, damp weather should not be ignored. After coming inside have a cup of hot cinnamon tea to prevent hypothermia. Cinnamon stirs circulation and with perspiration regulates body temperature to relieve aches. Chinese herbalists believe that cinnamon improves seasonal or other forms of depression because moving blood circulation relieves obsessive thinking. On cold, grey days, lift your mood with a pinch of cinnamon and cardamom in your tea or coffee. Cinnamon is especially recommended for people with diabetes because it enhances insulin uptake, another reason why cinnamon improves energy and mood.

On the other hand, extremely hot weather, radiator heat, or a sauna are a threat to people with chronic inflammation, fevers and heart palpitations. Dry heat that evaporates vital fluids may aggravate irritability, sore throat, skin blemishes, and constipation. Is your tongue red and dry? Do you have a chronic dry cough and thirst? Sweating, a useful detoxifying treatment that reduces heavy metals, is drying and heating. If you feel dry, be sure to drink adequate fluids and take cooling green foods and rejuvenating, cleansing herbs such as aloe vera juice.

Headache/Heat Stroke: Chrysanthemum Flower Tea

During uncomfortably hot weather enjoy deliciously sweet and cooling Chinese chrysanthemum flower tea to prevent a migraine headache, heat stroke, blurry vision and a feverish feeling. It is recommended as a soothing tea for screen-watcher eyestrain. Enjoy a floral bouquet: In a glass pitcher place a handful of the dried chrysanthemum flowers, available online and in Chinese food and herb shops, then add hot water. The small dried yellow flowers will bloom. There is no need to sweeten this delightfully cooling tea.

Occasionally weather conditions may provoke temporary palpitations and chest discomforts. We will cover natural ways to safely prevent and treat colds and flu in this chapter. But first let's briefly consider our ongoing internal temperature and its effects on heart health. Hypertension [AKA high blood pressure] ,for example, is a major health problem that most of us face at one time or another.

Hypertension and Heat

Extreme cold weather is able to temporarily raise blood pressure but so can our internal heat generated by lifestyle and stress. Most Western doctors agree that we feel no symptoms of hypertension. But do they consider subtle discomforts that seem unrelated to blood pressure? There are several popular Chinese herbal pill formulas each translated as "Hypertension Repressing Tablets" that treat dizziness, agitation, and ear ringing caused by hypertension. When was the last time your heart doctor asked you about those symptoms? At home caring for yourself, your heart patient or loved one, we pay attention to little ordinary discomforts like dizziness noticing when it happens and why in order to monitor progress and avoid problems.

The herbal ingredients in the Chinese Hypertension Repressing pills known as Jiang Ya Pian lower harmful blood cholesterol and help prevent hardening of the arteries, while reducing subtle complaints including vertigo and tinnitus. Read the ingredients. The formulas contain different ingredients, some including animal derived ingredients such as earthworm. Many find this objectionable, so I recommend making a simple tea using two of the pill's main anti-inflammatory vegetarian ingredients prunella vulgaris (AKA self-heal) and skullcap. Simmer a handful of each dry herb in two cups of water for about 10 minutes and drink it when it is cool without adding flavoring.

Prunella, a small blooming weed in your lawn, is antimicrobial and has been recommended to treat herpes. Available in Chinese herb shops and online, dried prunella twigs and flowers, sold as xia ku cao, make a tasteless, cooling tea suitable for bedtime. Regular use of prunella can moderate anxiety stemming from an overactive thyroid. I have also recommended prunella tea for relieving menopausal hot flashes, springtime allergies, and insomnia. Skullcap is calming and enhances oxygen for brain health.

The several Hypertension Repressing formulas with the same name contain herbs that cool liver inflammation that result in fever and dizziness. Jiang Ya Pian [AKA Jiang Ya Wan, HypertenSure] sold by Active Herb online is vegetarian except for powdered oyster shell. However these and other very cooling herbs are contraindicated for weak or pregnant patients. If your tongue is pale and you feel chilled avoid cooling herbs. For example Jiang ya pian should be used with caution by breast-feeding women because da huang (rhubarb) a strong laxative can pass through the breast milk causing colic and diarrhea in infants. Use it with caution if you have diarrhea, poor appetite or chronic digestive weakness of if you use anti-coagulant (blood-thinning) medicines. It may cause mild abdominal cramping in sensitive patients.

There are widely used Asian foods we will consider later such as Auricularia polytricha [AKA cloud ear, tree ear) mushrooms used as blood thinners that can be cooked with soups and grains. Chapter

17, "Embrace your remedies" includes the Ayurvedic herb arjuna a tree bark that reduces cholesterol, regulates hypertension and protects blood vessels. Arjuna is sold as capsules or powder you can add to tea. Health Concerns, a California company, makes a pill called IBP that contains grapeseed oil to reduce hypertension. A number of traditional tonics gathered from mountain forests and gardens are now sold in North American health food stores. However Chinese traditional doctors say nothing soothes, cools and calms our nerves like an earthworm. You might take up gardening and watch one.

Flu for Heart Patients

Each year in the United States there are millions of cases of the common cold. Adults have an average of 2 to 4 colds per year and children have even more. Most people get colds in the winter and spring, but it is possible anytime. Colds and flu are hazardous for heart patients because they increase an underlying phlegm condition and can aggravate heart irregularities due to weakness, shortness of breath, and coughing. However, the biggest threat to heart patients is a complication of colds or flu—pneumonia. Although a cold is in itself often not too serious, pneumonia makes it hard to get enough oxygen. This makes your heart work harder.

Colds and Flu Comparison/Contrast
Colds: Fatigue, body aches, stuffy nose, sore throat, possible slight fever, comes on slowly over several days, remains contagious 3 – 4 days and without natural treatment may take a week to resolve.
Flu: Sudden high fever, headache, coughing, sinus and lung congestion, remains contagious 5 – 7 days and can kill weak patients the same day or last for several days.

Prevention for Heart Patients

The American Heart Association warns that decongestants should not be used by the more than 100 million Americans with high blood pressure (higher than about 120/70) because decongestants raise blood pressure to unsafe levels. Always check with your doctor or pharmacist to make sure a cold medicine does not interfere with your heart drugs. Here are some simple home remedies you can enjoy while resting and drinking fluids during a cold.

Basil Leaf Tea – the heart patient's friend

In Mediterranean countries a common garden herb has long been a first choice against colds and flu germs, fevers, cough and sore throat. Basil leaves and basil essential oil are antibacterial. Sweat out a cold and protect immunity with fresh green or dried basil leaf tea. Eat basil in salads or by the handful. It helps soothe depression. The good news for heart patients is that basil reduces cholesterol, phlegm and a vague, heavy, listless feeling that makes pain and depression miserable. Anti-inflammatory basil has been used to help combat bowel inflammation and rheumatoid arthritis. Many naturopathic doctors prescribe basil in treatment of diabetes, respiratory disorders, allergies, impotence, and infertility because basil contains cinnamanic acid found to enhance circulation, stabilize blood sugar, and improve breathing.

Basil especially the extract or oil has antioxidants that protect the body against free radical damage associated with aging, some skin ailments, and most forms of cancer. Used in cooking or taken as a nutritional supplement, basil combats common viruses like colds, flu, and the herpes family of viruses. Here are common uses of basil to enhance breathing and combat colds and flu symptoms. They are simple and they work.

Folk Remedy Basil

1. Healing: Basil removes bronchial phlegm. Chew a few leaves or drink a cup of basil tea up to once an hour. The leaves strengthen the stomach and induce perfuse sweating. The seeds can be used to rid the body of excess mucus.

2. Fevers: Boiling leaves with some cardamom in about two quarts of water, then mixed with a little (optional) rice milk, brings down

temperature. Take ten drops of extract of basil leaves in one cup of warm water every 2 to 3 hours.

3. Coughs: Basil is an ingredient in cough syrups and expectorants. It can also relieve asthma and bronchitis.

4. Sore Throat: Gargle with warm water boiled with basil leaves.

5. Respiratory Disorders: Treat asthma, bronchitis, cough, cold, and influenza by simmering a handful of basil leaves with 1 tablespoon of fresh, peeled and chopped ginger in a quart of water for an hour. That makes a water extract. However you can also steep basil leaves for 10 minutes to make a tea.

6. Stress: Chewing 12 basil leaves twice a day is recommended by some herbalists to prevent stress. It will at least purify the blood, improve energy and improve breathing and breath odor.

Chinese Cold and Flu Remedies

TCM herbal cold/flu formulas such as Gan Mao Ling pills contain safe, natural anti-inflammatory antibiotics including honeysuckle flower. Use Gan Mao Ling at the beginning of a cold to sweat out a chill and stiff neck. Or add a packet of powdered herbs to juice called Flu Away instant beverage made by Yin Yang Sisters available online. Breathe Free another Yin Yang Sisters instant beverage clears sinus congestion safely its main ingredient being magnolia buds. None of these Chinese pills or beverages raise blood pressure or aggravate chest pains. In fact several Chinese tea sweeteners, such as Ban Lan Gen instant beverage made with (antibiotic) isatis root and cane sugar, taste pleasant and effectively kill epidemic germs and reduce fever and headache. People with chronic fever conditions do well to regularly add this to tea or coffee. Any sort of antibiotic foods or herbs eventually weaken digestion so it is wise to increase yogurt, kafir or probiotic pills as well.

Cozy Home Remedies

Give yourself a break. During a cold stay at home, rest, drink lots of warm tea with lemon and fresh ginger. To open sinus congestion and improve breathing sniff or apply with a Q tip a drop of organic tea tree oil into each nostril. Sweat out aches and chills by adding 1 – 2 tablespoons of dried ginger powder to a warm bath. Drink a cup of warm basil leaf tea. Another useful kitchen herb is oregano. A tea made with oregano leaves the cooking herb is antibacterial and antiviral without raising blood pressure. Then wrap up and stay cozy in bed. Your garden and kitchen will keep you safe during cold season.

Andrographis for fever, sore throat, and flu

An extremely effective antibiotic herb recommended for flu sold in capsules in North American health food stores and online is called Andrographis (AKA Andrographis paniculata, Indian echinacea). In Chinatown herb stores the same inexpensive dried twig is called chuan xin lian. Pills made from andrographis and isatis [banlangan] both herbal antibiotics are in a pill called chuan xin lian. Vitamin Shoppe sells Kold Kare pills made in Maine, which is standardized andrographis. Another popular Scandinavian cold remedy Kan Jang contains standardized extracts of both andrographis and Siberian ginseng (Eleutherococcus senticosus). Andrographis is an immune-boosting herb used to treat fever of colds and flu, respiratory and sinus infections, and certain cancers. Positive research results have been seen in relation to stomach, skin, prostate and breast cancer cells, in test-tube studies.

Andrographolides in the plant enhance immune functions such as production of white blood cells (scavengers of bacteria and other foreign matter), release of interferon, and activity of the lymph system. Although andrographis is safe for most people, its bitter taste may trigger a headache, fatigue, nausea or diarrhea. To avoid digestive side-effects you might take the herbal pill along with cooked food or ginger tea.

Anyone using blood-thinning drugs, blood pressure medicines, and chemotherapy drugs should consult their physician before using andrographis or other strongly anti-inflammatory or liver cleansing herbs because they may remove medicines from the body. At home I might add a tiny pinch of the bitter twig and a slice of raw ginger into my morning tea pot to head off a sore throat or cold. It can be used throughout flu season, but like any antibiotic it should be balanced with healthy digestive bacteria from yogurt, turmeric, naturally fermented vegetables and other sources.

A flu-shot or not?

Some people swear by flu shots and the medical establishment re-commends them especially for the elderly and for surgery patients. They are a money-making boon to drug companies. However, a grow-ing number of people avoid flu shots fearing ingredients including flu virus strains from previous years. The flu shot injection contains thimerosal, a source of mercury, as a preservative. On the other hand, the flu vaccine applied inside the nose contains the *live virus*, which means it could mix with a superbug in the nose (see the chapter on superbugs.) The combination of flu and superbug kills. Neither flu shot nor nasal application presents a perfect solution. Recent research points to brain damage resulting from certain vaccines. We need to keep up to date with related research done by brain specialists. You risk either getting the flu or getting sicker from the vaccine. The flu shot may not even contain the correct flu strain for the present year. Whether or not to use the flu shot should be seriously discussed with your physician considering the flu as a possible threat to heart health.

Cold/flu prevention for heart patients

Of course wash your hands frequently, encourage your family to do so, and place a hand sanitizer within easy reach. Did you know that cold germs as well as MRSA, an antibiotic-resistant superbug, colonize in the nose? At least one third of the world's population are carriers of MRSA without having symptoms. In chapter 6 we will see the disastrous effects of superbugs for heart patients. Warn family and friends to sneeze into their tissue or cupped hands then wash their hands. Wear gloves outside during cold/flu season. Open a window when taking a taxi because cold and flu germs live for hours after someone has sneezed. Fresh air may help to reduce them.

A favorite prevention treatment for sore throat and colds and flu is gargling with warm water and antimicrobial pure, essential tea tree oil. (See the Q & A for a product link.)

Heart patients

Insomnia is a particular problem for heart patients because disturbed sleep weakens vitality and aggravates heart irregularities including arrhythmia and chest pain. Choosing the right sort of sleep treatment is important. All over-the-counter herbs and natural remedies that sedate qi must be avoided. Hops, valerian, and passionflower (Passiflora incarnata) are too sedating to the nervous system and the heart especially for people at risk of heart failure.

Flower teas for improved sleep

Chamomile tea is safe for heart patients because it is digestive, however it can cause allergies for people sensitive to ragweed. Linden flower tea, a popular evening tea in France called tilleul, is cooling for liverish irritability and may improve high blood pressure as it soothes nervous irritations. Are you traveling? A capsule is easier to use than a tea: Here are two Asian sleep treatments that improve health and may ease certain heart discomforts. Avoid using sleep remedies during flying because the effects may be too strong.

Bacopa

Would you like to improve your mind as you sleep? Some commonly used heart drugs list reduced mental clarity and memory as side effects. Although not recommended specifically for insomnia, the herb Bacopa monniera has long been promoted in Ayurveda for its ability to enhance memory and mental clarity. Some people cannot fall asleep because their mind is busy with anxious mumbling like radio static. Bacopa may be useful for them because it helps calm anxiety while improving mental functions. (8) See in Notes at the back of the book "Bacopa and the brain." The recommended dose is 500 mgs twice during the day for adults.

An Ayurvedic Sleeping Pill

Tranquil Mind, an Ayurvedic herbal pill made by Banyan Botanicals located in New Mexico, contains organic herbs useful for sound sleep that also regulate hypertension. Among the excellent herbal tonics in this pill are Eclipta alba, a rejuvenating herb that improves the liver, blood, complexion and hair combined with ashwagandha root an adrenal tonic. (9) There is no need to take a knock-out sleeping pill when so many wonderful healing herbs exist that correct the physical and mental problems that prevent rest and sleep. Next is another beautifying treatment useful for a night's quiet sleep.

A Warm Oil Rub

One way to settle down for a good night's sleep includes a warming oil rub for your feet. As you bring circulation to your feet with the oil massage, tension leaves your mind, aches leave your back and you feel relaxed. Sesame oil is recommended to quiet nervous anxiety, followed by a warm bath adding essential oil of lavender. Listen to music, a meditation CD or watch your favorite relaxing movie. You may drift off and wake up at the end of the movie. If you delay bedtime until 1AM or 2AM it will be harder to fall asleep.

Improve Your Heart as you Sleep

Dietary researcher Dr. Ibrahim Adnan Saracoglu recommends the following treatment to reduce cholesterol and improve overall heart health as well as memory. Wait until you start to become sleepy and at least two hours after eating dinner then drink an 8 oz. glass of fresh carrot juice with 1 teaspoon of oil added to improve absorption of vitamin A. Healthy oil capsules are easy to use. They include vitamin D3, E, flaxseed oil or hemp oil among others. The combination of raw carrot and oil is helpful for people who cannot sleep because of troubled digestion and breathing. The carrot's vitamin A improves memory when taken at night because that's when the brain needs it most. If you have weak digestion and a tendency for diarrhea, use caution with raw carrot juice.

A Cool Head

Dr. Bernard Jensen, author of many helpful nutrition books, was a generous soul who shared his great wealth of natural health knowledge with several generations of avid fans, patients, and health experts. He lived into his 90s, spry, charming and healthy. Following an automobile accident that left him partially paralyzed and in pain from bone fractures, he fasted with carrot juice for four months, added raw goat milk during the latter part of the fast, and recovered. Although his books and teaching stressed diet and Western herbal advice, he had a practical view on many aspects of health and wellness. He advised everyone to keep a cool head. To protect the brain and reduce hypertension discomforts, he advised avoiding long exposure in a sauna. Following his advice, at home I apply to the scalp a cooling hair oil such as jojoba or one from India containing amla powder, a rejuvenating gooseberry, or black cumin seed to enhance hair growth. You will read about amla in chapter 17. Applying Asian herbal secrets your sleep can become a time for health, rejuvenation and beauty.

Heart Health Checkup

- How often do you have comfortable sleep and awaken refreshed?
- How many pillows do you use? More than one or two may indicate a breathing problem and possible congestive heart problems.

- Do you feel short of breath when lying down? Climbing stairs? People who are overweight or have asthma may develop heart failure discomforts more easily.
- Do you toss and turn in your sleep? It may be from chronic pain. Try to isolate the cause of your restlessness and address it with a natural treatment for pain. My book *Naturally Pain Free* offers practical advice.
- Do you have recurrent dreams? Dreams are a sort of mental detoxification. At times I have dreamt of driving and being lost or being late for an appointment. It seemed to signal an uneasy, irregular or slow heartbeat associated with fatigue and worry. You may be able to identify such physical themes associated with dreams. The body talks to us and the mind reveals its secrets if we listen. Their themes echo in our heart.

Q & A: Immunity against infections
What's a simple defense against infections? *Tea Tree Oil is antibacterial, antiviral, antifungal. Wash your hands with water and as few drops of tea tree oil. Apply it to cuts, toenail fungus, bruises, dilute and gargle to prevent/treat sore throat; apply with Q-tip into the nose for colds/flu prevention and sinus infections. An all round detoxifier:* http://www.absorby-ourhealth.com/product/tea-tree-essential-oil/?ref=4041

SIX

SUPERBUGS NEAR AND FAR

I am sitting by an elegant swimming pool in the Florida Keys. The sunshine is bright and I happy to be on a winter vacation with Michael. I can see an iguana lolling in the grass and in a nearby mangrove patch a lazy manatee is amusing tourists. I notice on my arm a pink spot, a slight depression in the skin, but nothing seems unusual. Next day I have a slight fever. My usual liver cleansing herbs can not cool me. Our local medical doctor takes one look at my arm and says, "MRSA." Methicillin-resistant Staphylococcus aureus (MRSA) is a bacteria, a kind of staph infection, that is resistant to many antibiotics. I use a medical skin cream and a deep-acting sulfa drug, which gives me a painful yeast infection but nips the germ affecting my skin in the bud. Michael was not so lucky. We had kissed and shared the bed sheets which spread the bacteria, and soon he developed systemic (internal) MRSA. He sat shivering and pale in a chair too weak to stand. After taking the sulfa drug he eventually was told he recovered. But we remain unsure of the long term effects.

MRSA can kill heart patients. Michael was diagnosed with MRSA one year before his heart failure, and he was still weakened from the sulfa drug treatment with side-effects, including bruising, body aches and anemia. The MRSA bacteria eats flesh, including the heart and lungs, and is antibiotic-resistant. It mutates to keep one step ahead of modern medicine. We were given a sulfa drug, frequently used during the 1940s, that had been discontinued due to harsh side-effects, because the bacteria did not recognize that older drug.

Stephen Jay Gould (1941-2002) professor of zoology and geology at Harvard University, author of over twenty books said, "The most outstanding feature of life's history is a constant domination by bacteria." Healthy bacteria in our gut keep us alive, some others are harmful. Heart patients have to be especially careful to avoid infections because of weakened immunity from a heavy load of medicines and invasive treatments often required of them. In fact the sedating nature of certain heart drugs may even retard recovery time. Common infections weaken the heart by causing inflammation, arrhythmia or by damaging heart muscle. In this chapter we will look at Superbugs such as MRSA (Methicillin-resistant Staphylococcus aureus) a strain of antibiotic resistant staph bacteria. Tick and mosquito-borne diseases, including Lyme Disease, are a fast growing problem and pose an especial danger for heart patients.

Superbugs are everyday infections such as sore throat (streptococcus) and skin rash (staphylococcus aureus) that, due to overuse of antibiotics in patients, our foods and food livestock, have become more deadly due to their immunity to antibiotics. We used to fear superbugs in hospital settings where many patients use antibiotics and the chances of passing an infection from patients to medical staff or medical equipment and hospital furnishings are very great. Now we know that superbugs are found everywhere at gyms, yoga centers, in cabs and subways, on public stair-railings, in beach sand, and places where people live, work and play. Superbug infections are passed skin to skin or by touching infected pets, clothing and gym or other equipment used by infected persons. It can colonize in droplets released in the air by coughing.

People at high risk have skin sores or wounds, hospital patients with skin infections or intravenous lines, people with pneumonia, HIV or compromised immunity; people with stents or joint replacements, diabetes and chronic skin diseases like eczema. Staph is a very common infection, one out of three persons have it on their skin. Estimates vary but as many as one third of the world's population may have MRSA. Each year, 90,000 Americans suffer from invasive MRSA infection. About 20,000 die. Many are children. Superbugs have become much more common in recent years and, with proposed cuts in health spending, both research and cleaning staff due to reduced immigration, hospitals and communities will be less able to keep up with prevention and treatments.

Superbugs colonize in dark warm places especially your nose and sexual areas. Do you live or dine with a nose-picker? A dangerous dinner guest indeed. Cough and flu season make superbugs even more deadly as superbugs become airborne. Since we lack experience with newer strains of these superbugs we lack antibodies. That means superbug infections hit hard not only against the elderly and babies but also young, strong, otherwise healthy people. Germs are not particular about who they infect whether rich or poor people, and they are winning the battle of survival, showing up in unexpected places including luxury settings. This chapter is your guide to a new age of microscopic illness. Everyone, especially heart patients, must take special precautions when visiting the dentist or having surgery. Pay attention to who you visit and who you invite to dinner. You or someone you know may already be a carrier without overt symptoms.

Staph is one of the most common causes of skin infections in the United States. Babies get it and we call it diaper rash. An American nursing journal article by a dermatologist reported that most everyday skin rashes can be avoided if people simply changed their bed sheets more often! Some rashes don't need special treatment, however, MRSA is found in different parts of the body. The symptoms depend upon where you're infected. It can cause mild skin rash that looks like sores or boils, but it can also infect surgical wounds, the bloodstream, the lungs, or the urinary tract.

Garden-variety staph are common bacteria that easily live unnoticed in our bodies. Based on a January, 2013 article in *Science Daily*, 20 of 22 nursing homes in Orange County, California have CA-MRSA (community-acquired MRSA) with the higher number of infected people being under the age of 65. Younger people are mobile and social and therefore more effective at spreading germs. A much higher percentage of infected people work in medical settings or live in high-risk areas of the world where population density is high and sanitation poor. For example, MRSA is reported to be incurable in India. Drug-resistant tuberculosis has reemerged in New York and other big cities, and MRSA mixed with flu germs quickly kills people.

Overuse of antibiotics for livestock has increased such infections. Food animals became a breeding ground for drug-resistant infections that were passed to us in their flesh. In a January, 2013 article in *New England Journal of Medicine* entitled "The Future of Antibiotics and Resistance," Dr. Brad Spellberg quotes Dr. Alexander Fleming who in 1945 called for stopping the overuse of penicillin in order to slow the development of drug resistance. Spellberg writes, "Nearly 65 years later, in 2009, more than 3 million kg of antibiotics were administered to human patients in the United States alone; in 2010, a staggering 13 million kg were administered to animals. The majority of the animal antibiotic use was meant to *promote the growth* of livestock. We cannot confront resistance unless we stop exposing the environment to massive quantities of antibiotics and their resulting selective pressure." Spellberg suggests better monitoring and shorter use of antibiotics for patients and elimination of antibiotic use for growth of livestock. Here is an example of how superbugs especially harm certain heart patients.

Superbugs and your heart

Douglas had been our accountant for several years before he moved to Arizona and we lost touch. He was middle-aged, recently divorced, and like many people worried about putting his kids through college. We met him in a Thai restaurant when he returned to New York for his daughter's graduation. He looked thin, tense and I was surprised when he ordered only salad saying that was all he could eat. After polite chatter we learned he had been hospitalized for a month and given a heavy load of intravenous antibiotics for six months. Astounded I asked what had happened and he replied, "My teeth."

The risk of dental work, stents and (PCI)

Ten years previously, Douglas had experienced chest pain (angina) that signaled a heart attack, and he underwent a commonly used operation called angioplasty. In about 70%–90% of cases, angioplasty involves the insertion of a stent. A percutaneous coronary intervention (PCI), often called balloon angioplasty, is performed using a slender balloon-tipped tube a catheter which is threaded through an artery in the groin (femoral artery) or wrist (radial artery) to the trouble spot in a heart artery. The balloon is then inflated, pushing back the plaque, widening the narrowed artery so that blood can flow more easily.

Douglas's doctor had inserted a stent, a tiny structure made of wire mesh, similar to a spring inside a ballpoint pen, that when expanded locks in place, and holds the artery open. A drug-eluting stent slowly released medicine over time to prevent the artery from narrowing again. In addition, his doctor prescribed an anti-platelet medication to prevent future blood clots within the stent and arteries. But that did not protect against future infection.

Ten years later Douglas developed a gum infection that he did not notice. The tooth decay germs migrated from his blood to endanger the stent. Germs gather wherever they can and a stent being plastic has no natural defense against infection so that the area surrounding his stent became a stamping ground for a strept infection that nearly killed him. Any dental work or surgery, especially one involving a plastic or metal part anywhere in the body, makes a patient more vulnerable to serious infection since the body's natural germ-fighting defenses do not work for plastic or metal and the tissue surrounding the stent, or joint replacement, can easily become infected and die. You can protect yourself daily against tooth decay and gum disease, while protecting your heart with a natural, wholesome antibacterial tooth powder, neem tree bark, in place of commercial toothpaste. Also gargle with warm water and 1 drop of essential tea tree oil.

Someday in the sunny future we may be able to "grow" our own body parts using stem cells as suggested in a February 2013 article in the UK Telegraph, "'Grow your own' hip replacements could become available within a decade, according to British scientists working on a new type of prosthetic that would become an organic part of the body." But we will still need to protect ourselves against superbugs. Heart disease is serious enough without worrying about catching a cold or flu, a toothache, or rash!

Stay Safe and Clean

Do you live or work with sick or elderly people who take many medications or otherwise have weak immunity? Or with careless people whose dirty habits put your health at risk? Have you had MRSA or another superbug that makes you and those around you susceptible? You may be a carrier. Here are a few basic hygienic lifestyle changes to implement immediately. Everyone advises to wash your hands frequently but that is not enough. Especially when working with sick people, use an alcohol based soap and paper towels. Rinse with tea tree oil. Use the disinfectant tissues and antiseptic dispensers provided in smart supermarkets, hospital and doctors' offices. Avoid getting germs in your mouth, eyes, and skin cuts by keeping your skin clean and your hands off your face. Use a disposable tissue to blow your nose. Swab it out with tea tree oil on a Q-tip when exposed to sick people or hospitals.

Do you develop a sore throat after being out among people who cough? You can feel safe using herbal antibiotic Chuan Xin Lian the Chinese colds/flu pill or andrographis capsules described in the previous chapter. Antibiotic-resistant superbugs do not identify traditional herbal remedies and therefore are not resistant to them.

A gentile habit

Today in quality Japanese restaurants we are given a scented hand towel before and after meals. Let's reinstate the finger bowl, formerly a common practice in polite society. Do your family, dinner guests, or patients wash their hands after using the restroom? Do they pick their nose? Eat with their hands? Before a meal, place on the table in front of them a finger bowl filled with water adding a scented alcohol-based disinfectant soap. You might add tea tree oil and essential oil of lavender to a few drops of glycerin soap and water. Another thing to remember, restaurant menus, door knobs and stairway rails are *never* disinfected and, according to the NIH, often have Salmonella or E.coli germs on them. (11)

According to the Mayo clinic, Escherichia coli (E. coli) bacteria normally live in the intestines of people and animals. Most varieties of E. coli cause relatively brief diarrhea. But a few particularly nasty strains cause severe abdominal cramps, bloody diarrhea and vomiting. Normally, you may be exposed to E. coli from contaminated water or food especially raw vegetables and undercooked ground beef, but it can be passed by infected people on to anything they touch. Healthy adults usually recover from infections with E. coli within a week, but young children and older adults can develop a life-threatening form of kidney failure hemolytic uremic syndrome (HUS).

One health expert advised, "When eating in restaurants, hold the top of the menu and live." Most people hold a menu on the sides and not the top. You may prefer to order your favorite dishes without consulting the menu. But, as a heart patient or someone with compromised immunity, to be safe carry in your pocket or purse a package of disinfectant skin wipes.

Dress to avoid infection

There is nothing weird about wearing gloves when taking the subway or out shopping yet very few people wear gloves except during winter. Watch almost any movie made during the 1930's or 40's and you see men and women wearing hats to work, women wearing gloves and carrying delicate handbags. Since those days women have become hard-working, tough, careless—they no longer wear gloves. It's a shame.

Tea tree oil, Nature's germ-fighter

Add some protection to your makeup. You may already wash your hands and face and change your clothes and shoes after coming home from a hospital or visiting a sick friend. But if you add this simple protection before going out, you can avoid most infections and improve your breathing as well. Add a drop of organic tea tree oil to a Q tip and swab the inside of each nostril. Remember: Supergerms and cold/flu germs live in the nose. If you have chronic stuffy nose, according to Mayo Clinic, it is most likely a fungal sinus infection. Tea tree oil stops the infection and protects us from contaminated air in public transportation and other closed public areas. Taking tea tree oil internally daily one drop at a time in hot water or tea can also reduce or eliminate bacterial, viral and fungal infections. Be sure to support your digestive health by taking yogurt or acidophilus daily so that necessary intestinal bacteria can live.

Silver

Years ago while visiting India I found herbal pills wrapped in silver paper and thought it was a preservative, but was told that silver and gold leaf papers have been used by Ayurvedic herbal doctors for thousands of years because of their energetic value, silver being cooling and gold energizing. Silver was used as a topical antiseptic in Europe starting in the late 1800s. Silver nitrate solution is required by law in most American States used for newborns as a topical eye drop to prevent eye infections. I was pleased to have my surgical scars covered with a bandage containing silver paper and told not to remove it for a week when I had my hip replacement surgery at Dartmouth Hitchcock Medical Center New Hampshire, one of America's finest up-to-date teaching hospitals.

Silver, an antibacterial agent for internal as well as external use, has recently become popular and you can find many brands of colloidal (liquid) silver for sale online and in some stores. Colloidal silver, a liquid silver processed in a way to maintain the correct balance of ions, may be sprayed on skin or bedding. Or you can take one teaspoon internally first thing in the morning or between meals. Take acidophilus at another time of day to insure proper digestion. During a hospital stay apply the liquid to skin scratches or irritations. Argyria, when excess silver in the body eventually leads to a blue-gray tinge to the skin, has been eliminated since newer and better products have been produced. (10)

You can feel safe from bacteria if you rinse your mouth with colloidal silver or take one teaspoon daily between meals. See the Resource section for sources in North America. One woman I know developed MRSA in the hospital and was given up for lost. When she took one teaspoon of colloidal silver every four hours she recovered. Her case is not at all isolated. Some day surgeons may insert silver in addition to the traditional heart stents and valves.

Asian Herbs to Protect Immunity and Energy

Later chapters detail many sorts of tonics that enhance energy and immunity that have been used for generations by traditional Asian doctors. Here as a preview is an herbal pill that many people may use as long as they do not have fever or allergies to the specific herbs in the combination. It is an example of a typical Asian herbal formula that combines different sorts of herbs that work together synergistically in order to support wellness. Some herbs are germ fighters and others are tonics and finally other herbs are added to reduce unpleasant side-effects like cramps or dizziness. Here is how it works.

Astra 8, made by Health Concerns in California, contains top quality herbal tonics, including astragalus which increases T cells our natural defense against illness, ligustrum added to enhance blood production and circulation, ganoderma a medicinal mushroom to support immunity, eleuthero ginseng to reduce stress, codonopsis to fortify the lungs and kidneys, schizandra to protect the liver, oryza sprout to help regulate digestion, and licorice root added to ease absorption of the other herbs. This pill has been recommended as a general energy and immunity tonic and can be of great use during times of stress, inclement weather, and exhaustion. A theme I stress in this book is, enhancing vitality is the best defense against illness.

Some people swear by vitamin C. It does enhance all other remedies you use and helps to boost adrenal energy and therefore immunity. What is the best form of vitamin C to use? Eating oranges is not enough, besides they contain lots of sugar. Liposomal vitamin C has been proven most effective and easily absorbed form of C. It is broken down into nano particles. For example, http://www.absorbyourhealth. com/product/liposomal-vitamin-c-best-price-net-1-gram-vit-c-every-teaspoon/?ref=4041

Super-Dooper Germs and Greed

In December, 2015 Reuter's broke the story of American drug companies selling combination drugs that where neither approved by our FDA nor the Indian government to Indian doctors. According to Reuters, the problem in India, where there has been an explosion of combination drugs, is those drugs have become a way to boost sales and increase market share. More and more companies have tacked on ingredients to existing drugs so they can peddle a new product to doctors and chemists. Many doctors also see them as providing quick-fix solutions that cover multiple possible symptoms with a single pill, said a physician employed by a pharmaceutical company. Dumping unregulated prescription drugs into a country like India with a large population has and will continue to create superbugs at an alarming rate. A percentage of India is mobile, traveling for business or pleasure. That means their homegrown superbugs are worldwide.

Lyme Disease and Your Heart

There are infections that only avoidance of a tick can prevent. The best known is Lyme disease, first named in the 1970s for the town in Connecticut where it was discovered. The incidence of Lyme disease in America has grown exponentially in the last ten years, mainly in New England with Vermont, New Hampshire, Maine, New York State, Connecticut, Delaware, and Minnesota reporting the most cases, over 200 cases per 100,000 people infected most often during summer. With climate change, Lyme and other tick-borne disease has spread to Canada, Eastern and Western Europe. The early stage of the disease may or may not include a bull's eye skin rash that goes away in a week or so. Then comes fever, aches, fatigue, lethargy common flu-like symptoms that may be treated with antibiotics. Then stage three can include arthritic swelling and pain often in the knee, nerve damage such as facial paralysis (Bell's palsy) and heart damage including possible arrhythmia and heart failure. Not a pretty picture! Treatment is with antibiotics depending upon the stage and location of the disease. Here is some simple advice offered by Vermont Public Health on how to avoid Lyme disease:

- Avoid Ticks: When outdoors, walk in the center of trails and avoid wooded areas. Repel Ticks. Use 20-30 percent DEET on skin/clothing. Treat clothing/gear with permethrin
- Remove Ticks: Bathe or shower within 2 hours after spending time outside in tick prone areas. Conduct a full body tick check using a mirror. Inspect pets and gear for ticks;
- Here is something easy and safe: Running your clothing in the dryer for 5-10 minutes on high heat after coming indoors should kill any ticks that have attached to your clothing.

Heart Health Checkup

Heart patients and their caregivers have to be extra careful about cleanliness because any infection is dangerous. MRSA is worse! How often do you wash your hands with soap and warm water? How about after using the toilet and before eating? Do you or someone near you have a rude snotty habit?

How often do you change your bed sheets and bath towels? Bed sores are not the only problem you can get in a hospital or homecare setting. MRSA has been found on the plastic curtains that separate patients in private rooms. Acne and rashes are very common and may result from dirty clothes and linens, supergerms, mites, dust and allergies.

Do you touch restaurant menus or eat fresh produce from a supermarket, before washing them, despite germy hands that have touched it before you? Do you grab the door knob in a public bathroom or taxi, the stair rail in the subway or public building, or exercise equipment at the gym or a yoga mat without regard to safety? Most of us do. It makes a case for carrying your own hand sanitizer wipes.

Do you warn your dentist that you are a heart patient? Heart patients require different pain medications, often extra antibiotics and extra careful hygienic treatment, especially if they have a stent, pacemaker or other internal medical apparatus.

Do you live in or visit New England during the summer? Beware of Lyme Disease. There is no scientifically tested home treatment and medical treatment with antibiotics has to be updated as the disease changes. I have found articles by people who have claimed to be cured of Lyme disease after using an alcohol extract made from raw teasel root. It warrants investigation. If you go near the woods wear long pants tucked into boots and a long sleeve shirt. Walk in the middle, not the side of the road or deep woods during summer. Check for ticks and a bull's eye rash when you get home; shower, wash your hair, and put your clothes into the dryer at high heat. New England folk remedies for preventing tick bites are amusing—everything from wearing fabric softener sheets in your pocket to walking fast to out-run them.

Q & A: Immunity

I want a tonic to enhance immunity: *Pine Bark Extract: Anti-in-flammatory, antioxidant, tonic*: http://www.absorbyourhealth. com/product/pine-bark-extract-200mg-100-capsules-95-opc-flavanoids-powerful-antioxidant-free-radical-scavenger-dr-oz-recommended-skin/?ref=4041

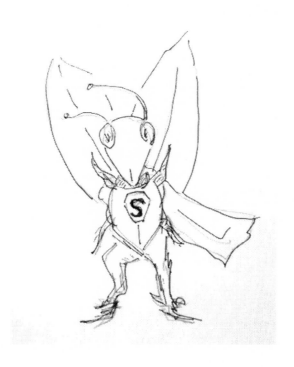

SEVEN

SAVE YOUR LIFE: EMERGENCY HELP

Maybe you and a companion are hiking, sitting in a subway car or an airplane or stuck in rush hour traffic and you feel a sharp prolonged chest pain. As the pain gets worse you wonder, "What if this is a heart attack? I've changed my lifestyle and diet, to the point of eating fresh garlic in salads, to thin my blood." The garlic has cost you several friendships. You look slimmer and bright-eyed, but now the center of your chest really hurts and the pain is spreading to your arm and jaw. Panic sets in. You start to perspire and sense your heart beating. Parts Two and Three of this book detail healing foods and powerful herbs that help prevent heart troubles from developing, but they are for long term, not emergency use.

After dialing 911, while waiting for an ambulance to arrive, what can you or your friend do as a safety treatment? Do not wait to decide whether or not the chest pain is a heart attack or simple angina a temporary stress pain that might develop when the heart is not getting enough oxygen. They seem the same but may end differently. Angina pain goes away.

Heart Attack or Angina?

Heart attack (myocardial infarction) happens when blood supply to the heart or part of the heart is cut off partially or completely, which leads to death of the heart muscle due to lack of oxygen. Heart attacks usually occur after periods of rest or being recumbent, and only rarely occur after exercise. That means it could happen early morning or when you awaken from sleep. TCM herbalists and martial artists who study meridian theory know that our organs are vulnerable at predictable times of day and night because the meridians affecting their function are more or less full of qi. The heart is vulnerable at around 10AM but meridians affecting digestion, adrenal energy and breathing during early morning also play a role in heart health.

According to the Mayo Clinic, someone having a heart attack may experience any or all of the following:

- Uncomfortable pressure, fullness or squeezing pain in the center of the chest
- Prolonged pain in the upper abdomen
- Discomfort or pain spreading beyond the chest to the shoulders, neck, jaw, teeth, or one or both arms
- Shortness of breath
- Lightheadedness, dizziness, fainting
- Sweating
- Nausea

A heart attack may cause any or all of the above symptoms for at least 15 minutes or the signs of the attack may be more subtle. Many people who experience a heart attack have warning signs such as back and leg aches, dizziness or others hours, days or weeks in advance.

Angina

Angina (angina pectoris) is a "miniature heart attack" caused by a short term blockage. Angina, unlike a heart attack, almost always occurs after strenuous exercise or periods of high stress. A key difference between a heart attack and angina is that angina starts to relieve a few minutes after resting, whereas a heart attack will not improve with rest. Pain in the chest can have many different causes and in an emergency you should not attempt to distinguish between them. Call for help when you experience chest pain especially if you have had heart problems in the past. During a heart attack you may have pale, cold, clammy, ashen grey skin, and feel an impending sense of doom. Take it seriously. Some people with diabetes have had similar discomforts that have gone away. But don't try to diagnose the pain by yourself. It is a good idea to cultivate a relationship with your acupuncturist well before any panic attack. Do not feel guilty if you are so shocked and afraid by your or your loved-one's heart attack that all you can do is call 911. That is what you are expected to do. But here are some natural options you may be able to use to great effect.

What to do about severe chest pain or the above symptoms

- Call 911 for help.
- Loosen your belt and shirt to help ease breathing.
- Sit up comfortably leaning back at a 45 degree angle with feet on the floor but knees up. Stay comfortably warm.
- Breathe slowing and deeply into the lower abdomen.
- Take your prescribed medicine if you have it. Do not eat or drink anything.
- Press the acupuncture heart-revival points (described below) located in the palm and at the tip of the little finger.
- If possible, take a dose of Suxiao Jiuxin Wan a Chinese "heart revival" pill to help dilate blood vessels and ease breathing. The recommended dose is usually 3 – 4 pills for mild chest pain and difficulty breathing and 10 – 15 pills for heart attack.
- Stay calm.

Acupressure for relieving chest pain

If you are a caregiver for your family member or a heart patient, learn where the following acupuncture points are and how to use them. They may come in handy for easing simple temporary chest pains as well as serious heart problems. The acupuncture meridian associated with the heart and its functions follows its internal branches and comes to the surface of the skin at the underarm. Its points are located on the inside of the arm closest to your trunk and down to the tip of the little finger. In the lower end of the heart acupuncture meridian located on the palm side of each hand and to the tip of each little finger there are points that may relieve chest discomforts and ease blood flow through the heart. In other words those points lead inflammation, congestion and pain away from the chest and to the pinky finger. Use strong stimulation for up to five minutes on the following two points using your fingernail, a toothpick or pencil tip without puncturing the skin.

Pinch Pinky

Waiting for the ambulance to arrive, the simplest acupressure treatment to help relieve chest pressure is to pinch both sides of the nail and tip of the pinky finger with the thumb and pointing finger of the other hand. Pinch hard and hold until you can breathe comfortably and chest discomfort is improved. That might be as long as five minutes or more. Here are two additional "heart-revival" acupuncture points Heart 8 and 9 that you might stimulate with your thumbnail. See the illustration.

Heart 8 (shao fu, lesser mansion)

Find the point by making a loose fist. The tip of the little finger is where to find Heart 8, between the 4th and 5th metacarpal bones inside the palm. This point has been used to treat sore throat, tongue stiffness, and pain along the inside of the arms. Also "heart qi deficiency" with symptoms of palpitations, fear, and hot palms.

Push Heart 8 with strong stimulation and gently turn your neck to relieve stiffness in neck and upper back. Your acupuncturist can help you find these points and give supportive treatments. For example, for suspected heart failure, Heart 8 may be combined with Kidney 3 (tai xi, great ravine) located in the depression behind the ankle near the attachment of the Achilles tendon. Find Kidney 3 by pinching the back of the ankle at the Achilles tendon with two fingers. Kidney 3 is on the inner side of the ankle. Kidney 3 is used in acupuncture to "tonify kidney qi" in order to treat difficulty inhaling, dizziness, chronic weak lower back and knees, and frequent urination or uncontrolled diarrhea. Tell your acupuncturist if you have "cock's crow diarrhea" watery early morning diarrhea that comes suddenly at around 5:30 AM or earlier. That indicates that your qi (vitality) is low.

Heart 9 (Shao Chong, Lesser Surge)

This is the last point on the heart meridian located at the top inner corner of the nail of the little finger. To locate the point see the top of the hand, pinch the pinky finger with the opposite thumb and pointing finger placing the thumb on the side closer to your body and pointing finger on the outside edge. Heart 9 is located on the thumb side at the cuticle. See the drawing.

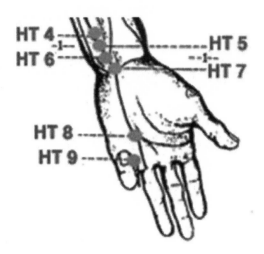

In acupuncture, the point called Heart 9 is used to clear excess inflammation and/or blockage from the heart meridian. An acupuncturist may take a drop of blood from it or needle it to treat anxiety, panic attacks, manic depression, epilepsy, etc. It has been used to restore consciousness for heart attack and stroke. It reduces a feeling of fullness below the heart, treating "blood and energy stagnation," and severe pain or distention in the heart area.

In general the tips of fingers and toes are the extremities of certain acupuncture meridians. They may be bled by a trained acupuncturist to ease pressure in the associated meridian or to achieve a strong internal rebalancing. For example, I once revived a young tour guide after she fainted from heat stroke, her first trip as a tour guide, in a northern Thailand jungle. I "sterilized" a sewing needle by dipping it into a match flame. A good trick to know if someone has heat stroke, but if stuck in a traffic jam having chest pains—pinch the tip of your pinky finger and call 911.

Pills for chest pain/heart attack: Chinese Suxiao jiuxin wan

Another thing you might do while waiting for an ambulance to take the heart patient to the hospital is for the patient to take a dose of Chinese over the counter herbs Suxiao jiuxin wan which are tiny pills that work like nitroglycerine to open blocked blood vessels and help resolve chest pain. They melt in the mouth. Some people regularly take a small dose (3 pills one or two times daily) of these herbal pills daily as part of their heart trouble prevention program. Medical camphor, a main ingredient, feels cooling to the throat and deepens the breath as it facilitates circulation and relieves chest pain. Asthma sufferers may find it comforting if it reduces wheezing for them.

Chinese Suxiao jiuxin wan (pills) for angina pectoris and heart attack: Keep the small ceramic bottle of pills at your bedside and in your wallet, or purse.

Suxiao jiuxin wan (AKA Su Xiao Jiu Xin Wan; generic name; Quick-acting Heart Reliever pill) is commonly used in China. An older, overweight friend who had developed shortness of breath while walking, a chronic heart failure symptom, before using Asian herbs regularly takes a small dose (4 – 5 pills) of Suxiao jiuxin wan in order to walk with ease in New York's polluted streets. He recently walked into a Chinese-run laundry in Manhattan, and the woman behind the counter smiled at him saying, "You use Chinese medicine." She smelled the faint aroma of camphor (like Vick's vapor rub) from Suxiao Jiuxin wan on my friend's breath. That's how commonly that medicine is used by Chinese people. Fifteen clinical trials involving 1,776 people were reported for suxiao jiuxin wan at pubmed (12.)

The conclusion of the trials was "Suxiao jiuxin wan appears to be effective in the treatment of angina pectoris and no serious side effects were identified." Another study cited at the website for University of Maryland Medical Center states: "suxiao jiuxin wan improved ECG measurements and reduced symptoms and frequency of acute angina attacks compared with nitroglycerin." The Chinese are slow to run strict clinical trials on herbs that have been in common use for hundreds of years. However, more research has been carried out on Asian herbs at NIH and at universities.

Suxiao jiuxin wan's herbal camphor (borneolum) dilates blood vessels. The other ingredient chuanxiong (AKA *Ligusticum chuanxiong* Hort.; *L. wallichii* Franch.) stimulates heart action and works along with the medicinal camphor to sweep blood vessels clean. According to TCM, the small pill that is dissolved slowly in the mouth or under the tongue, "Promotes qi and circulation. Relieves pain: like headaches, abdominal ache, chest pain, muscle pain, difficulty in menses (painful period), amenorrhea (no period.) It corrects blood stasis." It feels cooling for your throat and sinus. It is relaxing and improves breathing. It may lower blood pressure and ease circulation in the head, neck and chest.

If you take this sort of qi-moving pill regularly, do not take it with food, but only between meals. It may be taken at any time for severe chest pain. This pill is also useful for sex. It gets blood circulation to move where needed. According to the manufacturer other uses for Suxiao jiuxin wan include improved blood flow to the brain and it has antibiotic effects. (13)

Do not mix this medicine with other herbs, caffeine, or homeopathic remedies. You might keep some in the glove compartment of your car and your office desk. In Chapter 27. there is a checklist of supplements and herbal medicines you should keep on hand. The list of recommended remedies is based on research done by numerous heart experts and venerable healing traditions. You will understand how and when to use the remedies as you gradually read this book which can help you to decide which healing path to take.

Heart Health Checkup

Observe the palms of your hands. Are they red, pale, dry, warm or cold? Your hands contain the end points of meridians that impact your heart, lungs, and chest. If your hands tend to be cold and stiff, you can suspect that your circulation is challenged.

If hands tend to be warm, you may be a feverish, inflammatory person, or simply overheated by the environment such as radiator heat in winter or hot weather in summer. However if your hands tend to be warm/hot and red and dry you may have a problem with inflammation, dehydration or a related illness such as diabetes or congested blood circulation. Hot hands or cold hands are a long term tendency indicating imbalance.

However in an emergency situation, hands may suddenly change to a cold sweat. Your head may throb and throat feel dry and tight as your body reacts to stress.

Locate the acupuncture points on your hands described in this chapter and become familiar with how they affect your breathing and circulation when you massage your hands daily. Your hands are connected to your heart. They may give you the slack you need to survive a heavy incident, an accident or shock.

Another thing that protects the heart is the pericardium, a loose fibrous sack of tissue filled with fluid that protects the heart against external shocks. In Chinese medicine it has been called "the heart protector." It lubricates the heart, anchors it in place, and protects the heart from infections coming from other organs such as the lungs. Inflammation of the pericardium can mimic heart attack pain and may be caused by viral, bacterial and fungal infections such as HIV, herpes, mumps, and tuberculosis. Medical treatment is necessary.

Q & A: Panic

I am having a panic attack with pounding heartbeat, anxiety and sweating – *tightly grab your left wrist with your right hand, hold, inhale slowly and exhale downward slowly to your feet several times. With thumb and pointer finger of right hand pinch the tip of the left hand middle finger, the end point of the pericardium meridian, and hold as you breathe slowly.* If heart/chest discomfort does not resolve quickly, call 911.

Michael's Realtime One

Spending a week in a hospital is like being a prisoner. You're in bed most of the time, hooked up to an intravenous tube so you can go no farther than the adjoining bathroom. Nurses, pleasant enough, come by every so often, day and night, to take samples of your fluids. You wince when you're stuck with a needle, sleep because you're doped, and you remember when you were living. I was reminded of our two cats. Sure, they were tenderly cared for, mostly by Letha—fed prime cat food, combed and brushed, talked to and petted frequently. But in downtown New York or the Vermont woods they couldn't leave our apartment or condo—for their own good—and when driving in a car they were kept in a cage. A soft life but imprisoned.

We got the cats at a pet refuge in Vermont because of an invasion of voles in our condo in the woods. Sometimes called field mice, voles are stout, short, and hairy, and they run in packs. Since cold weather in the Green Mountains kills them, they burrow into your home at the first sign of autumn. Traps don't work. You can poison the creatures, but we don't harm animals, so our only solution was get a couple of cats, good hunters and their cat scent keeps voles away. At the refuge we were swamped by an array of friendly pussies, racks of them, each hoping to be adopted and find their "forever home." Except for a cage in a corner, from which we heard loud feline complaints. We were told by a staff member the female cat had been isolated because she didn't get along well, and that the refuge couldn't recommend her adoption. We sprang for her, and because of her stripes and lean, hungry look, we named her Tiger. Letha spotted a handsome male cat with long white fur, a distinguished look, blue eyes and a gorgeous fluffy tail. Obviously a ladies man, we named him Sir Fluff.

We no longer have voles in Vermont or mice in Manhattan. Tiger has earned her stripes. Fluff remains adorable and has become Letha's boyfriend. Our longtime friend, the author Ursule Molinaro, remarked that cats are people. Certainly they can communicate with us in ways sometimes subtle and, when hungry, by nagging and poking. Like us, cats may be driven to attempt the impossible or dangerous. In Vermont we have a back porch, about forty feet above the meadow that falls away until it rises again in green hills. It's a fine, healing view, and the nearby trees attract birds. Their chirping alerts Tiger who will charge at the screen door, taking it down a couple of times. If we hadn't reinforced the door, Tiger would have gone onto the porch and into mid-air, chasing birds. The ensuing fall might have used up her nine lives.

People can be just as foolishly driven by instinct, or by wishful thinking. Lying in a hospital bed, being occasionally tormented by this or that jab, I thought about my own life's path and what had brought me to being laid low. I had followed the American Dream conscientiously and had run across some of its nightmarish elements. I grew up a street fighter in Brownsville, Brooklyn, a tough neighborhood to this day. My maternal grandfather, a blacksmith from Russia, was the neighborhood storyteller on the lower East Side, and my mother grew up a book reader. So did I, thanks to the Brooklyn Public Library at Grand Army Plaza, which I bicycled to along Eastern Parkway. At twelve I forged an I.D. that gave me access to adult books, and I read fiction from Dickens and Jane Austin to Hemingway and Norman Mailer. I became a jazz addict, and I sneaked in at the be-bop clubs on 52nd Street. At sixteen I found myself at Cornell, dressed in my one button pearl grey suit with a rolled collar and black string tie. Presto! A frat boy in tweed jacket, jeans, and white bucks who was majoring in philosophy and taking Russian lit classes with Vladimir Nabokov. Later I tried law school, then joining Fidel Castro's rebels in the mountains of Cuba, and for a while teaching at NYU. But I'm neither a revolutionary nor scholar, so I became a freelance writer.

That worked for a time. I could get by on the advances for my next book, and one book was sufficiently scandalous that it was covered in the tabloids from New York to London and translated from Istanbul to Seoul. I had my 15 minutes of fame, being recognized on the streets of Manhattan by deliverymen. As the twenty-first century rolled in, the book business, overshadowed by the Internet, no longer paid regularly. So, knowing nothing about the stock market, in 2001 I started buying gold at $240 an ounce. It looked cheap. In 2008 when world markets collapsed I bought dirt cheap mining stocks, and by 2012, with gold nearing $2,000, I was a millionaire. Letha and I did spring and fall in Manhattan, winter in Miami, and summer in Vermont. Then came the gold crash in April 2013, which cost me at least a million, self-doubt, aggravation, and heart failure. You want to be your own man, a tough guy? Or a hunter cat? You're going to pay the price. . .

It's after July 4th, I'm out of bed, and Letha and I are in Dr. Alan Kono's office. A native Hawaiian, he fits fine into New England. He is a dedicated man, actively shuttling between Dartmouth Medical, where he is head of the heart failure unit, and a major Boston hospital. Although nearing the end of my hospital stay for acute heart failure, he wasted no time in telling me, "You could drop dead anytime." He was looking over the results of my catheter exam, an experience you would prefer to avoid. Stretched out on a surgical table in a darkened room, with a catheter tube plugged into my groin and traveling up into my coronary blood vessels, I couldn't move or see anything. But I could hear the hospital radiologists talking, looking at their X-ray screens, until one called out, "Okay, I got something." The term "catheter" goes back to Ancient Greek medicine, meaning "to sit," because Greek doctors maneuvered the narrow tube through the urethra into the bladder. In my angiography, the procedure gave a picture of the inside of the arteries, to see how badly they were obstructed. Several major blood vessels were clogged by plaque, in two arteries causing a constriction of 75% of the blood flow. My heart became starved for blood and failed, or nearly so.

A slight rupture in either vessel, known as a heart attack, would likely kill me. Despite the distinction made for diagnostic purposes between heart failure and heart attack, the two are kissing cousins. One sets you up for the other about half the time. The evidence of disease (termed atherosclerosis) is plaque build up (mainly the fatty substance known as cholesterol) in the blood vessels, straining the heart muscle and impeding the flow of blood to the bodily organs, muscles, and extremities. But cholesterol itself is not the villain. As you will learn from Letha, cholesterol is both absorbed from food and made by our livers and essential to our brains, nervous system, and digestion. We can't function without it. So what are the root causes of heart disease, and how can it be prevented and cured? Therein lies a great quarrel, a battle over our very lives.

Dr. Kono was concerned. He emphasized my perfectly awful test results. My left ventricle, the heart's main pumping engine, was failing. Further, the heart cells secrete an amino acid tagged BNP. The higher the number the harder the heart muscle works, and my number was sky high. My ejection fraction, which measures how well the heart is pumping blood, had fallen into the pits. I got the message, and the doctor calmly presented three corresponding avenues of treatment: first, cardiac drugs. These he would prescribe in any case until I saw him next. They were maintenance, to prevent the disease from progressing. Next came stents, surgically inserted into the clogged areas of arteries to open them and allow the blood to flow. Former President George W. Bush had the procedure done in August 2013, as a matter of course, though it caused some controversy. Finally, there was the doctor's suggestion: coronary artery bypass surgery. Think of it as blood's traffic detour: the highway is blocked so you abandon it and go around using side roads. With a new route set up, and the arteries sewed up, the heart satisfactorily pumps blood to far-flung bodily destinations. It should be a permanent fix. My Vermont dentist had a quadruple bypass, and he drills away like a much younger man.

Released from the hospital, escorted to the parking garage, I was given some time to think over my choice. Behind the wheel of my car, a free man in control of my destiny, Letha at my side, I knew my path.

PART TWO

FOODS FOR A HAPPY HEART

Flavorful teas, sour cherries, cooling greens, pungent cleansing
spices—these are flavors that comfort your heart

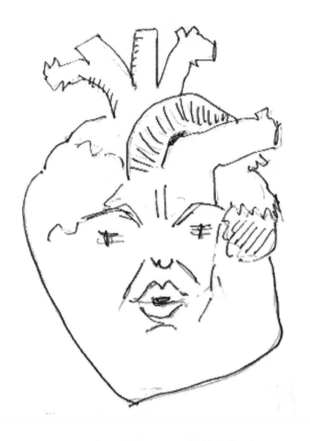

Your diet gives me a bellyache!
Think light, easy to digest and nourishing foods.

EIGHT

TEAS FOR YOU AND ME

Michael's early memories include drinking Wissotzky Russian tea from a glass in Brooklyn. Outside old men played chess in the park and argued politics in various languages. Today tea may come fruit flavored, puffed with tapioca or spiced. But real tea whether in a mug or delicate cup, served hot or cold offers many heart benefits. There are healthful teas made with stimulating garden herbs, middle-slimming and digestive ingredients, beverages traditionally used by monks to soothe frayed nerves, and natural tea sweeteners. However, we begin our tour of teas with a bow to the inventors of Camellia sinensis the tea plant and traditional tea culture.

Ch'a the Chinese character for tea begins from the top down with the radical for grass. We see two vertical blades growing in a level field at the top of the word picture. Below are a person's arms and below that a tree. The Chinese are a practical people. They describe tea not as the thing itself but a plant in relation to us in the world. A person in a field picks tea leaves from a tree. Lu Yu, known as "the saint of tea," wrote the first tea encyclopedia after the Chinese had used it as medicine for a millennium. The plant he described was not the same evergreen bush we know today. He opens *The Classic of Tea* (*Cha Ching*, A.D. 780) with "tea is from a large tree in the south" and describes tea trees in Szechwan that are so wide that two men must link arms to encircle the trunk. He writes the leaves resemble gardenia and smell of clove and the flowers are like the wild red rose turned white. He describes the best wild tea leaves as russet-colored, curled, grown in stony soil and that "Tea picked from sunless mountainsides or valleys are not worth the effort." He believes tea drinking should be an exercise in moderation and limited to three cups daily.

However, Lu Yu writes, "If one feels hot, is given to melancholia, suffering from aching of the brain, smarting of the eyes, troubled in the limbs or afflicted in the hundred joints, he may take tea four or five times. Its liquor is like the sweetest dew of Heaven." Today we enjoy tea to clear the senses, energize the body, and lift our spirits. Tea, used for pleasure and medicine for countless generations world-wide, has brought together diverse cultures. Here is one example.

Tibetan Tea

I enjoy the memory of drinking Tibetan tea: Late morning in Lhasa as I walk through the Barkhor, the market alley surrounding the Jokhang temple in the town center, I repeat, "Om Mani Padmi Hum" like Tibetans who have come to worship at the steps of the Potala Palace and pray for the return of their spiritual leader His Holiness the Dalai Lama. Out of a dark corner, a Tibetan woman smiles and beckons for me to follow her. Invited to share tea in a Lhasa home, I sit watching my hostess cream yak butter in a tall wooden churn then mix it with Chinese tea, pouring the rich beige liquid into my porcelain cup. She wears dark blue Chinese worker cotton clothing. Her face is round, warm and brown; she is Tibetan from the highlands and smiling tells me that her son was sent to China to learn a trade. She works in the local hospital in Lhasa that once had Tibetan herbs and now uses Chinese-made herbal patent medicines for curing local Chinese workers' and tourists' ills.

Looking around her stucco house I see thick woven Tibetan carpets beside bright, red flower print Chinese cotton on the beds and couch. Flowers are painted on wooden cabinets. Everything in Lhasa smells heady from yak butter and the juniper incense offerings that hang a heavy cloud in the air. I wonder how this rich brew I am drinking made of Chinese tea, churned Tibetan butter and salt, the required beverage of all visitors to the rooftop of the world, originally came to Tibet. Tea was packed in burlap bags and carried for months on the backs of donkeys up from Yunnan. The long story of tea has brought friends and mortal enemies together. Tea may be enjoyed with milk and sugar, lemon, spices, or plain. Each culture has added its signature. But tea the plant, and the beverage made from it will always heal whoever enjoys it. Here is a teaspoon of tea history.

How tea came to bless the world

Legend shrouds the origin of tea and, like acupuncture and Asian herbal medicine, its discovery is simultaneously claimed by the Chinese and Indians. Monarchs, monks, missionaries, and pirates have spread the lore and wealth of tea. Chinese Emperor Shen Nung around 2700 B.C. was a scholar, an herbalist, a creative scientist and patron of the arts. He believed that boiling drinking water was necessary for health-- an important discovery. While traveling through poor areas of south China during the 1980s, I observed that human and animal waste were used as crop fertilizer and that little had changed for the living conditions in rural China for a thousand years. Some people lived in huts with dirt floors. Each spring reservoirs overflowed from heavy rains and people developed chronic indigestion, intestinal parasites, and fever symptoms commonly known as "summer heat." Boiling water kills germs. Boiled water is healthy but boring so anyone would want to flavor it with a tasty herb.

One day on a trip to the south, the Emperor's cook was boiling drinking water and some leaves from the Camellia sinensis plant, what we know as tea, blew into the caldron. The pleasing aroma attracted the Emperor's attention. Tea was born. Drinking tea, rich in naturally astringent tannins, cures many digestive ills, including certain symptoms of "summer heat." The nature of tea is cooling yet stimulating because its taste is bitter. The energy of a bitter flavor is considered a heart stimulant in TCM. Tea is cleansing, increasing elimination of impurities in the body. In that way it clears the senses and energizes the nervous system. Tea helps our heart because it relieves water retention, indigestion, bloating and improves mood. The Emperor and his men discovered the first heart healthy herb to stimulate energy during long treks.

During the mid-Tang Dynasty (780 A.D.) Lu Yu published his tea encyclopedia the *Cha Ching* after spending many years studying herbs. An orphan he was adopted by the Abbot of Dragon Cloud, a

Taoist monastery in modern Hubei Province, China. But Lu Yu left the monastery to travel as a comedian with a performing group. He had learned a lot about herbs and tea because monks considered tea drinking to be perfect for a life of moderation and contemplation. At age twenty Lu Yu began his tea quest in southern China. Locals thought he was nuts because when finding a particularly wonderful tea plant he sang and danced around it. The *Cha Ching* includes Lu Yu's knowledge of planting, processing, tasting, and brewing tea.

By 900 A.D., tea drinking spread from China to Japan where the tea ceremony or *Chanoyu*, was created and tea became an art form requiring years of study. Fast forward to the 17th century when Holland and England began importing tea. Catherine of Bragana married Charles II in 1661 and brought her custom of afternoon tea from Portugal. She served tea in the afternoon to avoid starving herself and then binging on meats and sweets at night which troubled digestion and complexion.

London's East India Company advertised tea as a panacea for apoplexy, catarrh, colic, consumption, drowsiness, epilepsy, gallstones, lethargy, migraine, paralysis, vertigo and everything else. Tea opened new British territories in India and Hong Kong. In Budapest's tea parlors, between the great wars, poets and rebels sipped tea, wrote poetry and hatched intrigues. In America tea has enjoyed popularity as a weight loss supplement, cancer prevention remedy, and has been added to cosmetics. Recently, responding to tea's increased popularity and research on its benefits, growers are producing American teas in California and the southern states. Tea festivals and tea schools in North America, Canada and online support tea culture and sales.

How Does Tea Work?

Camellia sinensis is normally classified into five types: white, green, oolong, black, and pu erh a red, fermented tea. All are healthful. Some researchers believe tea's benefits come from its digestive tannins. Many scientists believe it is tea's polyphenols and rich source of flavonoid antioxidants that protect against oxidative stress. Antioxidants help prevent disease. Tea appears to help control glucose and insulin and keep the gastrointestinal system running well. Improving digestion and elimination can certainly help balance blood sugar and lift our mood. Every task becomes easier when we easily digest our meals and focus our thoughts. Besides, brewing tea is an art that requires patience and taste. Inhale your tea's aroma from a lovely tea cup and watch the leaves unfurl. The depth of color and the steam as it rises are delightful.

The Tea Mood Chemical

Tea contains L-theanine a unique amino acid that enhances attention and mental focus. Unilever Food and Health Research Institute in Vlaardingen, the Netherlands reported a study in the 2008 *Asia Pacific Journal of Clinical Nutrition* proving L-theanine modulates aspects of human brain function. (14.) Tea's beneficial effects on mind and stomach make it a perfect addition to any meal. But there is more. Teas have anti-bacterial properties that boost our immune system. Although drinking tea with milk and sugar compromise it because milk protein reduces some of tea's benefits in the gut and sugar adds empty calories and inflammation. Try drinking it instead with almond milk or coconut milk. Persons with heart disease and/or diabetes benefit by adding stevia to sweeten tea. It reduces harmful cholesterol. What are the best forms of tea for the heart?

All styles and flavors of tea made with the tea leaf, Camellia sinensis, contain L-theanine. The difference in flavor comes in processing. Tea leaves are dried, toasted, and some are fermented for varying times to create the many tea flavors.

- White tea has the least caffeine and a subtle flavor.
- Green tea has a small amount of caffeine, a slightly bitter taste, is cooling, diuretic, and digestive.
- Oolong, a semi-fermented tea, has more caffeine which makes it useful for slimming. There are many styles of oolong, some with a light flowery aftertaste, others more rich and pungent are smoked with charcoal during processing.
- Pu Erh, a richly flavored, red-colored fermented tea from Yunnan, warms digestion and reduces cholesterol and hangover.

- Black teas have a higher caffeine content than white and green teas and they stimulate the nervous system to counter low energy. Black tea has proven cholesterol-reducing properties. If you are sensitive to caffeine in black tea, drink it along with a capsule of eleuthero ginseng, an adaptogen that reduces oxidative stress and LDL cholesterol.

Pu Erh Tea and Statins

The unique thing about Pu Erh, aside from its rich, earthly and delicious flavor and formidable digestive power, is that it contains lovastatin, a natural chemical that results from careful processing that helps prevent heart trouble and stroke. Statin drugs, such as Crestor and Lipitor, commonly used for coronary heart disease have strong side-effects, including muscle pain, headaches, nausea, and liver problems. However, the natural statins in Pu Erh are not harmful. In fact Pu Erh is often served to accompany rich, fat meals in China. Pu Erh gets my vote for the best heart health tea.

The Well Known Tea for slimming

'The Well Known Tea" is the name of a popular Chinese slimming beverage that combines oolong tea with herbs that enhance metabolism and internal cleansing such as hawthorn, a circulation tonic that reduces harmful cholesterol. We will study hawthorn berry in Part Three: Heart Protectors. Also in The Well Known Tea is a useful diuretic poria (AKA fuling). No irritating senna is added. Many people avoid slimming teas because they contain unpleasant bitter tasting ingredients or strong herbs such as senna which can cause abdominal cramping, nausea, or vomiting. Do not use senna products without medical advice if you are pregnant or breast feeding.

Heart health herbal teas (non-Camellia sinensis)

Most of the following kitchen herbs can be made into tea by simply steeping them in boiled water for five minutes. Often the taste and effects are strongest when using fresh green herbs, but dried cooking herbs can be stored in a cool, dry place for up to six months. In some cases the growing process or dose are important so I have noted details. Rooibos or Red bush tea originally from south Africa has gained popularity lately. It is a mild-tasting non-caffeine tea you might enjoy morning and evening while taking heart supplement pills. It is high in antioxidants and feels slightly astringent, makes your mouth pucker, but is smoother than black tea. Health benefits of red bush rooibos tea include its use as a cure for nagging headaches, insomnia, asthma, eczema, bone weakness, hypertension, allergies, and premature aging. It boosts immunity and eases digestive discomforts. Quercetin, a powerful antioxidant found in rooibos tea helps prevent many heart conditions including hypertension.

Energizer teas

Certain cooking herbs, including some of your favorites, are energy stimulants. Making a tea with them increases their qi punch.

- Thyme is stimulating and drying for lungs so that it may improve chronic wheezing and asthma with watery phlegm. If you have a pale tongue and shortness of breath, make a mild tea using thyme. Add a pinch of fresh thyme to a cup of hot water. Add no more than 1/8 tsp of the dried powder.
- Sage is recommended as an energy tonic for chronic fatigue. It reduces excess sweating associated with fatigue and weakness. Excess sweating can result from exertion or chronic fever conditions and hormonal imbalance (night sweats.) Use sage the energizer when sweating is spontaneous such as after a meal or if sweating is a problem all day. It is not recommended for night sweats or fevers because it can feel heating and drying.

- Rosemary is a strong adrenal and heart stimulant tonic that improves brain function. Use only a small pinch in your tea cup. Otherwise if you are very weak it might result in palpitations, headache, or feverish feelings.
- Oregano is a powerful antibiotic often used in early stages of cold and flu. It's spicy flavor is pleasant and stimulating for energy. If used long term, add yogurt or acidophilus to your diet as you would when using any herbal or other antibiotic. See my recipe for "The New Martini" made with oregano in chapter 18.

Anti-cholesterol herbal teas

Here are everyday foods you can enjoy as teas. You may want to grow your own herbs on a windowsill and avoid pesticides.

- Basil leaf (AKA sweet basil, (Ocimum basilicum)) has been used throughout the Mediterranean for generations as a diaphoretic (increases sweating) cold and flu treatment. It also reduces harmful cholesterol. Sweet basil reduces stress, cleanses the liver, helps regulate blood sugar and is a good source of iron. Two cups of chopped fresh basil leaves or 1 tablespoon of dried basil leaf provides 10% of your daily value of iron, making it on par with spinach. Recent studies of holy basil (Ocimum tenuiflorum, previously Ocimum sanctum) prove it is valuable for lowering cholesterol and triglyceride levels. Basil contains vitamin C and anti-oxidants that protect the heart from free radicals, also magnesium known to reduce stress and harmful cholesterol. Don't add sugar or sweetener.
- Tart Cherry juice is a major pain killer and heart protector beverage that reduces uric acid in gout treatments. Research published in the *American Journal of Clinical Nutrition* (2006) revealed that tart cherries rank fourteen in the top fifty foods for highest antioxidant content per serving size – surpassing red wine, dark chocolate and orange juice. Tart cherries neutralize free radicals. Tart cherry juice concentrate,

available in health food stores and online, is easy to use. Just add one teaspoon to your favorite tea twice daily. If you have trouble sleeping, drinking ½ cup tart cherry juice before bed, a good source of melatonin, may help you. Also see the section on tart cherries in chapter 10. Do you have a garden? Grow your own organic cherry trees and grapes. Their stems boiled as a tea reduce cholesterol.

- From China, a popular tea for heart problems Jiaogulan, (AKA Southern Ginseng) available in herb shops and online, is for high cholesterol, high blood pressure, and improving heart function. It is also used for strengthening the immune system, increasing stamina and endurance, increasing resistance to environmental stress (as an "adaptogen"), improving memory by improving circulation and as an anti-aging agent,/

Nutritive Tonics

Many heart tonics will be covered later but here is a tasty berry packed with essential nutrients that makes a heart protector tea.

Tibetan Goji Berry

Tibetan Goji berries and Chinese lycium (AKA wolfberries, matrimony fruit) look alike and are often confused when sold in stores or online but they come from different climate regions and have different uses. The confusion arises because the same Chinese pinyin word Gou Qi Zi is used to describe both.

Make a tea with Tibetan goji berries because they are grown in the Himalayas without using pesticides. Add a handful of dried berries to a cup of hot tea, Camellia sinensis. The berries will brighten your eyes, lift your spirits and provide important nutrients to protect your blood and heart. I prefer to soften Tibetan goji berries with water as tea instead of eating them dry because they are chewy. Goji supports a healthy life in many ways such as:

- Protects the liver — less fatigue
- Increases metabolic activity — burns fat and aids digestion
- Boosts immune function – Lymphocytes, Interleukin 2, Immunoglobulin
- Improves circulation, protects the heart and reduces harmful cholesterol
- Improves sexual function and fertility — boosts libido and energy
- Promotes longevity — brings life support to the blood and all internal organs.

You can find lots of useful information about the health benefits of Tibetan goji berries and order them by the package or pound at gojiberry.com. Tibetan goji berries are organic (grown without pesticides) neutral (neither overly heating nor cooling) and extremely nourishing and not the same as Chinese lycium fruit. (17)

Diabetes Prevention

Heart disease is linked to hypertension, obesity and diabetes. Eating to control diabetes requires whole grains that burn slowly, for example oats are heart healthy. You feel full longer. Choose vegetables with a low sugar content. Here are two teas to lower blood sugar.

Corn Silk Tea

If you are lucky enough to live in a state that grows Non-GMO (genetically modified) corn or in Mexico or much of Europe, then corn is healthy for your digestion and immunity. Cooking this tea is easy: Boil the pale silk "hairs" from inside organic corn on the cob and drink the cooking water which controls high blood sugar. Use it for slimming as needed. It is mild tasting. Instead of a sweetener add a zest of lemon to brighten the taste. The used corn cob when boiled makes a diuretic tea.

Bitter Melon Tea

Everyone in the tropics knows bitter melon (Momordica Charantia.) It looks like a pale, smooth, deeply grooved cucumber sold on the streets and in food shops in New York's Chinatown. My friend from Trinidad, calls it karela the type of bitter melon grown in India. Karela looks like a very bumpy bright green gourd in East Indian groceries. It controls diabetes and helps reduce excess body fat, chronic fevers, and complexion blemishes. Eating it steamed or sautéed can reduce your sweet tooth. (18.)

When using pills, the usual dosage is 250mg or more twice daily with meals. Allow several weeks for benefits. There are no reported side-effects. But use bitter herbs with care during pregnancy. If taken with other anti-diabetic medications, you should monitor your blood sugar levels closely because there is a risk of blood sugar levels dropping below normal.

Cherry Grain Balsam Pear Tea is dried sliced bitter melon sold online comes in a box showing the Yangtze Basin a beautiful tapestry of green and yellow fields and blue skies in China's Jiangsu Province. The tea itself is no less spectacular. Described as clear and elegant in flavor it is known to Asians by a dozen names such as towel gourd, tiansigua, tianluo, and xugua. The light, relaxing, pleasant-tasting beverage contains no caffeine. For a stronger tea, steep 3 or 4 pieces of dried Balsam Pear Tea in a cup of boiling water for about five minutes. The slightly bitter flavor is cooling and cleansing for chronic thirst, agitation, cough, and phlegm congestion anywhere. In Chinese herbal medicine, Balsam Pear Tea especially acts on the liver and stomach meridians to cool and cleanse the blood. That means its ingredients, including saponins, vitamins B and C, reduce impurities that could lead to excess bleeding. For heart patients with diabetes or chronic stress, people who live in polluted areas, or who suffer from sweet cravings, this tea is a must.

Stevia

Is there a sweetener that improves heart health? Yes. The leaves of the Stevia rebaudiana plant, a small shrub native to certain regions of

South America, have been used as both a sweetener and a medicine since ancient times. Stevia is botanically related to artichokes and sunflowers, as well as medicinal herbs such as echinacea and yarrow. In the 1970s Japanese scientists developed a process to extract the sweetest compounds from the leaves. Stevia extract is 250 times sweeter than sugar. Because the extract is so highly concentrated, it should be used very sparingly otherwise, it can have a bitter, licorice aftertaste. Research has shown that stevia is beneficial for reducing harmful cholesterol. (19) In your tea, use just a drop or a pinch. Our tea adventure does not end here.

Cream Teas

There is a long British tradition of adding milk to tea, however many people are lactose intolerant. Later chapters cover the cholesterol controversy, the fact that our brain requires cholesterol in order to function properly. Dairy products are one source of cholesterol, but another brain-soothing possibility is coconut oil which adds richness, flavor, and helpful saturated fat to the diet. Vitamin D3, vital for immunity, and turmeric, an excellent anti-inflammatory herb, are absorbed more efficiently when consumed with oils. On cold winter days I enjoy a modified Tibetan style tea by adding ½ teaspoon of extra virgin coconut oil to a cup of hot tea. The moisturizing coconut oil soothes digestion and nervous tension. It helps beautify skin and hair. Whatever your tea style, your heart will enjoy the many benefits of the leaf.

You don't like the bitter taste of turmeric or hate the yellow stain it leaves on your hands, kitchen counter or clothing? Then take a capsule. I take at least 1 gram of turmeric with my coffee or tea. Inflammation is at the base of most chronic disease--arthritis, cancer and heart disease. It damages tissue and increases aging and cell death. Liposomal Curcumin by Absorb Health products is the most absorbable form of curcumin which is turmeric extract, a powerful anti-aging antioxidant that protects heart health and helps prevent cancers and cell death. It is easy to use daily in tea or raw honey and inexpensive. See the Resource Guide for suggestions for turmeric.

Heart Health Checkup

How many cups of tea do you drink daily?

Do you prefer green, red, black, or oolong teas? Do you enjoy tea to benefit your digestion, energy, or mood? Chinese Pu Erh tea is a digestive remedy that contains a natural statin to help curb harmful cholesterol. Red bush tea is not the tea leaf. It contains no caffeine and has beneficial antioxidants.

Do you have tea bags at work or in your car or other convenient places? Did you know that one way to avoid infection when at the dentist and to speed healing is to place a tea bag over the area of the gap where your tooth is pulled? Tea is astringent and contains chemicals that support good health. Next are a few recipes for cooking with tea.

Q & A: Teas for cholesterol, weight loss

I want a tea for reducing cholesterol from fat foods -- *Pu-Erh a fermented tea.*

I want a tea for weight loss -- *Oolong tea or a slimming tea containing hawthorn*

I want a weight loss pill -- *Garcinia, African mango and white kidney bean extract can enhance metabolism to improve heart health.* http://www.absorbyourhealth.com/product/weight-loss-power-pack/?ref=4041

NINE

COOKING WITH TEA

Welcome friends to tea time, traditionally served between four and five in the afternoon, but for me it is all day. I have a cooking suggestion to post in your kitchen: "When boiling water, add tea." Tea makes any meal heart healthy because tea is slimming, stimulating, mood-enhancing, and it reduces harmful dietary fats and cholesterol to help prevent heart disease.

Tea for flavorful good health

Here are a few of my recipes to give you an idea of how versatile tea is. Use brewed tea for thinning sauces and mixing beverages. Tea is a perfect addition to low-salt cooking. We begin with a healthful snack or appetizer.

Tea Nuts

Why spend on fattening, salty snacks made with preservatives? This spicy delicacy is ready in minutes and adds charm to breakfast cereals or afternoon tea. Makes 4 cups

Ingredients   .
- 1 pound pecan halves
- 1 egg white, beaten until fluffy
- ¼ teaspoon stevia powder
- 2 tablespoons dried tea leaves, rubbed until fine ground
- 1 teaspoon garam masala powder or cinnamon powder
- ¼ teaspoon sea salt
- 1 teaspoon vegetable oil

Preheat the oven to 350 degrees F. Oil a large flat baking sheet. Beat the egg white in a large bowl. Combine the dry ingredients in a separate bowl.

Add the pecans to the egg whites coating them evenly. Then toss the pecans in the bowl of dry ingredients and mix well.

Distribute the nuts on the pan so they don't touch and bake for 15 minutes until brown. Remove them and turn them with a metal spatula or spoon as they cool. When completely cold you can store them in an airtight tin or jar.

Homemade Garam Masala

You can easily find Garam Masala in Indian food shops everywhere, though the exact ingredients and flavor of the spicy powder will vary according to the location where it's made in India. Here is a simple classic recipe you can store in a cool, dry place and use for spicing cooking or teas. Makes 1 /4 cup

Ingredients:
- 1 tablespoon ground cumin
- 1 ½ teaspoons ground coriander
- 1 ½ teaspoons ground cardamom
- 1 ½ teaspoons ground black pepper
- 1 teaspoon ground cinnamon
- ½ teaspoon ground cloves
- ½ teaspoon ground nutmeg

Mix the spice powders well and store it in an airtight container in a cool, dark, dry place.

Tea Borscht

I often add tea to cooking water for soups, pasta, or vegetables. This evening I made a quick and easy borscht with bright colored fresh vegetables and tea. Serves 4

Ingredients
- 1 cup each, sliced pieces of beets, carrots, celery, red cabbage, red onion, peeled kohlrabi, and zucchini squash
- (optional) 2 pieces of *Auricularia polytricha* [AKA wood ear, tree ear, black fungus] soaked, rinsed and cut into slices. It is a blood-thinning Chinese mushroom.
- 1 teaspoon caraway seeds, to taste
- ½ teaspoon coriander seeds, to taste
- ½ teaspoon black pepper, to taste
- ½ teaspoon of "seaweed soup mix" a mixture of kelp and alaria available from theseaweedman.com.
- Brewed Pu Erh or black tea
- Apple cider vinegar (unpasteurized, unfiltered) to taste
- Stevia, salt and pepper to taste
- Sesame Tahini to taste (optional)

Simmer the ingredients for five minutes up to fifteen minutes in strong Pu Erh tea which is digestive and reduces cholesterol. Cover the pot and turn off the heat to let it steam until the soup is cold. Correct the seasoning adding 1 – 3 teaspoons of apple cider vinegar. The root vegetables should be firm. Liquefy the mixture in a blender adding (optional) 1 tablespoon or more of sesame Tahini for a rich, smooth finish. Serve the soup chilled with crisp cucumber slices.

We will study the heart benefits of medicinal mushrooms in detail later. In this recipe and when cooking pasta I use reconstituted tree ear mushrooms. Two species of *Auricularia*, a group of jelly fungi, are often used in Asian cuisine. Both are sold dried in Asian markets and are reasonably priced compared to many wild or cultivated mushrooms. For culinary purposes, they are identical.

Tea-bouli Salad

Classic Mediterranean Tabouli Salad is made with cracked bulgar wheat, parsley, tomatoes, scallion, and a bright garlic mint dressing. My version is quicker, easier to make and heart healthy because it contains a cooling gluten-free seed, quinoa, instead of wheat. I add tea during cooking. Preparation time: 10 – 15 min. Makes 2 servings:

Ingredients:
- ½ cup quinoa
- 1 cup brewed tea
- Extra virgin olive oil
- 2 cups total of chopped parsley, red onion, garlic, 1 medium tomato keeping the seeds, (optional basil leaf)
- 1 cup sprouted chickpeas or canned and rinsed
- seasoning: salt, pepper, organic lemon juice

Brown the quinoa with a little oil using medium heat for 2 minutes to enhance the nutlike flavor. Don't allow the oil to smoke. Add salt and pepper and the tea and turn heat to simmer for about 12 – 15 minutes. During that final 5 minutes gently stir in the chickpeas and then remove the pot from the heat. Cook the quinoa soft not mushy so it can be separated with a fork.

Meanwhile wash and chop your parsley, tomato, onion, garlic. I cut the parsley with scissors into a bowl adding vinegar to wash it. Set them aside until you want to mix the salad. When ready to serve mix into the cold quinoa the fresh greens, more olive oil, correct the seasoning and add lemon juice for zest. Serve as a side dish or with hummus.

Quinoa [pronounced Keen-wah] a seed that is cooked like a whole grain, is a species of "goosefoot" (chenopodium) related to small shrubs such as beets, spinach, and tumbleweed. Quinoa is less congesting and inflammatory than wheat. The seed in its natural state has a bitter-tasting coating making it unpalatable. But quinoa sold commercially in North America has been milled to remove the coating and cooking improves its health benefits. Cooked quinoa is anti-inflammatory, lowers harmful cholesterol and is fine source of fiber, calcium, healthy fats, and vegetarian protein that makes it a useful food for prevention of heart illness and diabetes. (20.) Ounce-for-ounce, quinoa provides over twice the amount of calcium as whole wheat. Allow the mixture to ripen for a day or two in the refrigerator before using.

Tea Pasta

When boiling water for whole grain or quinoa pasta I add heart healthy reconstituted tree ear mushroom a natural blood thinner, sliced onion, a dash of turmeric which is anti-inflammatory and adds color, and tea leaves. Here is an equally healthy sauce.

Low Sodium spaghetti sauce, vegetable juice or salad dressing

People with hypertension or chronic heart failure are sometimes advised to lower their intake of sodium. Table salt is a denatured processed food. Most of the unhealthy sodium in our American diet comes from canned and processed foods, including commercial sauces, salad dressings, V8 juice has 980 mgs of sodium, and breakfast cereals. A study in the British Medical Journal from 2013 reported that over the counter pain medicines may contain high levels of sodium that put patients at risk. (21.)

Here is my low sodium pasta sauce. See my photo: sweet tomatoes, a kohlrabi (like a purple or green turnip high in calcium) zucchini, fresh basil, garlic, dried Italian herbs, red onion, lemon juice, extra virgin olive oil, pepper, and tea (Camellia sinensis).

Ingredients:
- 2 cups sliced sweet tomato
- 1 zucchini squash sliced
- 1 peeled kohlrabi (optional, a good source of calcium)
- ½ sliced red onion
- chopped garlic to taste
- fresh basil (shown) and fresh or dried Italian herbs including oregano, sage, thyme
- 2 Tbsp. extra virgin olive oil
- juice of ½ lemon
- ½ to 1 cup of strong tea
- a dash of red chili pepper sauce to taste
- stevia powder to taste

Whip the ingredients together in a blender leaving some chunks. Add more tea and it becomes a spicy salad dressing or vegetable juice. I like my sauce sweet and tangy. Choose sweet tomatoes or add chopped sun-dried tomatoes (drying concentrates the sugar) or stevia.

One pinch of stevia equals 1 teaspoon of sugar. See the benefits of stevia in chapter 8.

Allow the mixture to ripen for a day or two in the refrigerator before using. Correct the seasoning. Add a salt alternative as needed. Seaweed contains natural sea salt and minerals to keep your bones and teeth strong and a smile on your face. If you miss a salty flavor add a dash of dried dulse seaweed which is high in potassium among other necessary minerals. Salt substitutes from the supermarket may contain a high amount of processed potassium that affects heart rhythm. So be careful reading labels. You can find more information about low sodium cooking and recipes at my website www.asianhealthsecrets. com Search for "Low Sodium Alternatives."

Cooking with tea protects the heart, lifts our mood, protects against chronic illness, and helps us to focus on the important things–food, love, family.

Heart Health Checkup

How much sugar do you consume daily? It is hard to know. For example one can of soda may contain the equivalent of approximately 14 teaspoons of sugar. Cola and soda drinks are one of overweight America's big sugar addiction leading to diabetes, heart disease, obesity, and certain cancers. Drinking tea and cooking with tea, at the very least, enhances digestion and mood. It may also improve weight loss. Other hidden sugars come in barbecue sauce, dried fruit, fruit yogurt, take-out foods, granola bars, and energy drinks. Why not make tea sweetened with stevia?

Q & A: weight loss, mood and metabolism
I want a pill that boosts mood, reduces sweet cravings and improves weight loss – *It is 5 HPT but don't use if you already take an MAO inhibitor anti-depressant medicine.* http://www. absorbyourhealth.com/product/5-htp-100mg-100-capsules-mood-appetite-support-supplement-relieve-anxiety/?ref=4041

TEN

EATING RED

Red is the color of romantic Valentines and several important heart-healthy foods. I could inform you about their natural chemicals, including antioxidants, polyphenols, and their ability to thin the blood to prevent stroke until I am red in the face. But put more simply, these red foods are good for your heart: Tomato, tart cherry, cranberry, red and purple grapes, and red pears cool inflammation that damages blood vessels. Cayenne and other hot peppers help reduce blood cholesterol, triglyceride levels, and platelet aggregation, while increasing the body's ability to dissolve fibrin, a substance integral to the formation of blood clots. (22.) Cultures where hot peppers are used liberally have a much lower rate of heart attack, stroke and pulmonary embolism. I add a dash of low sodium veggie/hot pepper sauce to low sodium tomato vegetable juice and cut it with water. You might add a dash of cayenne to your salad dressing.

I have included a few easy recipes. You can find more Heart Healthy Recipes at www.asianhealthsecrets.com. Try a refreshing watermelon, tomato, red onion and arugula salad. The red ingredients enhance circulation. You can use any of the following red foods, even peppers, to make tasty jellies.

Tomatoes

Ask any Italian about the health benefits of tomatoes! Numerous scientific studies find that women with the highest intake of lycopene-rich tomato-based foods have a significantly reduced risk of heart disease. Aside from lycopene, tomatoes are loaded with vitamins A, C and E and have very few calories. In a five year women's health study of nearly 40,000 middle-aged and elderly women, as the women's blood levels of lycopene went up, risk for cardiovascular disease significantly dropped to a 50% reduced risk compared to women with the lowest blood levels of lycopene. Why? Fresh tomatoes and tomato extracts lower total cholesterol, LDL cholesterol, and triglycerides and help prevent unwanted clumping together (aggregation) of platelet cells in the blood, a factor especially important in lowering risk of heart problems like atherosclerosis. Excessive clumping of our platelet cells result in blood vessel blockage. Tomatoes are truly a heart healthy food. No body system has a greater need for antioxidant protection than the cardiovascular system.

Choose bright red or orange tomatoes with smooth skin and consume them within one week. When cooking use the seeds and skin which are full of valuable nutrients. Conventionally grown cherry tomatoes typically have pesticide residues. Buy local and organic. Avoid tomato leaf. It causes symptoms of poisoning, including severe mouth and throat irritation, vomiting, diarrhea, dizziness, headache, mild spasms, and death.

Quick Tomato Aspic

Here is a sweet treat made in minutes without sugar. Store it in the refrigerator. Serve it with vegetable dishes, kafir or salads. Serves 4

Ingredients:
- 2 – 3 packages of unflavored gelatin (Knox Gelatine or vegan)
- ¼ cup cold low sodium tomato juice
- 2 cups thinly sliced fresh organic cherry tomatoes
- 1 cup boiling hot Earl Grey tea
- ¼ tsp stevia powder
- lemon juice

Mix the unflavored gelatin powder with the cold juice in a bowl, let it stand 1 minute until the gelatin is completely dissolved, Add the hot tea and sliced tomatoes, stevia and lemon juice. Pour the mixture into a sterilized glass container or dessert mold. Refrigerate it overnight to set the aspic. If you use one packet of gelatin instead of two it will be soft enough to use as jelly. Store the jelly up to 2 weeks in refrigerator or 1 year in the freezer.

Tart Cherries

Pretty and delicious tart cherries are super foods. For heart health, I recommend adding at least 1 teaspoon of tart cherry juice to tea twice daily. The sour taste is cheery, refreshing and reduces chronic inflammatory discomforts.

Tart cherries get their deep red color from disease-fighting phenols called anthocyanins. (23.) Slightly more than 3 ounces (100 grams) of tart cherry juice concentrate delivers four times the necessary amount needed to maintain a good antioxidant defense system. A quarter cup of dried tart cherries daily is enough to keep you healthy. Research published in the *American Journal of Clinical Nutrition* reports that tart cherries surpass antioxidants like red wine, dark chocolate and orange juice. Regularly enjoying tart cherries may also improve sleep. If insomnia is weakening your vitality, here's a nice little recipe to give you more ZZZs.

Baked Cherry Banana

Bananas are high fiber and contain phytochemicals that protect against stomach ulcers. If you are hungry at bedtime, consider a satisfying comfort food baked cherry banana.

Ingredients:
   1 ripe banana peeled and cut into several pieces
   1 tablespoon tart cherry concentrate
   1 teaspoon unsweetened shredded coconut

Coat the banana with cherry concentrate and dip the pieces in the coconut. Bake for 20 minutes at 350 degrees until it is soft. Enjoy this with a cup of warm water adding 3 tablespoons of tart cherry concentrate.

Cranberry

Fresh cranberry season is Labor day through Halloween. We enjoy cranberry dishes at Thanksgiving and cranberry juice is recommended medically for naturally treating urinary tract infection (UTI). The best way to eat cranberries is raw. Add them to salads or juice them. Instead of ice cubes add frozen cranberries to tall drinks and cocktails Cranberry is an excellent source of vitamin C enhancing health, immunity and fertility. Cranberry has proven health benefits throughout the digestive tract, including decreasing our risk of periodontal disease, stomach ulcer, and colon cancer. Recent research has shown that cranberry may optimize the balance of bacteria in the digestive tract because the relative amount of *Bifidobacteria* is increased. Have you noticed how cooling, sour tasting fruits benefit the heart? For example sour cherries and cranberry.

As mentioned already, oxidative stress and chronic inflammation increase our risk of plaque formation and atherosclerosis. Dietary intake of cranberries and cranberry juice in normal everyday amounts has been shown to prevent two enzymes in the atherosclerosis process. Also cranberries play a key role to decrease risk of high blood pressure. Three related compounds in cranberry—resveratrol, piceatannol, and pterostilbene—provide support to our cardiovascular system. (Pterostilbene, [tero still been] similar to resveratrol, is being studied at several American universities for its capacity to lower harmful cholesterol, triglycerides, hypertension, and high blood sugar for diabetes and heart disease. It is a longevity-promoting nutritional supplement available online. See the Resource Guide.)

Fresh ripe cranberries can be stored in the refrigerator for up to 20 days. Cranberries retain their maximum nutrients and taste when enjoyed fresh because their vitamins, antioxidants, and enzymes are unable to withstand the temperatures used in baking. I buy lots of fresh cranberries and freeze them. My tart cranberry sauce is made fresh, either raw or lightly steamed and mashed without adding sweetener.

Cranberry Kale Salad

Squeeze fresh kale greens with your hands adding a little olive oil, add sliced red onion and a handful of whole raw cranberries. Add fresh garlic and lemon juice to your vinaigrette. Cranberries go well with fruit smoothies made with oranges, apples, pineapple or pears. Add finely chopped fresh cranberries as a dressing for fruit salads. Sprinkle a handful of dried unsweetened cranberries over a bowl of hot or cold cereal.

Cautions: Cranberry may interfere with the blood thinning drug Warfarin (AKA Coumadin). Also some people with certain kinds of kidney stones may be sensitive to cranberry. People at risk of calcium oxalate kidney stone formation should avoid cranberries. For less common types of kidney stones such as stones containing magnesium sulfate and those containing calcium phosphate, intake of cranberry juice may actually help lower a person's risk.

Red and Purple Grapes

Grapes are anti-inflammatory, cardio-protective, and blood sugar-regulating for longevity. The science about grapes is enough to make a convert to Bacchus, the god of wine. Resveratrol found in the skin of red and purple grapes improves blood flow by stimulating production and release of nitric oxide which helps in dilating blood vessels and increasing blood flow. (24.)

In addition to providing vitamin C and manganese, grapes are filled with antioxidant nutrients into the hundreds. However most research has been done on whole grapes including *the seeds*. How often do you get red wine made from grape seeds? How can you get the full benefit of grapes, especially when all you can find in supermarkets are seedless grapes? You might take grapeseed extract pills available at most health shops and even big chain stores. But if you enjoy making your own health wine, try my recipe for "Retsina" made with whole organic grapes and myrrh. Avoid using myrrh or other blood-moving herbs during pregnancy.

Use only organic grapes. Conventionally grown grapes are one of worst fruits for pesticide residues. If you have space you might grow grape vines in the yard or in a lit basement. Use neem spray to keep bugs away. I have seen grape vines grown indoors using large 5 gallon pots placed in sunshine, next to a wall or bookcase and away from your radiator. The following heart benefits have been demonstrated for grapes and grape components:

- blood pressure regulation, including high blood pressure
- total cholesterol regulation, reduced LDL cholesterol and LDL oxidation
- less clumping of platelet cells and cell adhesion to blood vessel walls
- better inflammatory regulation in the blood
- increased levels of glutathione in the blood

Letha's Home Made "Retsina"

Delicious Greek Retsina is a clear pale yellow tart wine made from Savatiano grapes from the vineyards on the slopes of Mt. Parnes in Attica, Greece. It has a delicate aroma and is fresh and rich on the palate from being flavored during fermentation with resin from Aleppo pine. There is no perfect substitute for this excellent wine that goes so well with Mediterranean fish or any Greek dish. What if you have been advised by your doctor to give up alcohol?

My non-alcoholic Retsina health drink, a tonic for heart patients, is made from fresh whole grapes including the seeds, tea, and the astringent liquid extract of myrrh, an evergreen tree resin long praised for its ability to heal wounds, reverse decay and preserve health. Myrrh extract gives the fresh grape juice a tangy flavor not unlike a wine made with pine.

IMPORTANT NOTE: If your are pregnant use only the blender grape juice, tea and add lemon juice to taste. Do not add myrrh which cleanses internal organs including the uterus. Blood-moving herbs threaten pregnancy when used in higher doses. Myrrh is contraindicated when kidney dysfunction or stomach pain is apparent, or for women who have excessive uterine bleeding.

Ingredients:
- 2 cups organic grapes including peel, seeds and a little stem
- or organic grapes and the equivalent of 1 gram grape seed extract from capsules.

1 cup strongly brewed black tea
Myrrh extract to taste

Blend the grapes and tea to a smooth liquid, adding more tea as needed. Strain this liquid into an airtight bottle or decanter. When ready to serve chilled, add a dose of liquid myrrh extract as needed. If you have a very weak heart, tend to be dizzy or headachy drink the grape juice plain or add only a drop or two of the extract. Otherwise you can use up to one dropper full for each wine glass.

Myrrh is a resin from the evergreen (Commipihora myrrha.) The essential oil has a rich, smoky, balsamic aroma that is purifying, restorative, revitalizing, and uplifting. It has a high level of sesquiterpenes, compounds that effect the hypothalamus, pituitary, and amygdala, the seat of our emotions. Myrrh purifies and heals. Frankincense and myrrh, both powerful healing herbs, were precious gifts brought by the three kings of Orient who were astronomers and doctors following a star to find Jesus.

TCM classifies myrrh as bitter and spicy and is said to have special efficacy on the heart, liver, and spleen meridians, as well as "blood-moving" powers to purge "stagnant blood" from the uterus. (I have recommended it along with aloe vera juice for women who have irregular periods and endometriosis.) Myrrh is often recommended for rheumatic, arthritis and circulatory problems and is an ingredient in numerous Chinese herbal anti-cancer treatments.

Red Chili Peppers and Your Heart

Ask someone from the American Southwest, central America or Mexico about the health benefits of chili peppers! They will say they like it hot! Cayenne and hot peppers protect the cholesterol in blood from oxidation, which is the first deadly step toward atherosclerosis. That means hot peppers literally melt the stuff that silently, slowly blocks arteries and puts blood flow at risk. Scientists have reported that chili peppers are a heart-healthy food with potential to protect against the No. 1 cause of death in the developed world. However, a good diet is a matter of balance not binging on one or two ingredients.

Cayenne's bright red color is from a high content of beta-carotene or pro-vitamin A. Two teaspoons of cayenne pepper provide 47% of the daily value for vitamin A essential for healthy mucous membranes in nasal passages, lungs, intestinal tract and urinary tract and serve as the body's first line of defense against invading pathogens,. However don't try it because it burns all the way down. Sweet red peppers contain substances that significantly increase heat production and oxygen consumption for more than 20 minutes after they are eaten. The comfortable heat helps you lose weight.

Sprinkle cayenne into your cooking and serve sliced peppers with salads, soups. Make a salad of fresh watermelon, tomato and sliced sweet red pepper. Steam salmon in pineapple juice on top of sliced red onion and red bell peppers. Brighten your dishes with lively red foods and live longer and better. For healthy aging and longevity, increase optimal nutrition with the fewest calories.

Christmas in Connecticut

Our favorite Christmas movie is *Christmas in Connecticut,* a romantic comedy from 1945 that stars Barbara Stanwyck as a single woman famous as a food writer for Sidney Greenstreet's magazine *American Housewife.* Her column describes her elaborate meals prepared at her farm in Connecticut and her baby, but she actually lives in a tiny New York studio apartment and can't cook. Her restaurateur friend, delightful Hungarian-born S.Z. Sakall (AKA Cuddles), furnishes the recipes. The plot thickens when Greenstreet, a gourmet, invites himself and Dennis Morgan, a war hero, to celebrate Christmas at Stanwyck's farm. Stanwyck agrees to marry her dull suitor (Reginald Gardiner known for playing caricature upper-crust English twits) in order to use his farm. With many plot twists that marriage is foiled. The action and dialogue are quick and witty, including insults hurled in Hungarian by Sakall. It all ends sweetly with a Stanwyck-Morgan clinch.

I am in much the same situation as Elizabeth Lane, the Stanwyck character. I write about cooking from my minuscule Manhattan kitchen in a closet without counter space for preparing foods You may also be limited by time, space, or experience. Luckily all the heart healthy red foods can be simply prepared in a pot on the stove or in a blender. I hope you enjoy them. Do your best and let the red foods do the rest.

Heart Health Checkup

How many red and purple foods do you eat daily? Do you drink red wine, red tea, or fruit juice cut with water daily? Do you eat cherries, berries, or add a little cayenne pepper to foods for zest? Do you have hypertension, diabetes, a spare tire or a heart condition? Have you had a stroke? Sour cherries, Tibetan goji and other berries are good foods to build blood and reduce inflammation in blood vessels which is at the core of atherosclerosis (hardening of arteries.) Next are powerful heart herbs from Asian cuisine you can add to your salads and soups.

Q & A: Cholesterol regulating pill
I want a pill to control high cholesterol - *Pterostilobene similar to resveratrol reduces cholesterol, triglycerides, high blood sugar reducing hypertension and diabetes.* http://www.absorbyourhealth.com/?ref=4041&s=pterostilbene

ELEVEN

FISHES AND SUCH

I currently describe myself as a vegan with a gourmet past. My daily serving of seaweed tea satisfies fish flavor longings. Supplements are convenient but there are heart benefits from eating the real thing. In New York, my favorite source of fresh fish is at Chelsea Market in our neighborhood. There you can find salmon from Iceland, wild Florida shrimp, silvery sardines and polpetto baby octopus from Spain I steam or marinate in a mignonette sauce made with vinegar, shallots, and cracked pepper. For jellyfish I go to Chinatown. Do you wonder what makes a fish dish healthy? Cardiologists praise oily fish as a source of omega 3 oils that replace hard to digest omega 6 oils found in meat and cheese. Try to have some fish every week. Benefits of eating fish and fish oil supplements include: Decreases triglycerides and blood pressure, increases HDL healthy cholesterol, reduces inflammation in arteries, reduces blood clots, stabilizes or reverses plaque and helps to counteract heart arrhythmias.

In the 1970s researchers found that Greenland Eskimos, who had a diet rich in fish oil, had a low incidence of heart attack compared to people in the West. But how much stress can an average Eskimo have? Fear of Polar bears? When the same low heart attack incidence was found among Japanese, who also eat a fish oil rich diet, I became convinced. Recent experts say if you have plaque, eating fish and fish oil supplements (sources of EPA and DHA fatty acids,) slows the rate at which plaque advances and protects against plaque rupture decreasing the risk of heart attack, sudden death, atrial fibrillation or arrhythmia. Medical sources advise for prevention the dose is 1 gram daily. Patients with heart disease, a stent, bypass or history of heart attack can benefit from higher doses.

Fish is served everywhere these days even at MacDonald's although their "Fish Filet Patty" may qualify as "and such." It is made with pollock, wheat and corn flour, salt, whey, dextrose, dried yeast, sugar, cellulose gum, colored with paprika and turmeric extract, and spice extractives and fried in vegetable oil laced with a petroleum by-product so it may be reused many times. Always check with your food provider for purity and safety.

Why are fish so important in a heart health diet? And which ones offer the best benefits? Aside from providing omega 3 oil that helps keep blood vessels healthy and supple, eating 2 – 3 meals of fish per week has been recommended for preventing and treating depression and mood swings. The oil in fish improves blood circulation and heart action, therefore, oxygen levels in the brain. Oily fish such as salmon, tuna, and sardines deliver heart- and brain-healthy fats.

Which are the best fish to eat and which ones will survive for the next generation of fish-eaters? The Monterey Bay Aquarium in cooperation with the Harvard School of Public Health (HSPH) and Environmental Defense Fund (EDF) maintain a website www.seafoodwatch.org that provides an updated listing of healthy, sustainable fish called the Super Green list. (35.) Seafood contaminants include metals such as mercury which affects brain function and development, industrial chemicals, including PCBs and dioxins and pesticides even DDT. These toxins usually originate on land and make their way into the smallest plants and animals at the base of the ocean food web. As smaller species are eaten by larger ones, contaminants are concentrated and accumulated so that large predatory fish like swordfish and sharks end up with the most toxins. You can download a guide to safe fish in your area here: http://www.seafoodwatch.org/seafood-recommendations/consumer-guides Included in the online guide are: "Best Choice", "Alternatives" and "Avoid." For example, as of March 2017 below is the list of Best Choice for New York state. However in Manhattan or any large good fish store you can get wild fish from around the world. Avoid farmed fish raised in tanks because there may be chemical pesticides used for them:

Arctic Char, Barramundi, Bass, Bluefish, Catfish (US) Clams, Mussels & Oysters, Crab: King, Snow & Tanner (AK) Croaker: Atlantic (beach seine, Lionfish (US) Mahi Mahi, Prawn: Freshwater (Canada & US) Rockfish (AK, CA, OR & WA) Salmon (New Zealand) Sardines: Pacific (Canada & US) Scallops (farmed) Seaweed [I suggest: theseaweedman.com]

Shrimp, Swordfish (Canada & US) Tilapia (Canada, Ecuador & US) Tuna: Albacore (troll, pole and line) Tuna: Skipjack (Pacific troll)

Top Fish Choices for New York are missing mackerel, coho salmon, and sablefish. Check for foreign sources that come from clean, low industrial areas. According to a 2008 report in the *New York Times* among the sea creatures with the lowest known levels of mercury are shrimp, oysters, clams, sardines, anchovies and herring, as well as the less exciting hake, tilapia, crayfish and whiting. Several of those fish also have good amounts of omega-3 fatty acids, which may help prevent heart disease. They include pollock, salmon, sardines, anchovies and herring.

Seafood containing omega-3 oil and have been popular choices among Asians and European fishophiles for a long time. They include oysters, octopus [AKA pulpo] and jellyfish. Lately you hear ads about a pill supplement made from a protein found in jellyfish that improves our memory. Looking deeper, unfortunately, we find that experiments done by the supplement manufacture injected the protein into mice brains. Jellyfish is a popular traditional Chinese festive food often served for New Year's feasts. It is high protein and high fiber.

Jellyfish appetizer

Here is my recipe easy enough to remember without taking a brain supplement. Packaged jellyfish cut into long strips is sold in Chinese and Vietnamese markets and every sort of food is sold online.

Ingredients:
- 1 pound salted jellyfish strips
- sliced scallion, carrots, cucumber
- vinaigrette dressing

Soak the jellyfish overnight in water to remove excess salt, drain the water then blanch the jellyfish in boiling water for a quick moment. Toss all the ingredients with the oil and lemon vinaigrette dressing. Serve as an appetizer.

Polpetto appetizer

You can pretend you are enjoying this dish in Italy where octopus is often prepared for Christmas dinner. I buy whole small wild polpetto baby octopus from Manhattan's Chelsea Market. Spanish cooks make octopus or polpetto tender by keeping it in the freezer for 2 days then thawing it in the refrigerator during the day they cook it. They cook it as detailed below then boil cubed potatoes in the polpetto cooking water and serve the dish with sautéed onion, black olives, paprika, olive oil and lemon juice. A simpler recipe is cooked polpetto in a prepared Mignonette sauce.

Serves 2:
Ingredients:
- 2 or 3 polpetto
- 1 sliced shallot
- olive oil
- dried Italian herbs
- Old Bay Seasoning powder for cooking fish, contains celery salt and paprika
- Mignonette sauce made with minced garlic, shallot, and vinaigrette

Sautee the onion in olive oil in a large deep ceramic pot. Add Italian herbs, Old Bay or other fish seasoning and water to boil. Holding the head, dip the polpetto three times into seasoned boiling water so that the tentacles curl. Then snip off the head with kitchen scissors and drop the polpetto into the boiling water turning the heat to medium. Simmer with the lid on for 30 -40 minutes until tender. Turn off the heat and allow it to steam covered for another 15 minutes. Pour off some of the water. You can serve it this way with or without the cooking water. If you pour off the water and save it as soup stock you may want to add the Mignonette sauce. Cut the polpetto into bite-sized pieces with a kitchen scissor. Serve hot or cold.

In Chelsea Market's Lobster Place I looked up at a young man, obviously a chef from the way he was ordering fish. We exchanged recipes for polpetto. He said, "Cook it either 15 seconds of ½ hour." So at home I browned garlic in olive oil, added polpetto cut into pieces and sautéed it for a few minutes, added some Italian herbs and 2 tablespoons of water, covered the ceramic pot and let it steam. Delicious and fast.

Store cooked polpetto it in a glass jar the refrigerator for up to a month or more.

Christmas Bouillabaisse

This is a simply elegant fish soup. It sounds ambitious but can be cooked within an hour in one pot in my miniscule Manhattan kitchen. I serve it with warm crescents and champagne at Christmas. The traditional Bouillabaisse from Marseille always has red snapper and shellfish. This year I got a small snapper cut into three pieces and asked the fish seller to keep the head and tail on. But I often substitute a salmon fillet for snapper. I added shrimp, mussels, and polpetto. It was a success. The trick is to assemble the ingredients, which takes the longest time, and add them in stages. Cooking the soup itself is fast and easy.

Ingredients:
- 1 wild salmon or char fillet cut into pieces
- 1 pound wild Florida shrimp, cooked, peeled and deveined
- ½ pound mussels
- 1 pound polpetto (optional) cooked and cut into pieces
- 1 cup of sliced fennel herb keeping the fennel bulb and feathery greens
- 1 tablespoon chopped orange peel
- 1 sliced sweet or yellow onion
- olive oil
- Old Bay Seasoning for cooking fish
- 1/8 teaspoon saffron
- ¼ cup red spaghetti sauce
- peeled sliced garlic to taste
- dried herbs, including oregano, basil, rosemary, parsley and 1 bay leaf
- Himalyan pink salt and white pepper

If you are using shrimp and/or polpetto they should be cooked separately and added the last minute to the soup. To prepare the mussels, soak them in cold water, remove the weeds and discard any mussels that open and do not close when you touch them.

Sautee the onion and fennel herb in olive oil until they are transparent. Add the Fish cooking Old Bay seasoning, red sauce, garlic and herbs and simmer for only a moment. Add the fish, cover with water for soup and simmer for about 10 minutes. Finally add the peeled shrimp, optional polpetto and uncooked mussels. Cover and simmer for 5 more minutes then turn off the heat to let them steam. Do not overcook the ingredients. Adjust the flavors and serve it warm.

Oysters

Do you like oysters but avoid them because they are hard to open and serve? Here is a great simple trick: Scrub raw oyster shells with a food brush. Place them in a pot adding one inch of water and ½ cup of beer or wine for flavor. Cover the pot, bring the water to a simmer turn if off, let it steam a moment until the shells open. Then they are done.

Fish Supplements

If you do not have time or a kitchen to cook fish, consider using supplements that contain deep ocean squid oil which provides omega 3 without a fishy burp you might experience from eating fish oil capsules. In the chapter Eastern Flavors, my vegan friends will be happy to read about shiso leaf a variety of perilla another rich source of heart healthy omega 3 oil.

Fish to Avoid

The large fish live longer and, therefore, contain more mercury. Children and pregnant women are most at risk because mercury stays in our body like it does in fish. When shopping check the fish's origin and the environmental news. In 2014, a list of fish to avoid include bluefin tuna, Chilean sea bass, grouper, monkfish, orange roughy, and farmed salmon [AKA Atlantic salmon.] Atlantic mackerel, crabs and scallops, though a source of omega-3's, have higher levels of mercury. They are on the list of fish that women and children can eat up to twice a week, along with catfish, cod, flounder, mussels, shad, sole, squid, trout and whitefish. The federal Food and Drug Administration FDA and the Environmental Protection Agency EPA advise pregnant women and children to avoid king mackerel, shark, swordfish and tilefish, and limit their consumption of some tuna. The New York city health department advises women and children to avoid completely Chilean sea bass, grouper, Spanish mackerel, marlin and orange roughy.

Seaweeds

Seaweeds, already mentioned in my recipes, offer wonderful nutrients, including natural sodium and essential minerals. Kelp, nori, and dulse are tasty food accents in cooking. Alaria a form of kelp has been found to reduce radiation in the body. I buy my dried seaweed by the pound from theseaweedman.com in Maine. Ecklonia cava, a brown algae harvested off the coasts of Japan, Korea and China, has been indicated for heart health, lowering blood pressure, also recommended for diabetes and weight loss. Following the radiation catastrophe in Japan during 2013, I called one of my favorite companies selling nutritional supplements to ask about their source of chorella a fresh water algae typically harvested in the China sea near Japan or Taiwan. I was informed that their chorella did not come from Japan and was tested for purity, including radiation toxicity. You have to find sources of nutrition you can trust.

Heart Health Checkup

What fish or sea foods do you regularly eat?
How often do you eat fish or seafood?
Have you tried squid, jelly fish, shellfish or krill oil for their omega 3 benefits?

It is a good idea and convenient to take turmeric supplements and oil-based nutritional supplements such as vitamin D3, vitamin E, A and flaxseed oil, evening primrose or other oils along with other oily foods to help insure absorption. Avoid frying foods. An easy way to cook fish is to steam it in a little pineapple juice or a spicy vinegar instead of cooking with oil.

Q & A: Mercury in fish

I love to eat fish but want to protect against pollution and environmental poisons – *Eat a cleansing diet including organic green vegetables in the cabbage family and take purifying supplements to detoxify the body from toxic estrogens from pollution, chemicals, food additives etc. for example:* http://www.absorbyourhealth.com/product/estrogen-balance-power-pack/?ref=4041

TWELVE

EASTERN FLAVORS

A number of delicious Eastern foods are widely-used health tonics that improve heart function. You know them from popular restaurant dishes: Thailand's mix of spicy, sour, sweet and pungent flavors are found everywhere. My favorite Thai dish when I visited northern Thailand and in our Manhattan neighborhood restaurants is refreshing, tart, and crunchy green papaya salad. Papaya's enzymes, minerals and high fiber provide many health benefits and green papaya is even more digestive than the ripe fruit. Its skin and fruit contain high levels of the digestive enzyme papain that works much like the enzymes produced by the stomach. Regularly eating papaya can improve diabetes and indigestion. Papaya's high fiber and water content promote regularity and a healthy digestive tract.

All parts of the papaya are low calorie and medicinal. The fruit and leaf provide papain. The dried leaf, for example added to tea, provides protein with papain and the fresh or dried seeds simmered a few minutes as a tea work like digitalis to calm the heart and muscles. The fiber, potassium and vitamin content in papaya all help to ward off heart disease. An increase in natural potassium intake along with a decrease in sodium is one of the most important dietary changes possible to reduce the risk of cardiovascular disease. Choline is a very important, versatile nutrient in papayas that aids our sleep, muscle movement, learning and memory. Choline also helps to maintain the structure of cellular membranes, aids in the transmission of nerve impulses, assists in the absorption of fat and reduces chronic inflammation. All important for the heart.

Served along with Japanese sushi you may find a deliciously spicy, fan-shaped, dark green shiso leaf used as a garnish. It, like nuts and fish, provides a good source of healthy omega 3 fats. Do you enjoy Chinese hot and sour soup? It contains a dried medicinal fungi that looks like black crinkled paper. It is dried cloud ear mushroom sold in Chinese supermarkets, a blood thinner extremely useful for people with high cholesterol. Here is how to use these exotic foods in your kitchen. They are easily available in Asian food markets and online.

Shiso leaf

Shiso pronounced "shee-so" [AKA beefsteak plant, Japanese basil, perilla] in the mint family can be used as you would basil or mint. It has green or purple leaves with a slightly prickly texture and pointy, jagged edges, and it has a unique and vibrant spicy, citrus taste. Use it raw or steep it as tea. Shiso leaves have anti-inflammatory, antioxidants and allergy-fighting properties to give the immune system a boost and the complexion a radiant glow. The omega-3 fatty acids found in shiso as well as its natural anti-inflammatory properties are thought to reduce the risk of heart disease, heart attack and stroke. Shiso is also rich in vitamin A.

The green leaf is more tender and flavorful than the purple variety, which is used to color pickled umeboshi plum. You can order fresh shiso leave online or sprout the seeds to produce a bushy plant.

Shiso goes well with: rice, noodles, tofu, salads, mushrooms, tomato sauce, ginger, sesame and soy sauce, fish and fruits such as citrus and berries. Here is a fast recipes you can enjoy fresh in summer and frozen into ice cubes year-round.

Simple shiso pickles

These refreshing pickles lower cholesterol and provide heart healthy Omega 3 oils.

You can use sliced baby carrots, radishes, cucumbers, pearl onions, celery, salad turnips, beets or other vegetables with this marinade.

Ingredients:
- ½ teaspoon stevia powder
- ½ cup apple cider vinegar
- 3 tablespoons mirin (optional - Japanese cooking wine)

- 1 tablespoon herbal (low sodium) salt substitute or kelp seaweed
- 5 Japanese cucumbers, or 3 large cucumbers (approx. 2 cups of sliced vegetables)
- 8 green shiso leaves

Have very clean hands and sterilized, air-tight glass storage jar when you make homemade pickles because they ferment naturally without preservatives. Whisk together to dissolve the stevia, vinegar, mirin and salt substitute in a ceramic or glass bowl. Scrub and slice the cucumbers as thinly as possible.

Gather the shiso leaves like a deck of cards, cut off the tough stems. Roll them into a tube and with a sharp knife slice them chiffonade-style. Add the cucumbers and shiso to the marinade and stir. Cover the vegetables with the marinade. The cucumbers will become smaller as they marinate.

Put the mixture in the refrigerator for at least 4 hours or overnight. Mix it a couple of times, then the cucumbers will take care of themselves. Serve this pickled salad icy cold.

Blood Thinner Mushrooms

Auricularia polytricha [AKA tree ear, wood ear, black fungus] "mushrooms" sold dried in Chinese food markets, are actually two species of *Auricularia*, a group of jelly fungi that grow on trees. They are often used in Asian cuisine for their crunchy bland flavor. For culinary purposes, they are identical. See my simple pasta recipe below. The dried ear-shaped cap is medium sized, dull in texture, and dark brown to black. The wavy lower surface has a contrasting powdery gray color. There are no typical mushroom stem or "gills" underneath the cap. A native of Asia and some humid Pacific Ocean islands, most Asian countries successfully cultivate *A. polytricha* today.

The Chinese add *A. polytricha* to dishes because they think it improves breathing, circulation, and well-being. Recent studies of the medicinal effects of *Auricularia polytricha* have identified a chemical that tends to inhibit blood clotting. Since blood vessel diseases, strokes, and heart attacks are associated with clotting, moderate use of this mushroom as food may be very healthy.

Auricularia auricula [AKA cloud ear, Judas' ear] is a smaller fungus, with a brown to black cap surface, and is dull brown underneath. It is found growing on dead wood worldwide. I first heard about this medicinal fungus from Dr. Andrew Weil who spoke at an alternative medicine conference about a man who was being tested for heart trouble at a clinic. During a lunch break he had some Chinese hot and sour soup that improved his test results. The cloud ear mushroom in the soup was a blood thinner that Weil said, "worked like [the drug] Coumadin but without side-effects."

Both cloud ear fungi are imported dried from Asia packed in plastic bags. I buy my cloud ear packaged in separate little boxes at Kam Mann supermarket at 200 Canal Street in NYC Chinatown. A wood ear will rehydrate in hot water in 15 to 20 minutes, and swell two to five times its original size. It looks like a swollen, shiny black orchid. Only two or three pieces are needed in a dish with four servings. After soaking a couple pieces of the dried fungi in warm water, or the contents of one small box of them, clean it under running water with light finger pressure to remove debris. Cut off any fibrous material adhering to the base of the mushroom.

These medicinal fungi are enjoyed for their crisp texture and color rather than taste. *A. auricula* is usually sliced in ¼-inch strips for cooking. Cook them at medium heat for a few minutes. For soups, stir-fried dishes, or salads, add the slices as the last stage of food preparation. I store washed, soaked cloud ears in the refrigerator for up to two weeks sometimes rinsing them to refresh them. Otherwise they tend to become sour. Discard any fungi that smells bad.

Here is a recipe featuring two strong blood-thinning ingredients—garlic and cloud ear. If you take drug-thinning medicines or aspirin and/or if you want to use cloud ear regularly, you may have to check with your doctor and adjust the dosage.

Simple Cloud Ear Pasta

Every country has some sort of comfort food pasta. I use multigrain spaghetti, buckwheat noodles, bean thread noodles or pasta made from quinoa, a seed, and cook it this way.

Ingredients:
- Pasta
- 1 – 2 pieces of cloud ear mushroom, soaked and sliced
- Garlic and turmeric powder to taste
- Olive oil
- (optional) red hot pepper flakes, chopped parsley

Add no salt to the water but do add about 1 teaspoon of olive oil so the pasta does not stick together. Sprinkle in some turmeric powder, which has many health benefits—digestive, anti-cancer, anti-inflammatory for blood vessels and joints. When the pasta is almost done add sliced cloud ear mushroom and raw garlic to the cooking water. Allow it to cook for a couple of minutes so the cloud ear is cooked through but still a little crunchy. Drain, rinse the pasta so that it is less sticky. Add back about 1 tablespoon of water in the cooking pot, chopped raw garlic, a little oil and the pasta. (Optional) red pepper flakes and chopped parsley. Toss the pasta to refresh the ingredients and serve it immediately.

A World Tour in Restaurants

You don't have to live in New York to enjoy world famous Eastern cuisines. Most big cities have a Chinese neighborhood with Japanese and Thai stores and restaurants nearby. I have enjoyed ambling through Chinatowns from Montreal to Boston, from New York's boroughs to Philadelphia to San Francisco and Los Angeles. Older Chinese communities tend to stay compact sharing their foods, herbs and native language. More recent migrations from China, Thailand, Japan or India tend to spread out into the general population.

Asian cuisine is famous for its spicy flavors, many teas and regional dishes. Some lesser known mild tasting Chinese foods such as sautéed sliced lotus root and pea shoots are sources of high fiber useful for weight loss and reduce plaque. Thai foods are pungent, sweet and spicy with tasty sauces and rich creamy curries made with coconut milk. Coconut is a source of protein and immune-enhancing lauric acid a saturated fat praised by alternative cardiologists. Coconut oil is nourishing and cooling.

Do you love Japanese food? That cuisine uses lots of fish, seaweed, and green tea–all of which are heart healthy foods. Cordyceps an immune-enhancing Chinese medicinal mushroom and astragalus root, both valuable energizing health tonics, are sold in American health food stores such as Vitamin Shoppe. The contents of such capsules may be added to soup recipes. You can find my list of preferred sources of herbs and supplements at the back of this book and at the "Product" page of my website www.asianhealthsecrets.com. But it is most fun to roam through quaint streets, visit the shops, see the people, smell the incense and taste the cuisines when you visit ethnic neighborhoods. If you live here or plan to visit New York, here are a few high spots among Asian supermarkets that sell herbal medicines.

Hong Kong Supermarket

Hester street is a place where you will find Chinese street vendors selling fruits you have never seen. Formerly a Jewish neighborhood on the New York's lower east side, it now speaks mostly Cantonese. Hong Kong Market is located at 157 Hester Street between Bowery and Elizabeth Streets and easily reachable with B or D subway trains that stop at Grand Street.

When I enter this supermarket I walk around in Heaven to take it all in. The produce section is huge with stacked fresh fruits and vegetables everything at great prices such as delicious little red yams for under a dollar a pound, lots of Asian greens, melons, mushrooms and unusual vegan ingredients you won't find anywhere else. I am often in Chinatown to teach a class so I buy dried mushrooms and fungi, a zillion sauces, and lots of dried cooking ingredients, also Guilin gao, duck and quail eggs, herbal medicines, fancy honey and such. The meat section has everything from familiar cuts to black chicken, parts of everything that squeals, and all sorts of dumplings. The shoppers are busy and crowded, many of them Chinese, always a good sign that prices are reasonable and honest. Hong Kong Supermarket is close to my Mandarin language class through ALESN.org at Sun Yat Sen school also on Hester Street so I usually visit it and the street vendors outside for my weekly shopping. Delightful.

New Kam Mann Supermarket

This food and variety store, located at 200 Canal Street between Mott and Mulberry streets, has been a Chinatown favorite since the 1970s. You can find sales people who speak English here. Reachable by the N, R or number 6 Lexington local train stopping on Canal Street, it has three floors. Downstairs are a good selection of teas and natural sweeteners, dishware, tea pots and cooking appliances, dried noodles and traditional items like incense. The main floor has dried sea foods, an herbal medicines section, including several varieties of ginsengs, aisles with lots of cooking ingredients, refrigerated fresh noodles and buns, a vegan health food section selling mushrooms, cloud ear and other fungi and a small butcher shop in the corner window selling Peking duck. I never get to the top floor to look at clothing and beauty products being too busy on the main floor buying Chinese bean-filled buns, lotus pastry and spices. Their website newkammann.com, though not representative of their wide array of foods, does offer a few items, including teas, gifts and beauty products, a caviar facial pack if you are feeling decadent.

Manhattan's Little India

My favorite East Indian stores in Manhattan are around Lexington and East 28th street reachable by number 6 Lexington local subway. There are great small shops like Butala Emporium selling quality herbal remedy pills, cosmetics, also some clothing and decorative household items and Hindu sculptures of gods and goddesses. Their website is indousplaza.com. Of the area's many good restaurants my favorites include Chennai Garden by Tiffin Wallah at 127 East 28th near Lexington. They have a daytime vegetarian buffet that is worth the trip. It also pays to follow your nose and try a wide variety of south Indian vegetarian places. The largest supermarket in the area is by far Kalustyan's which takes up half the block at 123 Lexington Avenue between East 28th and 29th streets. Several large rooms have too many spices and foods to name on the main and lower floors and a bright, airy deli upstairs sells foods and a large selection of teas and coffees. Their website kalustyans.com is useful and gives you an idea of their global food items from India, East Asia and the Middle East. Our great ethnic neighborhoods are a trip abroad without the usual hassle.

Heart Health Checkup

You might use tongue diagnosis observations from your Heart Health Checkups to see if you should avoid or enjoy pungent flavors. Here is a brief refresher. A large tongue shows digestive bloating, water retention or a high sodium and/or sweet, rich diet. Increase sources of potassium such as papaya. A narrow tongue, especially when there is chronic thirst or dryness, shows dehydration. Increase moistening green foods. A red tongue, along with chronic hunger, burping, or constipation often indicates inflammation that can affect the heart and blood vessels. Add cooling supplements such as 1 gram per day of turmeric and possible blood thinner foods and herbs.

Q & A: Mushroom pills

I want a mushroom supplement from a clean source that is thoroughly checked for pollution and contamination -- *Combination Medicinal mushroom capsules for cancer and heart health protection*: http://www.absorbyourhealth.com/product/medicinal-mushroom-power-pack-2/?ref=4041

THIRTEEN

DESERT COMFORTS

My favorite meditation fills me with crisp desert air charged with sunlight that reaches my all-knowing heart. It is my healing space. I inhale bright blue light that floats above the Sandia mountains. At sunset the Rocky Mountain range of my childhood home turns pink. Endless sky turns multicolored as the sun dips below the Rio Grande valley's rolling hills towards Santa Fe. What does the desert need most? Water. Beige sand and subtle colors turn pink and yellow as flowers bloom after rainfall. The heart needs water to naturally reduce hypertension. Lacking adequate daily drinking water, the body retains sodium as a water storage mechanism and that raises blood pressure. How much is enough drinking water? Some cardiologists recommend at least 8 -10 eight ounce glasses of water daily possibly more for heart patients. Individual needs vary. You observed your morning urine in the Heart Health Checkup in Chapter 3. Clear, pale yellow, odorless and abundant urine with ease of flow indicate adequate hydration.

Desert Plants for Heart and Blood Vessels

Healing energy from the sun and sand in desert plants rid body and mind of impurities and irritations. Respected since ancient times, they assure our survival. This chapter details slightly bitter, cooling and detoxifying remedies that protect internal tissue, including the heart and blood vessels. Cooling, cleansing prickly pear, sometimes called cactus pear, makes a tasty snack and refreshing, healing beverage. Aloe vera, native to Africa, grows in hot desert climates and blooms after four years when mature. In Biblical Psalm 45 we learn that Jesus' garments "smell of myrrh, and aloes, and cassia. . . He is delightful to the senses and the spirit." Myrrh, aloe and cinnamon were used throughout the ancient world to prevent spoilage and in Egypt to preserve the dead.

Hearty night-blooming primrose protects blood vessels. Its oil helps lower blood pressure and eases chronic inflammatory pain by reducing harmful acidity. We will learn more about the importance of alkalinizing supplements and their role to protect blood vessels in a later chapter. For the present time, let's consider a cactus and aloe vera for reducing acid reflux pain and other side-effect of certain heart drugs, including muscle spasms and indigestion.

Nopalea

You can often find sliced green nopales cactus in Latin American or Mexican food shops. The spikes are removed, slicing them off with a knife so that the cactus can be stir fried or added to dishes. The mild flavored cactus reduces blood sugar for treating diabetes.

Nopalea, a delicious beverage made from nopale cactus [Opuntia cacti] fruit enzymes, grape seed extract, and concentrated fruit juices, provides vitamins and minerals necessary for cleansing and maintaining digestion at optimum efficiency. Nopalea reduces toxins and inflammation throughout the body correcting the underlying origins of chronic pains and heart disease.

I add an ounce of the fuschia-colored juice to a half glass of water and taste Coolaide from my childhood. Immediately I get recipe ideas for Nopalea ice cubes and popsickles for adults and kids. A treat for people with diabetes, pain, low energy. The juice ingredients are zillions of fruit enzymes, including cherry and papaya but mainly juice from nopale cactus, a desert panacea–pure, clean, safe, filled with sunshine from the Sonoran desert. I inhale clean air.

When was the last time I breathed so well? The walk I took through the southwest desert with my sister. My spine cracks into place in my middle back. Soon I am turning my neck around, my entire body is falling into a better place as I relax and breathe. My chest opens up and heart feels more at ease. Pain leaves as the body detoxifies and energy is refreshed. I can hardly wait to enjoy the benefits of this cactus drink for my complexion, energy, and joints after using it for a month. It is said that daily use of Nopalea helps the body to achieve optimal cellular health. To reduce sugar content add some water. It has no preservatives.

Inflammation and your health

Inflammation and dehydration are an underlying cause of many heart problems. Digestive inflammation increases pain, allergies, breathing difficulties, bloating, cramps, heartburn, and ulcers, also affect blood sugar contributing to diabetes. Widespread body cell inflammation causes overall fatigue especially for the heart.

You can find contacts online to buy Nopalea. People in Latin America and Mexico have been eating nopale cactus as part of their everyday diet for generations. Now we can enjoy the fruit as well. Sold in many supermarkets the pink fruit of nopale cactus is called prickly pear. As we have seen in previous chapters, there are many anti-inflammatory foods that benefit the heart and this one tastes delicious and is very easy to enjoy. Here is my home recipe for an inexpensive prickly pear drink.

Letha's Prickly Pear Cocktail

Whip this up in your blender, enjoy it as is or add it to a smoothie containing valuable cooling fruits and green vegetables.

Ingredients:
- 3 – 4 peeled, diced prickly pears; it has seeds which you can eat
- 1 tablespoon tart cherry concentrate
- ¼ cup fresh or frozen unsweetened cranberries
- 1/8 teaspoon cinnamon powder
- 2 cups brewed cold white tea
- (optional) 1/2 tsp. mashed clove of garlic as a blood thinner
- (optional) stevia for sweetening
- Serve this fresh and chilled in a Martini glass. Garnish it with fresh parsley or mint leaves.

Aloe vera

I love desert aloe vera. It is clean, cool and fresh, the scent of high desert filled with sunlight and sage. Smear the thick pulpy gel that lies under the crisp green peel on sunburn to ease burning pain. Drink pure organic aloe juice or gel in water to sooth an upset stomach, bad breath, constipation and some food allergies. Aloe is an alkaline food that resembles the healthy tissue of internal organs, free from impurities and acids that age us and create misery. Many times, I have recommended aloe as a daily beverage for people who want to lose weight, control diabetes, ease inflammatory joint pain or correct indigestion or menstrual problems. This slightly bitter tasting healing plant also protects blood vessels by reducing stress and inflammatory damage, a truly healing plant.

I drink it plain and leave it out of the refrigerator so that it turns pleasantly sour. Another nice way to enjoy aloe is to add up to ¼ cup of the juice or gel to mango, papaya, grape or prickly pear juice. Those juices are quite beneficial in themselves. Remember them, aloe vera, and fruit pectin powder added to water when it is time to detoxify your body from the side-effects of medicinal and street drugs. We will cover that in depth in Part Three along with natural alternatives for statin drugs' many unpleasant side-effects. If you have sensitive digestion or tend to have diarrhea, start by adding no more than 1 tablespoon of health food store aloe juice or gel, for example Lily of the Desert brand, to tea or juice then increase as needed. Do not exceed ¼ cup of aloe daily. You should soon notice smoother, easier digestion and elimination, fewer inflammatory symptoms ranging from acne to menstrual cramps, no bad breath, and less chronic thirst or gnawing hunger.

You won't feel the good job that aloe is doing for your heart and blood vessels, but you will feel refreshed mentally and spiritually. Aloe, because it is alkaline and heals wounds, rejuvenates the entire body from the skin to vital organs, blood vessels and blood.

Are there risks when consuming aloe vera? Yes when used to excess. Internal use of any bitter herb which may be laxative should be avoided by small children and pregnant women. Interestingly, one traditional treatment used by Chinese doctors to help patients with elevated blood pressure to avoid an oncoming stroke is to give them a strong laxative and/or diuretic that reduces fluid volume of the blood and thereby quickly lowers blood pressure. However, during pregnancy a strong laxative can easily cause miscarriage. Other side-effects of consuming aloe vera are usually caused by taking the harsh capsule of the concentrate and not the juice or jel.

Cautions: Oral aloe used as a laxative can cause cramping and diarrhea for people who have weak digestion. This may cause electrolyte imbalances if aloe is consumed for more than a few days. Aloe gel, for topical or oral use, should be free of athroquinones (primarily the compound aloin) that can be irritating to the gastrointestinal tract. People allergic to garlic, onions, and tulips are more likely to be allergic to aloe. Don't take aloe leaf pills, which are harsh, especially if you have intestinal problems, hemorrhoids, kidney problems, diabetes, or electrolyte imbalances. Adding 1 teaspoon to 1 tablespoon of the juice or gel to water is a gentle way to soothe heartburn and acid reflux.

Drug interactions: If you take medical drugs regularly, talk to your doctor before using aloe. It could interact with or replace certain medicines treating diabetes, high blood pressure, laxatives, steroids, and licorice root. Laxatives such as aloe can reduce the dosage and effectiveness of certain medicines. For example aloe vera gel taken orally helps people with diabetes by lowering blood sugar levels and may also help to lower cholesterol. It certainly has fewer side-effects than blood pressure medicines! But you have to determine for your individual use the best dosage to promote comfort without reducing absorption of vital minerals.

A High Desert Cleanse

As a semi-fast for enhanced energy and weight loss you might add 1 – 3 tablespoons of aloe juice or aloe gel in water or concord grape juice along with cleansing herbs once a day. This may improve weight loss and is easier than an actual fast. If your digestion is weak, have it along with a small meal. At the same time take 2 capsules of grapeseed extract which is detoxifying and (optional) 3 pills of mineral rich organic alfalfa. This is a general anti-inflammatory, anti-cholesterol cleanse done for a few days or up to a week several times a year.

Reducing harmful and poorly digested foods should be a regular part of any heart health lifestyle.

You can modify this recipe to reduce hypertension this way. Add aloe to tea and take the recommended dose of grapeseed extract along with hawthorn an herb we will cover later. The aloe soothes heartburn you may experience from using irritating foods and new herbs. Deep cleansing with natural herbal supplements has many benefits. I have found that periodic use of bitter greens along with alkaline deep-cleansing supplements such as aloe can lead to a burst of creative new ideas.

Heart Health Checkup

Do you have arthritis, allergies, headaches, skin rashes, bad temper or gout? Do you have thinning hair, brittle fingernails, bloodshot eyes? These are all signs of harmful inflammation. So are diabetes, cancers, and heart disease at base inflammatory illnesses.

Inflammation, however, is not the only problem that may be eased with cooling cleansing foods and herbs. The herbs in this chapter improve liver function, blood quality and therefore circulation. What do you think that does for your brain? When was the last time you started or even thought about a new art, business or other creative project? Do you lack energy, ideas, memory? Your medicines may be dulling more than you know. An article from 2010 entitled "It's Not Dementia, It's Your Heart Medication: Cholesterol Drugs and Memory" in *Scientific American* confirms some of our worse fears about heart drugs:

> Cholesterol-lowering statins such as Lipitor, Crestor and Zocor are the most widely prescribed medications in the world, and they are credited with saving the lives of many heart disease patients. But recently a number of users have voiced concerns that the drugs elicit unexpected cognitive side effects, such as memory loss, fuzzy thinking and learning difficulties. Hundreds of people have registered complaints with MedWatch, the U.S. Food and Drug Administration's adverse drug reaction database, but few studies have been

done and the results are inconclusive. Nevertheless, many experts are calling for increased public awareness of the possible cognitive side effects of statins—symptoms that may be misdiagnosed as dementia in the aging patients who take them.

No critic of statins dares use the word Alzheimer's. Dementia is an old fashioned word for what used to be considered an incurable, debilitating disease of the elderly. Now we call it Alzheimer's. Medical complications resulting from invasive treatments and terrible side-effects provoked by heart medicines have been expressed by countless heart patients on health websites. This book can help you to face the challenge of drug side effects from a patient's and caregiver's point of view not from stacked research data or drug company claims.

Q & A: Antioxidant effective for hypertension

I want an antioxidant pill that reduces hypertension - *Grape seed extract is quickly gaining popularity as a powerful and versatile antioxidant. It has been linked to improved hypertension, decreased inflammation, and increased bone density.* http://www.absorbyourhealth.com/product/grape-seed-extract-200mg-100-capsules-95-flavanoids-highly-potent/?ref=4041

Michael's Realtime Update Two

Down from Killington Mountain, off US 4, Letha and I are visiting Jim who bakes and sells delicious tarts. Raspberry is a favorite with his customers, but I like the lemon flavored tarts just as well. From his bakery in a small frame house in the Vermont countryside, dominated by a massive oven, Jim sells to stores in New England and by appearing in catalogs and online to diverse customers. We have known Jim, a portly fellow with a cheerful manner, for years, and we watched his business grow. His tarts are so tasty you could become addicted.

Jim's surroundings are quaint and peaceful. The bakery is reached via a back road off the highway, which runs east to west through a deep valley green with foliage in mid-summer. Nearby stands a traditional Episcopal chapel, in which Jim is the organist, and the chapel's lush garden. There is a water fountain inviting guests and their pets to quench their thirst. This is far from the hustle of Manhattan, farther still from the wars and plagues of much of the world. Still, Jim, middle-aged and otherwise healthy, suffers from a form of heart disease—atrial fibrillation. This is the most common type of abnormal heart rhythm, the heart beating rapidly and irregular, occurring in sudden episodes or more chronic. Aside from complaints such as shortness of breath, the condition is dangerous, a precursor to stroke. Letha has devoted a chapter to the ailment, but I wonder why Jim has come down with it.

A genial, generous fellow, perhaps he is a secret worrier. He runs a small but active business that sells a perishable product, which is a source of aggravation. My Dad was a business partner in a large commercial bakery in Brooklyn that sold to restaurants and cafeterias. He would bring home fancy cakes produced by his favorite baker, and as a kid I developed a sweet fang that keeps me rounder than I like. Dad, with the business in trouble, died of a heart attack at fifty-three. But here in Vermont life runs as tranquil as the brook we admire outside the bakery.

Now we're driving up VT 100 toward Pittsfield, a typical small town with a few white clapboard buildings, a white church steeple poking at the moody sky, and a red brick library that has an annual book sale. Nothing changes year to year. The quaint cemetery is more populated than the town. We pull off and walk along a dirt road called Lower Michigan. It meanders and has nothing to do with that state.

This pleasant stroll, past an old farmhouse with an older barn, passes a wooden house being built and rebuilt by the owner, who keeps Chinese ducks and lets them wander around. Black and white, ungainly, you may know them better as Peking Duck in a Chinese restaurant. We suspect that, come summer's end, these fellows will meet a similar fate.

Only a few weeks out of the hospital, I'm breathing and walking just fine. The air is clean, mellow, the smells and sights green and life-giving. My heart and yours, dear reader, needs this re-creation to heal from a busy, stressful, yet sedentary life. We also need to be good-hearted. One step Letha and I take is to feed a flock of domestic geese at the Grist Mill, a restaurant with a large water wheel on Killington Road. Big, white, these geese are pets who swim in graceful order in the pond, and not only won't they be served up as a meal, they will eat almost anything. We feed them leftovers, especially grains or bread, and as soon as we get out of the car chaos erupts: The flock of six honk away, making a great hullabaloo as they rush across the lawn to us. We feed them quickly, trying to keep our fingers out of their snapping beaks, and making sure the one with a broken wing gets enough to eat. They squabble, their manners are atrocious, but they are loveable.

We all need love, which according to song and story in many languages comes from the heart. We need to give love from the bottom of our hearts. Disappointments happen, and our hearts, ourselves, and our friends and neighbors may need to be bolstered against "the slings and arrows of outrageous fortune," to quote the Bard. There is a medical term for emotional damage done to the heart: Vital exhaustion (VE) is defined by cardiologists as a condition in which you are stressed to the point of exhaustion. Energy is gone, irritability increased, you feel overwhelmed, defeated. There is danger of a cardiac event. We have all been in such a place, and though we can pull out of the depths of despair (or just the nagging kind), some surrender. As Edgar Allen Poe wrote, "There is no dying without a dying of the will." The great poet and teller of tales, the first American author to try to earn a living through his writing, gave up and died at age forty.

For myself, there's a secret of survival. I've had a lot of schooling, plenty of exciting travel in dangerous places, maybe too much romance, but at heart I'm still a rough-'n'-tumble kid from a tough Brooklyn neighborhood. I need to be true to *me* to keep my ticker going okay. So, though it's a nuisance, I pop my prescribed pills, heart healthy vitamins, Letha's recommended herbs and supplements. But I'll do without a stent—that's for the ex-president—and no bypass— that's for my dentist. I want to go further than them.

PART THREE

HEART-PROTECTORS

Body/Mind/Spirit Natural Treatments for your Heart
Sea Treasures, Roots and Tree Bark

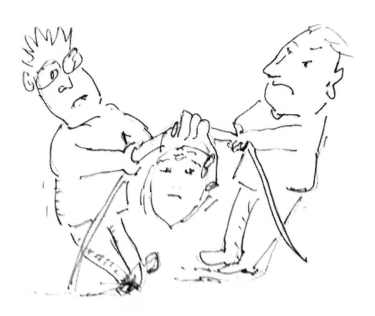

The cholesterol wars

FOURTEEN

THE CHOLESTEROL WARS

Medical research of drugs for preventing heart disease, especially when resulting in official health guidelines, is playing ball with your health. The old chicken or egg question for us now reads, "What comes first, which is most important -- cholesterol or inflammation in your arteries -- for causing blood vessel damage, heart disease and stroke?" Answers vary and both sides are armed with statistics. Some statistical analysis stack studies upon studies so that the controls become ever more obscured. Such computer-generated hocus pocus is used to prescribe treatments for us. We are easily beguiled by numbers.

Stiff Upper Lip and Statins

We love the Brits. They are so polite and orderly when standing in a proper Q lined up at airports. Do their organizational skills at times go too far? Sir Rory Collins of Oxford University, armed with studies funded by drug manufacturers Mercke and Pfizer, greatly influenced official British medical guidelines in 2014 suggesting that the use of statin drugs to reduce cholesterol could greatly save lives. The official response was that statin drugs were recommended for nearly every adult regardless of whether or not they had heart symptoms. Today Professor Collins has revamped his statement saying earlier studies did not properly investigate dramatic statin drug side effects, including muscular pain, nausea, memory loss and reduced testosterone leading to ED erectile dysfunction. Some experts and many patients are concerned that statins increase obesity and inactivity due to intense muscle pain that prevents exercise. But it gets worse.

Statins and Type 2 Diabetes

Statin drugs decrease both insulin sensitivity and secretion. According to current British medical sources, "Statin therapy is associated with a 46 per cent increased risk of Type 2 diabetes after adjustment for confounding factors, suggesting a higher risk of diabetes in the general population than previously reported." Ask doctors about statins and diabetes and they typically say the test results are inconclusive. Is it worth the risk? In 2014 a number of the UK's leading doctors vowed to ban prescribing statin drugs to their patients. Among them was Dr Malcolm Kendrick, author of *The Great Cholesterol Con*, who wrote, "Ironically diabetes triples the risk of heart disease for men and multiplies it by five for women, so the very drugs given to prevent heart disease may well be causing it in, potentially, millions of people."

In the USA: Statins and Aspirin

On this side of the pond, Dr. Michael Roizen, MD, chief wellness officer for Cleveland Clinic, has said, "Even though the National Institutes of Health NIH recommends that 35 million Americans take statins, considerably more than that actually do. If all the benefits we think statins provide actually prove to be true, perhaps statins should be taken regularly by *almost all* of us, as aspirin is, and started at about the same time, age thirty-five or forty." Roizen does qualify his statement by saying we lack long term studies on side effects and admits that reducing cholesterol too low may cause neurologic or immune dysfunction. Considering that many of us will live into our eighties, taking statins would be a very long, expensive drug habit.

On the other hand, John Abramson, senior lecturer in the department of healthcare policy at Harvard medical school, has said, "The trials on statins did not show that they prevented deaths. They also prevented only a small number of heart attacks and strokes. . . . The full data on the efficacy and the side-effects of statin treatment is not publicly available because all the trials were funded by drug companies and they had not released the figures."

In the United States regardless of age, people with a high cholesterol reading in blood tests are routinely prescribed statins in an attempt to help prevent heart attack and stroke. The rationale for this broad and increasing use of statin drugs for Americans who are lacking symptoms of heart disease is purely statistical. In England statins are given to people with a 20% risk of cardiovascular disease. However during Spring 2014 the NICE the UK's National Institute for Health and Care Excellence advised that the risk percentage should be cut in half reduced to 10%. But juggling the numbers does not mean that twice as many people will be protected by statin use. Given the dangers and side-effects expected from statins that measure of safety is hardly the case. (26.)

Whether the origin of heart disease should be blamed on harmful cholesterol or inflammation, in *Heart to Heart,* we will treat both as significant concerns and act accordingly with diet and natural medicines that support health and well-being. As we know there are good and bad dietary fats that can clog blood vessels. Most of us suffer from blood vessel inflammation in one form or another resulting from stress, environmental chemicals, radiation from computers and cell phones, emotional upset, bad habits like smoking, eating junk foods rich in sugars, and processed foods or those loaded with omega 6 oils.

Dr. Dwight Lundell, MD., heart surgeon with fifty years experience, founder of Healthy Humans Foundation in Arizona, and the author of The Cure for Heart Disease and The Great Cholesterol Lie, believes, "Mainstream medicine made a terrible mistake when it advised people to avoid saturated fat [like coconut oil] in favor of foods high in omega-6 fats. We now have an epidemic of arterial inflammation leading to heart disease and other silent killers."

Cholesterol Bottom Line

It is doubtful that the cholesterol controversy will be easily or soon resolved given the official dictum for reducing cholesterol medically and the more recent alternative cardiologist claims that cholesterol is very necessary for health, memory and wellbeing, and should not be curbed. A case in point is made by alternative cardiologists who advise that cholesterol is necessary for healthy brain function and for our immune system. A number of studies indicate that people with higher total cholesterol have stronger immunity. Cholesterol is something that you can track with blood tests. Most doctors test for total cholesterol. According to many cardiologists it should between 180-250 mg/dL.

Pro-cholesterol people advise that most importantly for immunity a suitable LDL (so called bad cholesterol) level should be between 80-140 mg/dL, but not any lower. Alternative cardiologists also stress that your cholesterol fractions and subtypes are quite important. They measure the size of cholesterol globs. Small dense cholesterol can more easily break off and jam blood vessels causing stroke and heart attack. The trouble is that most doctors do not test for these fractions or subtypes, even if you ask for the tests. Alternative-minded cardiologists advise that cholesterol levels should be checked by one of the newer generation blood lipid tests, such as the Vertical Auto Profile (VAP) test or the Lipoprotein Particle Profile (LPP) test, and there are certain ranges you want your scores to be in for a number of different categories. (27.)

In addition to the recommended healthy cholesterol level ranges (Note 27 at the back of the book), your doctor, if urged, can review your test results to see if your LDL unhealthy cholesterol is mostly made up of large, fluffy particles that are not dangerous, or small, dense particles (known as "LDL-pattern-B") that are dangerous. If it turns out that your LDL cholesterol is mostly of the small, dense therefore dangerous variety, they may recommend to address cholesterol levels much more aggressively than if your LDL cholesterol is mostly large and fluffy.

This means if you are taking a statin medication purely for cholesterol lowering you might consider quitting them gradually and with medical guidance. A smaller size dose taken daily is better than skipping days with pills because the heart does not like to be surprised. Crestor is a second generation statin drug following Lipitor known to have resulted in liver damage.

Natural statins are found in several foods including, as we have seen, PuErh tea and a supplement that has become popular as a pill red yeast rice, originally a Chinese food coloring added to soup. It contains lovastatin. In Chinese medicine, red yeast rice is used to lower cholesterol, improve blood circulation, and help digestive problems.

Some doctors say age is a factor and recommend for men under age 75 with diagnosed cardiovascular disease or significant risk factors for heart disease a statin drug may be prescribed. As heart patients reject or stop taking statins, as statins prove ineffective for preventing stroke, official recommendations and restrictions are changing. For many users the side effects far outweigh the benefits. In the following chapter, I summarize a natural approach to maintaining healthy cholesterol for prevention of heart disease.

The cholesterol controversy has been with us a long time. Remember the dietary attack on eggs and other saturated fats during the 1950s? Now coconut oil is back in favor. Some doctors conclude that cholesterol acts like a bomb ready to explode. Others consider it a healing balm, a necessary fact of life. Is there a middle way? We can enjoy certain fats. Certainly everyone agrees upon the benefits of consuming the omega 3s contained in oily fish, krill, squid, non-processed wholesome foods, fresh fruits and vegetables, and to avoid fried junk foods containing transfat. We need to develop the habit of looking at labels, cooking and eating in a pleasant low-stress environment, enjoying the company of friends and delicious meals made with love.

Beta-blockers

Another controversial category of heart drugs are beta-blockers commonly used in the treatment of high blood pressure and congestive heart failure. They work primarily by blocking the neurotransmitters norepinephrine and epinephrine (adrenaline) from binding to beta receptors, thereby dilating blood vessels, which reduces your heart rate and blood pressure. Put simply they keep blood vessels open. Until recently, the European Society of Cardiology (ESC) recommended using beta-blockers in patients undergoing non-cardiac surgery. But abusive medical research has come to light and slowly begun to change the way European cardiologists approach use of standard heart drugs.

A now famous case of flawed medical research was reported in the *Guardian*. The research paper, originally published in the online version of the *European Heart Journal* and reported in the *Telegraph* in 2008 refers to research done by Don Poldermans, a cardiovascular researcher in the Netherlands, who was fired for scientific misconduct in 2011. Some of the strongest evidence for the European Society of Cardiology's (ESC) guidelines on beta-blocker use in patients undergoing non-cardiac surgery came from Poldermans' research. The Erasmus Medical Center in Rotterdam stated he was fired because he was careless in collecting the data for his research. What is the result of sloppy research leading to skewed heart health guidelines? A spokesman from WebMD said that British researchers published a paper stating that by following an established guideline UK doctors put patients at risk. It took two years before the European Society of Cardiology withdrew the beta-blocker recommendation after the Poldermans scandal had unraveled. (28.)

Beta-blockers and Non-Cardiac Surgery

What does this confusion about heart drugs guidelines mean for you? What if you need to have non-cardiac surgery, for example, dental, appendix or hernia surgery? Surgeons advise us to stop blood thinning medicines before surgery. What about beta blocker drugs or others that keep your blood flowing? Hospital surgery teams are often organized by which doctors and nurses are available at the time needed for surgery.

Make sure your surgeon and dentist know about your heart medicines.

An Apple a Day vs. Statins

Here is cheerful news. A study published in the *British Medical Journal (BMJ)* reprinted from *CardioBrief* 2011, found that simply eating an apple a day might help prevent cardiovascular-related deaths in those over age 50 to a similar degree as using a daily statin drug. When the UK researchers took into account the *side effects* of statin drugs they reported, "Prescribing a statin to everyone over the age of 50 could lead to over 1,000 extra cases of muscle disease (myopathy) and more than 10,000 additional cases of diabetes..."

Perhaps pectin in apples helps detoxifies the body as well as a heart drug. Pectin powder taken daily has been recommended in cases of environmental radiation poisoning when taken for a month at a time several times a year. Pectin powder added to water has also been recommended to reduce harmful cholesterol and heavy metal poisoning as well as a therapy for diabetes and heart burn. It is easy to add a teaspoon of mild-tasting natural pectin powder to a cup of green tea.

I end this brief introduction to the cholesterol/inflammation/statin drug controversy with a recipe. In later chapters we will consider cholesterol lowering foods, targeted heart supplements and treatments to help eliminate underlying heart problems. But for now start the day as I do with green tea and an apple. If you like sweets, here is a safe choice:

Apple Pie

Raw apple is fine high fiber, dried slices are fun, although they contain concentrated sugar, but baked apple is soothing for a sensitive stomach. My apple pie contains no sugar, salt or fat, takes minutes to prepare and an hour to bake. It can be refrigerated for a couple of days if it lasts that long. Preheat the oven to 375 degrees.

Ingredients:
- 4 small or 3 large organic apples
- 1 handful dried organic raisins
- cinnamon, clove, cardamom powder, (optional black pepper) to taste
- 2 tablespoons Tapioca flour or 1 tablespoon of instant Tapioca granules
- juice of ½ organic lemon and (optional) ½ teaspoon lemon zest
- 1 prepared Graham cracker pie crust

When in Vermont, I buy my apples from my farmer friend Charlie Brown. His smile is bright, his cheeks rosy from eating his apples sold at Rutland's Farmers' Market. You may find quality organic apples in your supermarket, but they have been handled by countless people, shipped, refrigerated and possibly covered with wax.

To remove dirt, chemicals and wax, soak the apples in warm water with 1 tablespoon apple cider vinegar for a few minutes and carefully scrub the apples. Remove the seeds and stems. Slice them into a large non-metal bowl. Stir the apple spices and Tapioca flour mixing well to cover the sliced apples. Allow this to stand for a few minutes.

Pour the apple spice mixture into your prepared pie shell. I use Graham crust because it sweetness is enough to satisfy without added butter. However, if you want to avoid a processed foods, you can make your own low fat crust this way. Coat the bottom of a glass baking dish with a little olive oil and in a bowl mix raw oatmeal flakes, shredded raw coconut mixed with a little water and oil as a crust. Pat it down to match the shape of the baking dish. Then cover it with the apple mixture.

Cover the spiced apple filling with airtight aluminum foil and bake for one hour. When you remove it from the oven to cool, remove the foil and mash down the apples slightly with a fork so that the juice mixes with the chunks. If it looks dry add a few drops of lemon juice. Enjoy!

Heart Health Checkup

Are you currently taking heart medication? If so do you experience: Muscle stiffness, difficulty walking or exercising? Memory loss, poor concentration? Reduced sexual vitality and libido? Blood sugar problems including diabetes? Fatigue, anxiety and/or depression? Look again at the Note #7 at the back of the book for side-effects of common coronary heart disease medicines from rxlist.com.

Do you have your medicines organized so that you can easily take them throughout the day? Do you also take supplements such as vitamins, minerals, heart supplements Okayed by your doctor?

Do you regularly consume these blood thinners—garlic, aspirin, vitamin C, cloud ear mushrooms, or other? You will read about Serramend a natural, safe blood thinner in chapter 23.

Q & A: Joint Pain, inflammation and heart health

I want to reduce joint pain and inflammation while I protect my heart and blood vessels. *Cissus quadrangularis is recommended from human trials for joint health and pain reduction. It has been used for centuries in Ayurvedic medicine. Pine bark extract is an antioxidant, anti-inflammatory, immuno-stimulant shown to improve ADHD. Krill oil is an absorbable form of Omega-3 fats found to decrease C-Reactive protein levels, the key marker of inflammation; decrease triglycerides levels; decrease symptoms of arthritis, and more. Curcumin is a powerful anti-inflammatory and anti-viral agent.* Here is a combination pill: http://www.absorbyourhealth.com/product/healthy-joints-power-pack/?ref=4041

FIFTEEN

THE NEW CARDIOLOGY

By now you may be wondering what road to take in order to avoid dependence on heart drugs, stents, heart surgery and their complications—especially considering the quagmire of conflicting research data, extreme diets, and scare tactics used by special interests. You already know the basics. We live under more stress now than ever before. Women, city dwellers, the unemployed, the over age fifty, junk-food snacking, non-exercising, shrinking nearly gone middle class is hard hit. If the answer to survival were to simply walk for an hour a day, eat apples, and stop smoking, lots of people would live longer. As simple as that would be, it is most likely not enough. Life happens, and it is difficult to avoid injuries to health and happiness. There are side effects to heart drugs that deplete essential nutrients the body needs in order to function. They reduce the slack, that extra energy we need to defeat challenges. We need to increase our nutritional quotient and enhance the odds for survival. In a word—our heart needs fuel.

One trend among the new cardiologists is an attempt to use nutritional supplements as adjunct therapy or drug substitute treatments. I will cover their approaches in the following chapters. Lacking satisfactory long term studies of both recent standard heart drugs as well as their nutritional substitutes, we must judge for ourselves, with expert medical guidance, how to best use an individualized natural approach. One thing is for certain--If you are already taking heart medicines, do not quit them suddenly or all at once because your body is used to them. Stopping them may have disastrous results. You might be able to use both natural and chemical treatments simultaneously for a while. Consult with your heart specialist, continue testing, and do not reduce the dosage of medicines until the natural therapies are working to your advantage.

An estimated half of patients prescribed heart drugs quit using them for various reasons including their cost and side-effects.

Comments from disgruntled statin users young and elderly are found on the Internet. Cholesterol is brain food for the young and may protect the brain against aging. Do your heart drugs reduce your memory, physical movement, sex life and immunity to illness? Cholesterol is a link in the production of testosterone. Vitamin D is also synthesized from a close relative of cholesterol: 7 dehydrocholesterol.

Cholesterol the Calming Brain Food

Nowhere is the importance of cholesterol as evident as in the human brain. Low cholesterol levels have been linked to violent behavior due to adverse changes in brain chemistry. Low cholesterol levels have been linked to depression and suicide. According to Dr. James Greenblatt, MD, the Chief Medical Officer and Vice President of Medical Services at Walden Behavioral Care in Waltham, Massachusetts and Assistant Clinical Professor of Psychiatry at Tufts University School of Medicine, "Although cholesterol-lowering medications might lower the risk of heart attacks or strokes our obsession with lowering cholesterol completely ignores the potential psychological consequences that may occur with low cholesterol." The majority of research leads to the conclusion that low cholesterol leads to higher rates of depression. (29.)

Cholesterol and Memory

The human body is composed of trillions of cells and cholesterol is one of the molecules that allow for cell interactions to take place. Cholesterol plays an essential role in the brain, which contains 25 percent of the cholesterol in our body, because it is critical for synapse formation that allow us to think, learn new things, and form memories. In fact, some authorities believe that low-fat diets and/or cholesterol-lowering drugs may contribute to Alzheimer's disease. (30.)

Dr. Stephanie Seneff from the non-profit Weston A. Price Foundation goes so far as to suggest that heart disease is the result of cholesterol deficiency, the complete opposite of the conventional medical view. *"Yoi!"* as my Hungarian grandmother would say.

I wonder if Gramma, who lived to be 93, was on to something by cooking with bacon drippings. She never heard of olive oil back then. Years ago I saw pigs roaming in rural Hungarian village streets. Gramma's cooking fat was natural, fresh and available. We have lots more healthy dietary choices today. For example, grapeseed oil. The worst oils may be cottonseed and corn oil because in many American states they are GMO genetically modified. GMO foods are linked to leaky gut and a variety of digestion/absorption problems. Palm oil used in everything from cookies to face cream seriously deforests large areas of the world leading to soil erosion, death of many animal species and ultimately to climate change.

A number of alternative medical doctors recommend dietary fats such as fish oils supplements and coconut and olive oils for cooking as sources of necessary cholesterol to support healthy memory, vision, and heart health. But oil is only part of the picture. The right dietary factors have to be in place at the right time to reduce heart stress. The noted cardiologist and holistic health author, Dr. Stephen Sinatra, MD, who stresses the importance of the *size* of LDL recommends taking niacin, vitamin B3 the kind that causes flushing, to make LDL fat globules "fluffy" so that they cannot easily cause blood vessel blockage.

One main thrust of this argument concerns making the heart itself stronger. That is possible by increasing heart muscle energy and immunity with targeted supplements that act as energizers inside the cells. Another aspect of reducing heart stress, according to Sinatra, involves reducing unhealthy inflammation in blood vessels that make them brittle and more likely to crack as happens during a heart attack. In short, the heart gets more energy to work efficiently and less inflammation to damage heart tissue and blood vessels.

Dr. Sinatra's Awesome Foursome and then some

The Sinatra solution is dietary supplements to prevent and reverse inflammation of the inner lining of blood vessels no matter what the cause. Sinatra recommends squid oil supplements, some butter, and not to avoid all fats. Sugar is Sinatra's enemy especially sugar in processed foods, corn sweeteners, and pastry, white flour and nearly all refined grains because they turn into inflammation. Sinatra's supplements whether for weight loss, vision, or heart health contain squid oil said to be more easily absorbable than fish oil. Let's look closer specifically at Sinatra's heart energizers he calls the "Awesome Foursome."

On his informative website, Sinatra writes, "For reversing cardiovascular disease (CVD) supplementation with the "awesome foursome," is the most targeted way of sustaining your heart's energy needs at the cellular level and providing nutrients necessary for metabolic processes." Sinatra's "awesome foursome" are coenzyme Q10, L-carnitine, D-ribose, and magnesium, which according to him, "individually and collectively help increase energy, or ATP, production in your body by supporting mitochondria within cells." Adenosine triphosphate (ATP) transports chemical energy within cells for metabolism. Cells require large amounts of ATP to contract and relax the heart, maintain cellular ion balance, and synthesize proteins and fats. (31.) Magnesium is important for keeping blood vessels open and flexible. The most absorbable form is magnesium threonate. (see the Resource Guide section.)

At around age forty, our production of CoQ10 and L-carnitine generally starts to decrease so that most people associate lack of energy with middle age. Sinatra's answer is to supplement the heart's energy with his "awesome foursome" especially if you have coronary artery disease (CAD) the buildup of plaque that affects blood vessels. With CAD, the heart continually overworks to pump blood through inflamed and congested blood vessels and ultimately expends energy much faster than the body can produce it. Sinatra believes the usual medical drugs, for example statins and beta blockers used for stabilizing people during emergency situations and improving symptoms, actually *inhibit* the production of CoQ10. So that taking a CoQ10 supplement can counteract pharmaceutical side effects of energy depletion.

Each of the foursome plays a fundamental role in cellular metabolism according to Sinatra, "especially in supplying the heart with the energy it needs to preserve its contractile force and can safely and effectively be ingested in tandem with beta-blockers, calcium channel blockers, nitrates, and ACE inhibitors. Not only will taking energy-enhancing supplements help alleviate negative side effects associated with these drugs, but it might eventually reduce, or even eliminate the need for such medication."

This is good news for heart patients. Michael took certain of Sinatra's supplements along with his blood pressure drug and natural remedies and there are no unpleasant side-effects. But are there added benefits for people who do not have a heart illness? Sinatra believes that supplementing our heart energy with supplements that enhance ATP can be a "fountain of youth." Chinese herbalists agree that a strong heart supports courage, a bright complexion, ease in breathing and improved memory and concentration. There may be an advantage in using part or all of the awesome foursome to stay in shape and correct chronic fatigue. In particular Ribose (AKA Beta-D-ribofuranose, D-ribosa, D-ribose, Ribosa) is a sugar produced by the body. Ribose has been used to enhance athletic performance by boosting muscle energy and to improve symptoms of chronic fatigue syndrome (CFS), fibromyalgia and coronary artery disease. Ribose helps prevent symptoms such as cramping, pain, and stiffness after exercise in people lacking certain enzymes due to inherited disorders. It is safe to use daily.

TCM doctors teach us that the heart is the ruler of our emotions, that if the heart is healthy our *shen*, the spirit that dwells within the heart, is able to rule body and mind as an enlightened Emperor. Our emotions will less likely to cause illness even under extreme circumstances. Caregivers get a big dose of worry, anxiety, and exhaustion. D-Ribose powder, a natural sweetener, added to foods may help reduce the physical and emotional overload. Also look back at chapter 3. to see how homeopathic remedies such as pulsatilla, gelsemium or ignatia amara can help relieve caregiver stress. Homeopathic remedies, recommended by a professional homeopath, can key into our particular needs to effectively treat emotional as well as physical symptoms. By supporting emotional balance we support heart health.

Asian natural doctors use herbs, we will see later, to energize and rejuvenate the heart. Your cardiologist may not have heard of heart healthy herbs except garlic and possibly hawthorn. Some doctors have recommended combining hawthorn with magnesium threonate and grape seed extract to tone and protect blood vessels and help maintain healthy blood pressure. Herbs work in a different manner than Sinatra's foursome. Herbs work more like health foods to nourish and regulate the heart tissue and rhythm, blood vessels and circulation. Based on medical testing, heart doctors sometimes use unusual terms for heart tissue and function such as a stiff heart or an overworked heart, which may not respond well to a stimulant. Check with your doctor about your specific condition.

Without ATP, our cells die. Toxic exposure from drugs, chemical pollution from insecticides and pesticides, mercury and heavy metals, radiation, vaccines and some pharmaceutical drugs contribute to mitochondrial instability and vulnerability. The mitochondria act like batteries in our cells. Our exposure to poisons cause mitochondrial die-off, tissue impairment and pathology. Vaccines and some pharmaceutical drugs contribute to mitochondrial instability and vulnerability. We experience this as chronic fatigue. Most people need CoQ10 and magnesium threonate for the simple reason that we live in such a toxic world. CoQ10 may slow the aging process in large part due to its membrane stabilizing activity. (32.)

Magnesium helps to reduce the ill effects of stress and poisons in our foods and environment. It is worth repeating that the right source of magnesium helps keep blood vessels supple and open to regulate blood pressure and prevent hardening of the arteries and hypertension, heart disease and stroke. Unfortunately magnesium supplements are not easy to digest or absorb. Foods often lack adequate minerals because the soil has become nutrient poor. Magnesium threonate allows magnesium to be absorbed more easily than other kinds of magnesium. It can reduce stress, toxins and improve memory.

Symptoms of magnesium deficiency include headaches and migraines, dizziness, confusion, cardiac arrhythmia, nervousness, spasm pain in the neck, face and shoulders, gastrointestinal cramps, nausea and vomiting, urinary and uterine cramps, tight calves and foot cramps. Does that stiffness and vague chronic pain sound like you sitting at your computer? Stress uses up our magnesium, so does caffeine, and makes our comfort and sleep difficult. Do you drink coffee and/or caffeine tea all day? Aside from easing cramping and chronic pain, a certain form of magnesium threonate, improves brain function and circulation. Importantly, magnesium threonate crosses the blood-brain barrier which allows it to have effects on cognition. One study with magnesium threonate showed an 18% improvement in short-term memory and a 100% improvement in long-term memory It also improves anxiety responses.

It is easy to take magnesium threonate at the time your memory most needs it when the brain is quiet and you feel sleepy at night. At bedtime have a glass of fresh carrot juice, add 1/2 teaspoon of coconut oil. The carrot provides vitamin A the brain needs and the oil enhances absorption of the A. Then take your dose of magnesium threonate so that your brain can be rejuvenated, your senses cleared and your memory improved while you sleep. You can find my recommended product sources at the back of this book and among the "Products" section at www.asianhealthsecrets.com.

In Woody Allen's all's well that ends well movie *Hannah and her sisters* he has divorced Hannah (Mia Farrow) and married her sister Holly (Dianne Wiest.) The amicable movie divorce is far from the real-life divorce of Woody and Mia. At movie's end Woody quips, "The heart is a very resilient little muscle." Life should be as smooth as a feel good movie. The heart may be resilient but it needs help. Here is your observation for this chapter.

Heart Health Checkup

TCM has indirect ways of noticing heart health. Illness has an odor, a color and sound. A Chinese herbalist will take your pulses. The heart pulse is the top of twelve pulses found on the palm side of your left hand. TCM doctors look at your tongue for color, shape, movement, and markings. A bumping high pulse and red dry tongue shows inflammation. An irregular heartbeat might signal poor energy, a tired heart, or under-functioning digestive organs and troubled circulation through the abdomen or chest. The heart is not separate from the rest of your body and mind.

Chinese herbalists listen to your voice. Is it high and squeaky from anxiety, sharp or tense indicating muscle stiffness and inflammation? Is it low and breathy and fading indicating low vitality or stumbling stuck qi? A popular vocal style used by some young professional women is a high pitched sound that comes from nowhere, it sounds ungrounded and unpleasant. I don't know if it is an attempt to sound feminine or heart-related stress. More information is needed. Put a number of your different observations together such as your energy, breathing, facial hue. There are even more subtle ways to observe stress: Illness has an odor. Is there the characteristic burnt and bitter body odor of heart (Fire Element) inflammation? Or does the person smell a bit like garbage from liver constriction? Is there a trace of rather stale sweet smelling fragrance from diabetes? Is the facial coloring inflamed, purple or blotchy showing inflammation or pale or sallow indicating chronic fatigue and poor circulation? Use your senses and overall impression of vitality. This is not rocket science, but a way to become more sensitive to your body and your patient.

None of these old fashioned clinical observations impress the cardiologist armed with test results. Tests based on animal or human studies only predict what is likely to occur given a large population. The results must be duplicated for the large selection under controlled circumstances. It would be easier to predict results if we were clones. Our informal observations – we all make them—can become more appropriate and beneficial for a daily health routine. If signs indicate inflammation, eat cooler foods, add moisture from green vegetables and Pu Erh tea to the diet. If your Heart Throb or patient looks at you with droopy eyes, sighs when breathing, complains about cold weather then his/her qi is low and may benefit from an herbal or supplement tonic, cooked warm foods and stimulating spices. A warm bath and loving massage improves sleep and mood. Here are things to check for yourself:

- At what times of day and evening do you feel most tired?
- Do you have chest pains after exercise or upon waking?
- Are your hands and feet often cold and clammy?

Look again at chapter 7. if you have recurrent or intense chest pains that last more than a few minutes. Chronic fatigue may feel like depression, a negative attitude, or aches that slow your game. Traditional Chinese medicine has charted the hours of day and night that we are most likely to feel certain discomforts or illness. The 2017 Nobel Prize winner in physiology and medicine also "discovered" this old Chinese notion of natural circadian rhythms to be the case—he found the gene. Energy is not a constant: We respond with internal organ function when their meridians are full or empty of energy at the corresponding times. Doctors (and martial arts masters) trained in the Chinese Meridian Clock use this knowledge to help them predict vulnerability of internal organs. For example, they believe if you feel chest pain or are worn out around 10Am to noon, if that is when you crave a stimulant, then your digestion and heart are weak. They verify with pulse and tongue diagnosis. Morning is the time when healthy heart energy should feel strong and steady. It may be the best time to take heart related herbs. If you feel withdrawn or collapse into a nap during afternoon and early evening from around 4PM to 7PM, if your legs ache, your urine is excessive and sexual vitality low, then adrenal energy (AKA kidney/adrenal Qi) is low. Rest, nourishing food and adaptogenic (stress-reducing) tonics are in order.

Are you tired all day? Is your sleep disturbed? Do you have chronic pain from fibromyalgia? Aches feel worse from lack of sleep and weak circulation. Mood, our ability to think clearly, deal with stress and react appropriately suffer. Heart and adrenal tonics detailed in this book often improve such discomforts. You see old-fashioned diagnosis is subjective and inexact compared to modern testing, but it promotes beneficial holistic treatment. That is important for protecting our energy daily. Enhancing vitality, immunity and mood naturally provides the slack we need to combat extraordinary stress. For some people that might mean a walk in the park or twenty minutes of meditation. It is uplifting and feels purifying. In the following chapter we will see how herbal heart tonics and energy supplements work better when the body is free of toxins. Improving overall wellness supports our "resilient little muscle."

Q & A: Heart Strength

I want a simple food I can use daily to strengthen my heart -- *D-Ribose powder helps increase ATP Production, our natural source of energy. It is heart-protective and decreases workout recovery time. Add it like sugar to sweeten tea or coffee.* http://www.absorbyourhealth.com/product/d-ribose-powder-auto-renew/?ref=4041

SIXTEEN

BEWARE TOXINS

Dietary fads are fueled by health advocates who jump in with scare tactics like we are all going to drop dead by eating grains. It's true, processed foods like white rice and white flour are low in nutrition which stresses the pancreas, but whole grains have been around since ancient Egypt. Consider the big picture. A few years ago we stressed complex carbohydrate foods including whole grains in order to lose weight, regulate blood sugar, and generally stay healthy. You have to be selective. Oats, quinoa, air-popped non-GMO corn, barley and seeds like millet digest better, contain fiber and are, therefore, safer for the heart. Natural fresh, organic non-GMO foods are wholesome. Over-refined foods increase inflammation hazardous to blood vessels already inflamed from stress, radiation and pollution and start a dangerous chain reaction. To fully live life, travel and experience new, exciting people, places and foods we ought to have ways to avoid getting sick.

Your Gut and Mood

There is a factory for health and wellbeing that helps your heart stay strong. It is your gut. Both brain and intestine are created from the same tissue during fetal development and are connected via the vagus nerve. In other words mental health is connected to bacteria and microbes living in your gut. Gut bacteria produce mood-boosting neurotransmitters including serotonin, dopamine, and gamma-aminobutyric acid (GABA). In fact, the greatest concentration of serotonin, the feel good neurotransmitter, is found in your intestines and not your brain. (34.) It gets even better and more complex. As late as 2015, scientists at University of Virginia discovered a link between the brain and immunity when they discovered lymph nodes in the brain. It has been suggested, therefore, that neurological illnesses occur due to under-functioning of the lymph system that reaches the brain. Does that mean that the brain backs up with poisons if we lack the right gut bacteria? As with most medical laboratory research, it will take a long time for scientific findings to impact use of medicines and diet. The short answer is: How can you protect your gut/brain/immunity connection? Deep cleansing has many benefits. Start with smart food combining, a few specific dietary restrictions and regular purification.

Intestinal Parasites and Your Heart

Why am I writing about parasites in a heart health book? Cleansing for heart health begins at home in the gut. The site of our immunity, as well as our absorption of nutrients, is the gut. No matter what medicines, herbal remedies or health foods you consume, if digestion and absorption are impaired you will not benefit from your health regime. Many people have intestinal parasites without knowing it because the problem is built into their regular diet. For example, mixing meat and dairy foods or fish and dairy foods supports an internal environment in which harmful gut bacteria, yeast and parasites thrive. Drink unsafe water or eat food prepared by unclean hands–even in fine restaurants–and you've got parasites. Ice in cold drinks is not made with sterilized water. Remember that when you travel.

Start clean to stay strong. You have no idea how many people touched your foods and if they washed their hands. Wax coating fresh produce is no protection against germs. A world traveler of long standing, I have dined in places you would never go and dealt with digestive complaints that harm vitality. My favorite short term (up to two weeks) gut cleansing treatment is a daily cup of strong coffee adding drops of bitter wormwood and black walnut hull liquid extract and a dash or clove powder. Or for long term home treatment add neem tree bark powder to coffee. To help maintain a healthy gut some people eat yogurt with turmeric powder. You can also support healthy gut fluora with good combinations of probiotic bacteria in capsules easily available from your health food store. I naturally ferment vegetables for their healthy bacteria, and have one serving daily.

Bitter tasting neem leaf can be taken in capsules and is anti-bacterial, anti-viral, anti-yeast and anti-parasite. Neem tree bark powder, full of useful antioxidants, is less bitter than the leaves and can be added to coffee similar to New Orleans chicory coffee.

Radiation

We can't avoid our toxic world. One of our biggest threats is radiation from exposure to cell phones, computer WIFI, digital clocks, micro-waved foods, refrigerators, medical and dental Xrays, especially cat scans, room sized airport scanners, etc all of which scatter brainwaves and weaken immunity. Dietary mistakes, environmental and food chemicals increase the sizzle. The Environmental Protection Agency warns we are routinely exposed to radiation amounting to 200 millirems of household radon per year and pregnant women should be exposed to no more than 500 millirems per year. Repeated high doses of ionizing radiation result in the death of our cells. If a sufficient number of cells are affected the function of organs is impaired. Our exposure to electro-magnetic sizzle can only get worse. In the near future we will deal with the effects of computerized cars that drive themselves and wrap around virtual reality entertainment systems that emit electro-magnetic waves into our brain from all directions. We can already wear a cell phone like a wrist watch. Someday will we be able to implant a cell phone, like a hearing aid, in our ear? Where does it come from, this craze to feel connected with a high tech umbilical cord? How can we protect our heart from radiation exposure?

Grounding Radiation

Exposed to free radical stress our blood thickens and positive charges accumulate in the body causing chronic inflammation a marker for most chronic and degenerative disease. Grounding our internal radiation effectively helps alleviate that inflammation. Grounding reduces pain, improves sleep patterns and gives us a sense of wellbeing we can only feel when connected to earth as nature intended. Grounding helps to thin our blood by providing red blood cells with a surplus of electrons so they can repel each other and avoid becoming "sticky" which leads to blood clots, heart attack or stroke.

How do we ground harmful radiation? Just as any lightning rod would we send the radiation back to earth, by walking barefoot on damp grass, sand, soil in your garden, or the beach. Be careful to avoid Lyme disease! (See the chapter on superbugs) You can also help to ground radiation by walking barefoot on your wood floor, tile or unpainted brick. Research has demonstrated it takes about 80 minutes for the free electrons from walking barefoot in your grass to reach our bloodstream and transform our blood cells.

If you can't go outside there are ways to ground yourself indoors. First identify the sources of harmful rays and pollution. Much of our worst exposure is unconscious. I see college kids working with their laptop covering their lap spewing radiation into their vitals, gabbing on cell phones and smoking. You even get fallout from other people's cell phones because the rays cover a distance of about six inches from the emitting antenna. (33.) Most vulnerable are the very young. Don't carry a cell phone in our clothes. Text if you must.

Let's create a safe room where wellness and peace may flourish. At home isolate your computer area. Most radiation from computers comes from the screen and for laptops from the machine itself. Cover the computer screen with a protective material available online and ground yourself by putting bare feet on a grounding pad at your desk. Grounding pads are available online and can be placed under your computer, keyboard or under your feet. Large grounding pads fit under your bed sheets. Put your computer desk near the center of the room so radiation does not bounce off the wall.

Surround your desk and computer area with cacti, a known deterrent to radiation. Avoid or regularly clean heavy drapes and upholstered furniture in your computer area that might absorb dust and radiation. Use a speaker phone instead of holding the cell phone to your ear. At a comfortable time in the evening turn off phones, computers, and other electronics. After the nuclear meltdown in Japan a few years ago many people around the world became aware of the radiation threat. Grounding toxic radiation in the body helps regulate sleep rhythms, helps you sleep better and therefore improves weight loss and heart health. Most houses and apartments are grounded for protection against lightning.

To ground yourself, use a grounding sheet in bed or ground yourself with your computer chassis while you work. That is easy to do if you have a yard and work by the window. You can ground the computer by attaching a copper wire to it and put the other end of the wire out the window and into the earth. Some big old fashioned computers are already grounded. Attach one end of the copper wire to your computer chassis which is grounded (not your laptop) and place the other end with the clip inside your sock while you work. You are grounded because the computer is.

Here's what I do in our small second floor New York apartment. I ground myself or my computer keyboard and mouse pad by attaching a grounding alligator clip to each end of a long copper grounding wire from a hardware store. One end of the exposed copper wire attaches to me in my sock and the other end clamps onto the cold water pipe under the sink. If your cold water pipe is plastic, clamp the alligator clip on to the brass tightening nut.

Another way to do it is even easier: Take two "plug to gator" cords. One end will have a grounding plug the other end is an alligator clip. The plug has three parts, 2 flat and one round metal prong which is the grounding prong. Flatten the two flat prongs and plug only the round prong into a surge protector. Use the gator end to attach some copper wire that you roll into a disc. Attach that disc to you, one on the bottom of each bare foot, or what ever you want to ground. When I ground myself with a copper wire while sitting at my computer, I feel calmer, quieter and I sleep better at night. It attracts qi and inflammation downward when you put it at the bottom of your feet.

Note: Do Not use any grounding device during a thunder storm. Remember grounding thins the blood and may affect heart drugs in other ways so, if necessary, check with your doctor about dosage for blood thinner medicines.

An Anti-Radiation Food Additive

Fruit pectin absorbs lots of poisons. You would have to eat lots of apples to get enough pectin. But luckily fruit pectin is available as a powder for people who like to can fresh fruits or make jelly. It has been suggested to take 1 teaspoon of fruit pectin powder in water daily for 3 – 4 months several times a year. Pectin sends poisons to the liver to be eliminated. This can easily be added to a routine springtime and autumn detox program to help curb allergies and aches at the very least.

Household and Personal Chemicals

Don't pollute your body or home with harsh chemical detergents. Environmental chemicals can stress your heart, general vitality and immunity. You can do a lot of cleansing with simple safe ingredients such as baking soda and peroxide or baking soda and white vinegar used for washing floors, home appliances and clothing. Most people are smart enough to have their old metal teeth fillings replaced with safe non-toxic white ones. But we are still exposed to lead and other heavy metals every day in the air and water.

Chelation therapy has been used by heart patients. It is medical intravenous EDTA (AKA Calcium Disodium Edathamil, Calcium Disodium EDTA) used to treat lead poisoning and brain damage caused by lead poisoning, to evaluate a patient's response to therapy for suspected lead poisoning, to treat poisonings by radioactive materials such as plutonium, thorium, uranium, and strontium, and for removing high levels of copper and calcium. EDTA is also used intravenously for heart and blood vessel conditions including irregular heartbeat due to exposure to chemicals called cardiac glycosides, "hardening of the arteries," chest pain, high blood pressure, high cholesterol, and blood circulation problems such as Raynaud's syndrome. Other intravenous uses include treatment of cancer, RA rheumatoid arthritis, osteoarthritis, and macular degeneration, diabetes, Alzheimer's, multiple sclerosis, Parkinson's, and skin conditions including psoriasis. Discuss chelation therapy and supplements with your heart doctor because there are drug interactions with insulin, blood thinning drugs and diuretics.

Here is the simplest way to help remove heavy metals from your body: Perspire. A sauna may be too hot, or too long an exposure of heat for heart patients. But working up a sweat as you walk or exercise is a good idea. Dr. Bernard Jensen, a famous nutritionist, long ago recommended adding ¼ cup ginger powder to warm bath water, then wrapping up in a terrycloth bathrobe and heavy blanket to sweat out pains and impurities. That keeps your head free from excess heat.

A Toxic Lifestyle

A typical scene you often see on the street or in restaurants is a couple, obviously attached or married, sitting opposite each other while reading their text messages. People these days read screens not faces. Psychologists now call automatic email updates toxic. Remember when the typical person on call was a doctor? Now with automatic email updates everyone is on call all the time. At the beginning of 2016, a report in the UK *Telegraph* suggested that technology enabling people to be at their email's constant beck and call has created a culture where people must feel they are constantly available for work. As a result, an "unwritten organizational etiquette" has become ingrained in the workplace and employees have developed anxiety. Experts have recommended that switching off the 'Mail' app on our mobile phone may alleviate anxiety in and out of the office. At home to improve sleep, unplug your phones and computers and get away from electronic devices.

Heart Health Checkup

Lead poisoning:

Do you have abdominal pain, fatigue, constipation, loss of appetite, kidney failure, calcium deposits in eye affecting vision, and/ or hardened skin (scleroderma)? They are signs of lead poison. It is a hard fact to swallow that most of us suffer from some degree of lead poisoning because of air pollution and old water pipes from the street to your apartment. A water filter may help.

Radiation poisoning:

A small amount of radiation can be a good thing. It is found in the soil, plants and our body. But too much exposure is dangerous. Non-ionizing radiation is mostly emitted through waves like sound waves, radio waves, and ultraviolet (heat) waves. It's what makes things like cell phones, light bulbs, microwave ovens and diagnostic ultrasound machines work. Although non-ionizing radiation can be harmful in very high doses, this type of radiation cannot change the molecular chemistry of a person or thing. Ionizing radiation such as cosmic rays from the sun and stars, and radon (an element found in soil) and manmade sources such as X-ray machines and radiation therapy for cancer treatment is powerful enough to split an atom and change the molecular chemistry of a person or thing. It's this type of radiation that can lead to radiation sickness, even months following exposure, and death. Symptoms of radiation poisoning from a slight exposure include nausea, vomiting, falling blood counts, and a predisposition to infection and bleeding.

As part of a heart healthy detoxification program that includes foods, herbs, purified or spring water, herbal baths and sauna treatments, it may be wise to add a form of affordable, easily available chelation therapy. Cardio Chelate pills contain EDTA that support optimal cardiovascular health. Taking the Cardio Chelate capsules of course is not as strong as intravenous EDTA, but you can feel some of the positive effects such as enhanced energy and circulation. Start slowly and take the recommended dose two hours before or one hour after a meal for improved energy, breathing, and to help reduce chronic pain. Do not mix EDTA with oral hydrogen peroxide treatments in order to avoid side-effects. I will cover numerous other enjoyable ways to detoxify the body and improve circulation such as foot soaks in Part Four.

Q & A: Detoxification from heavy metals

I want a natural product for a deep detoxification treatment at home –

Heavy Metals: *Borax is a mineral used in Chinese medicine TCM as an anti-inflammatory treatment recommended for reducing heavy metals, yeast, parasites, and joint stiffness and pain. In North America borax powder, Twenty Mule Team Borax, a detergent enhancer and water softener, has warnings against internal use. However, certain alternative health websites recommend adding a small amount of the powder to a bath and as a natural hair wash that strips out hair product chemicals. That can affect hair color.*

Excess synthetic environmental estrogens from pesticides and pollution:

Chemicals found in cruciferous vegetables tend to balance hormones and reduce harmful estrogens that may lead to chronic inflammation and cancers. http://www.absorbyourhealth.com/product/estrogen-balance-power-pack/?ref=4041

SEVENTEEN

EMBRACE YOUR REMEDIES

This book, a love story about long time caring, gives you the opportunity to vitally connect with your personal healing options. Our treatment choices, curative foods and herbs available from online and direct sources, are listed at the back of the book. Your best remedy choices are directly influenced by your observations detailed at the end of most chapters. That is especially true in this chapter where, as an example, I have simplified your choice to three Ayurvedic herbs that support healthy heart action. They are arjuna tree bark, guggul tree sap, and amla an Indian gooseberry.

There is a ton of information and research on each of these Ayurvedic herbs since they have been in use for thousands of years. Since they are better known originally in Asia and are being studied in laboratories worldwide, we often feel swept away by too much scientific information without really feeling connected with the herbal choice. Being bombarded daily with reports of new great superfoods does not help. We feel, "Oh not another miracle food!" To remedy the ennui, with each herbal description I offer here a few questions intended for self-observations along with a brief visualization of the herb's energy, a kind of herbal meditation, so that you may connect spiritually and emotionally with the treatment. Please feel free to discover your own images.

When we pass through life events like a ghost or a running bull without allowing expression to our feelings, we do not know what is actually influencing vital choices. When we lose touch with our inner voice, we may accept invasive treatments without thought or question despite the known risks. Doctors no matter how dedicated rarely have time to explain complicated heart tests, drugs or treatments to uninformed patients. They speak in code. A heart health conversations between you and your doctor can break down into confusing numbers that are useless without proper foods, herbs, and lifestyle habits to prevent illness. In other words the test result numbers are aimed to get you to take heart drugs, have stents and surgery—or else!

Again, it's important: If you already take heart drugs and want to add or substitute herbal treatments, begin slowly with the herbal medicines, continue your medicines with your doctor's knowledge and continue medical testing to monitor your progress. As your heart tests improve you might be able to increase the herbs and reduce the drugs along with your doctors' participation. The required heart and blood tests can guide you with herb dosage. But the ultimate choice of your foods and herbs will be a personal connection you will feel with the herb, its use, origin or other emotional connections. We cannot fully appreciate a remedy by using only the analytical half of our brain. The herb may work fine, but you remain passive. Make friends of your healing herbs.

As you read through the following herbal chapters, seek an herbal expert who can regularly monitor your progress according to traditional Asian tongue and pulse diagnosis. People ask me daily for herbal advice online. They send me photos of their tongue and a long list of symptoms and questions. Often I can help, especially when their symptoms are obvious, but it requires follow-up with local health professionals. Herbs enter and leave the body much like foods so that most treatment discomforts are temporary. Watch your dosage and report side-effects. Don't try to change everything at once. Trust yourself to know how quickly to proceed.

The following descriptions may introduce you to new herbs that become your best herbal choice. You might use them to make simple teas to be used before meditation. The right remedies will speak to you. Find an herbal guide who can advise you about your best time-tested, highly respected single herbs and herbal combinations and how to use them as medicines. For now, let's engage your imagination:

Arjuna

Arjuna, a warrior prince, is the hero of the *Mahabharata*, an ancient Sanskrit epic narrative about a war of succession in Haryana north India. His name means "shining brightness." He is young, handsome and slender with a bronze complexion and wavy black hair, and wears golden armor studded with pearls and coral. He overtakes his enemies with an invincible bow Gandiva and arrows. His muscles shine in sunlight. His teeth are white and jaw square with a noble face, a strong brow and piercing fiery black eyes. He is decked in fabulously rich gold jewelry and a headdress and he has the traditional red mark of beauty on his forehead. In legends Arjuna is the chosen one, the one closest to God, who always aims for perfection. With his stance rooted squarely on the ground and his spirit reaching for the sky, he shows us the correct way to be a hero, a good man, son, and husband.

Lord Krishna is Arjuna's charioteer in battle. Love tempers his bold white horses keeping them true to course. Arjuna is loyal to the god of love. He is the iron muscle in the arm of love, the golden one who gives us strength and shields us from harm.

Arjuna tree bark

Named for a god, tan, hard and dense arjuna tree bark is astringent. The powdered herb added to tea makes your mouth pucker. It strengthens the heart muscle, a bow and arrows in your chest. Terminalia Arjuna the scientific name is described as astringent, sweet, acrid, cooling, and aphrodisiac, a cardio-tonic, urinary astringent, and expectorant that protects against infections and helps heal ulcers, cirrhosis of the liver, excessive and unpredictable sweating, and hypertension. Ayurvedic physicians use arjuna to relieve angina (chest pains), hypertension and plaque buildup in the arteries. It dilates blood vessels and strengthens heart muscle contractions and brings more oxygen to the heart. (36.)

According to medical sources, Arjuna is a mild diuretic, with antithrombotic (blood-thinning, anti-blood clot), prostaglandin E2 enhancing and cholesterol-lowering activity. There is clinical evidence of its beneficial effect in coronary artery disease alone or along with statin drugs. Among many published scientific studies is one from January 2005 in Journal of *Ethnopharmcology* which reports beneficial effects of arjuna (Terminalia arjuna, TA) for prevention of ischemic heart disease. (37.)

Ischemic means the heart is not getting enough blood and oxygen to stay healthy. Arjuna has anti-ischemic activity by helping to keep blood vessels clean. It increases our potential to correct excess blood lipids. It also reduces left ventricular mass and increases left ventricular ejection fraction. That means it effectively helps the heart to receive necessary blood flow and to push blood out to the rest of the body.

According to Dr. Stephen Sinatra women are more prone to have certain chronic heart problems because we have smaller blood vessels than men therefore limiting the amount of blood that passes through clogged blood vessels. In fact heart symptoms in women are often misdiagnosed as heartburn, indigestion or jaw pain. An enlarged left ventricular mass is also associated with "broken heart syndrome." See the later chapter on a woman's heart. The beautiful youthful warrior, Arjuna, may be your best defense against chest pain. Arjuna works equally well for men and women to reduce angina (chest pain) and cholesterol problems. (38.)

Heart Health Checkup for Arjuna

Do you have frequent or long lasting chest pains?
Do you feel short of breath climbing stairs?
Are your muscles weak and tired after exercise?
Do you have hypertension, higher than 120/70?
Do you smoke?

Arjuna has been used to treat heart disease since ancient times, however, it may interfere with your heart medicines and in some cases replace them. Therefore it is best to consult an experienced Ayurvedic herbalist about its use and dosage if you combine it with heart drugs. People in India add the powder to tea or milk daily as a heart protector. If you want to use it for chest pain or to improve cholesterol it may be best to do what they do in India. Add ¼ tsp. of the powder to a cup of tea first thing in the morning for up to a week. If you have no stomach upset or other discomforts you can continue and be sure to check your progress with regular medical testing. If after about six months your doctors are surprised by your health improvements you can tell them you have a noble warrior protecting your heart.

Arjuna and Punarnava for Heart Failure and Belly Fat

Let us not forget cleansing herbs that act as tonics. The Tibetan monk and private physician for HH the Dalai Lama, Yeshi Dhonden, recommends using arjuna and punarnava for prevention/treatment of heart failure. Punarnava [AKA Boerhavia diffusa , hogweed] according to Ayurveda, is bitter, astringent to bowels, cooling and purifying. It helps maintain efficient kidney and urinary functions with its diuretic, laxative, stomachic, diaphoretic, anthelminthic (expels parasitic worms), anti-spasmodic and anti-inflammatory action. Punarnava is useful in biliousness, blood impurities, leucorrhoea, anemia, inflammations, heart diseases, asthma, alternatives etc. Avoid punarnava during pregnancy.

It helps in treating obesity. It is hepato-protective, used in treatment of jaundice and other liver problems. It provides relief from joint pains and inflammation, works as a blood purifier, gives immunity to the body, and improves functioning of lungs. Some researchers have suggested that it has antibacterial properties. (39.)

In conclusion punarnava is excellent anti-inflammatory and diuretic used as a heart tonic and kidney tonic. Punarnava is used to treat jaundice, general fever and obesity and one of the best natural herbal cure for respiratory diseases. Recent studies have shown its effectiveness in fever like malaria, jaundice and constipation complaints. Due to its high diuretic properties it is very beneficial for recovery from chronic swelling.

In effect, Dr. Dhonden's recommendation for heart failure is:

1. Strengthen heart action and reduce cholesterol with arjuna

2. Reduce fluid buildup, obesity, and kidney and liver damage with punarnava. The combination provides an excellent one/two punch to get heart action going easily and correctly.

Punarnava has fresh dark green leaves and little purple flowers. It's name in Sanskrit means "brings back to life. It refreshes and renews, invigorates and lifts the burden of illness and worry. You might add ½ teaspoon each of arjuna and punarnava powder to a little unsweetened apple sauce daily to brighten the day, strengthen the heart, and reduce belly fat.

Guggul

Guggul cleanses/reduces fat, cholesterol, fibroids, and sluggish metabolism. Guggul extract, a sticky yellow aromatic resin also known as Bdellium, comes from the stems of the mukul myrrh tree, a small thorny plant that grows from northern Africa to central Asia, though it is most common to northern India. This fragrant resin, respected in India's traditional medical system of Ayurveda, is used for treating obesity and "blood fat disorders" which means guggul cleanses away harmful blood lipids, body fat, phlegm and dense cholesterol. Guggul is reverently named in Sanskrit "one that protects against diseases." Since so many symptoms of aging are aggravated by impurities trapped in body and mind, guggul may be considered a precious rejuvenating treatment. It can be heating or irritating so watch for your tongue color and texture changes. Avoid its use during fever and pregnancy.

I imagine guggul as a lovely tree spirit, a wood nymph who clears the air of cloudy mists, blows away dead leaves, sweeps a path in murky woods and makes the waterfalls glisten in sunshine. Her bright gaze melts damp, gnarled branches and scatters slugs that fester beneath leaves. She dispels sadness, cuts short self deception among gloomy, dispirited people and reveals the method to discover truth and harmony. Her fragrance is woodsy, spicy, and enticing in its clarity like early morning light falling through leaves to warm the forest floor. Together guggul and arjuna make a perfect combination for self realization, bringing clarity and strength. Open a spice jar of black guggul powder or a bottle of guggul capsules. Allow the enlivening bitter/sour charcoal-like fragrance to play with your sense imagination. How do you imagine guggul?

Guggul tree gum

Guggul has a long history of use in India as an aid for weight loss, arthritis and rheumatism, and for inflammatory skin disorders such as acne. It reduces hemorrhoids and water retention. Guggul is promoted in the West primarily as a remedy for helping to lower cholesterol and improve the circulatory system. Research suggests that guggul may improve overall healthy cholesterol levels. It contains guggulsterones that inhibit the synthesis of cholesterol in the liver. These compounds also appear to inhibit cholesterol from oxidizing.

Guggul benefits the circulatory system in other ways as well. It appears to have anti-platelet and anticoagulant activity to inhibit the formation of blood clots in the circulatory system—as a stimulating, cleansing blood thinner. Because of this, caution should be used when taking guggul with aspirin, NSAIDs and blood thinners.

Guggul helps lower lipoprotein (a) and C-reactive protein, two blood factors known to have a link with inflammation and heart disease. Because of these benefits, it is clear that guggul can be a valuable aid in preventing heart disease. Guggul may be helpful for weight loss because it acts as a thyroid stimulant increasing metabolism and fat-burning action in the body, including helping to lower triglycerides. Excess body fat, overall excess weight and high triglycerides especially pose a threat to women's heart health.

Guggul extracts have a definite anti-inflammatory action. (40.) Its guggulsterones support healthy lipid metabolism encouraging bile production required for digestion and absorption of fats and vitamins in the lower intestines and support the liver's ability to process, metabolize and excrete cholesterol. Guggulu is indicated for hypertension by keeping blood vessels clear and elastic. It strengthens the heart as well as digestion, and our immune system. It has been shown to increase helpful HDL and lower harmful LDL cholesterol. And because guggul helps rid the body of thick fibrous toxins it improves breathing, smoker's cough, it cuts short upper respiratory tract infections and relieves pain and swelling in joints and muscles. Avoid using guggul during pregnancy.

A little known study published in 2008 in *Pharmacologyonline* Newsletter "Stability study of a herbal drug" shows guggul's effective use for reversing oxidative stress, improving myocardial ischemia and even for neurodegenerative diseases and its use as an anti-dementia drug. Guggul's use as a deep cleansing rejuvenating panacea is not over-rated. However it is such a powerful cleanser that long term overuse may result in dry skin, emaciation, weakness, and dizziness.

Guggul and Red Yeast Rice

One way to avoid side-effects of guggul and take a measured dose is by using a standardized capsule available in health food stores which contain guggul and red yeast rice. The yeast grown on red rice is fermented with a specific type of yeast Monascus purpureus and contains sterols, isoflavons and healthy fats. The fermented red rice paste is a soup ingredient used for many years to reduce cholesterol. The yeast acts as a natural statin by reducing an enzyme HMG-CoA reductase much the same way a statin drug does. The health food store capsule is convenient to take and may substitute for statin drugs for some people. The dose is important and citrinin, a processing byproduct of red yeast rice that is toxic, should be removed from the capsule. If the dose of red yeast rice is higher than the recommended amount, you can expect some of the same side-effects as a statin drug. For example, headache, joint aches and liver damage. To avoid such side-effects some brands of red yeast rice add natural sources of plant sterols and a liver-cleansing agent such as artichoke leaf extract.

Heart Health Checkup for Guggul

Do you carry too much extra body fat especially around the waist?
Do you have asthma or thick fibrous mucus congestion?
Do you have breast or uterine fibroids or fibrous or fatty cysts in the skin?
Do you have intestinal parasites? Do you travel to areas where they thrive?
Is your energy too often logy or sluggish especially in humid weather?
Do you easily get depressed or develop a headache when it is dark and rainy outside or when you feel too heavy from slow digestion? Do you have a pale tongue with thick coating?
Do your joints ache, swell and feel painful?

Short term use of guggul for one or several weeks is safe for many people. However guggul can affect the actions of heart medicines in some cases minimizing their activity. It is a deep powerful cleanser of fat, phlegm and cholesterol. Guggul may also alter hormonal balance especially estrogen. Avoid guggul if you are pregnant or have an active estrogen sensitive cancer. Avoid using guggul along with estrogen replacement medicines and contraceptive drugs. Tamoxifen (Nolvadex) is used to help treat and prevent estrogen sensitive cancers. Guggul could theoretically affect estrogen levels in the body and might decrease the effectiveness of tamoxifen (Nolvadex). For other drug interactions with guggul and heart drugs and blood thinners see note (41.)

Barring medical drug interactions, who can safely use warming, stimulating, cleansing and rejuvenating guggul for a short term period? People who suffer from chronic pain, including arthritic and rheumatic pains, back pain, headaches, body stiffness, and fracture recovery. Guggul can generally be used by people with a tendency toward obesity, congestive cardiovascular disease, digestive weakness, low libido, sterility, impotence, skin diseases, low body temperature, reduced immunity to seasonal illness, cancer, low thyroid function and low energy. It is a fine remedy for many elderly persons that can be taken regularly to offset the negative effects of slow metabolism.

Avoid guggul if you tend to be very thin, dehydrated, too hyper, overheated, and insomniac or when your nerves and thyroid may be overactive. How can you tell if your thyroid is overactive? You can't stop talking, running around doing things unable to think calmly and sleep deeply. It is difficult to concentrate, decide or stick to one thought at a time. You may feel overemotional, dramatic, out of control. You may feel and look flushed or feel dizzy or have thinning hair and chronic hunger and thirst.

The tree spirit guggul burns with a bright purifying fire that lights the way to health and happiness.

Amla

If you are aging too rapidly, feel overheated, and fear that stress is taking its toll on your energy and looks, if you are losing your thick hair, lustrous skin, and clear vision—amla may be the cooling rejuvenation treatment that you require. Amla is an Indian gooseberry. I imagine alma as a fast, green dragonfly buzzing through shady corners with sylvan wings like Puck doing magic, giggling at illness, knocking out fatigue and flying rings around aging. According to Minnesota Dragonfly Society, they are fearsome hunters. In his book Dragonflies of the North Woods Kurt Mead writes, "If dragonfly larvae were eight to sixteen inches long, as they probably were 300 million years ago, we would dare not swim in fresh water for fear of being attacked." Any moving, living thing can be prey for dragonfly larvae, and they swallow their prey within 1/100 of a second. Adult dragonflies capture live prey on the wing. The larvae live beneath the ice in suspended animation. It's a lovely image—clear glass covering the delicate dragonfly, wings extended in graceful dance inside a frozen pond. Green, fresh and strong against winter's ice.

Amla (Emblica officinalis, Amalaki or Indian Gooseberry)

Amla is a green, sour fruit that is a noble opponent for heart troubles. Don't confuse the Appalachian gooseberry with east Indian amla or amalaki, known as "the Great Rejuvenator." Amla the Ayurvedic herb is cooling, detoxifying and astringent, helpful for digestive problems and enhancing cellular regeneration. Amla is well-known for its antibacterial and antioxidant properties for supporting good blood circulation as well as nourishing the brain and improving eyesight. Amla may improve diabetic retinopathy because it supports health blood vessels.

Ayurvedic doctors use amla as an overall rejuvenating tonic for the liver, spleen and lungs, especially for people who tend to be overheated, dehydrated and stressed. Amla regulates elimination, enhances fertility, helps the urinary system, acts as a body coolant by flushing out toxins. It increases vitality, improves muscle tone, strengthens the bones and teeth and causes hair and nails to grow. Amla is a known heart and blood vessel rejuvenator. (42.)

We have learned a lot about the heart and how it works so far in this book. But there is more: We should reduce heart and blood vessel stress as much as possible. Having a strong heart muscle is not enough. Our polluted, warlike world is aging, health-defying, and down right dangerous. The heart and all its arteries are lined with inner skin cells called the endothelium. These endothelial cells help regulate blood pressure, blood flow, and ensure that nutrients and oxygen get to all our vital tissues.

Oxidative stress can reduce the production of nitric oxide which protects the lining of the arteries. Nitric oxide tells the arteries when to relax in order to improve blood flow. Without adequate nitric oxide production, oxidative stress damages precious endothelial cells that line the arterial walls. In laboratory studies with cultured endothelial cells, amla has been shown to increase nitric oxide production, and thus support the health of the arteries. Amla has also been shown to support healthy and normal antioxidant activity in the blood. It destroys oxidized molecules, slows the oxidation process, and enhances the body's natural defenses against oxidative stress. In a January 2009 article originally from the *Indian Journal of Clinical Biochemistry*, republished in PubMed, amla, spirulina and wheat grass were compared for their overall antioxidant activity, and especially for vitamin C and E and polyphenols. Amla (AKA amalaki) pushed the other super foods off the playing field.(43)

How do we know amla improves the heart and blood circulation? One indication is by noticing our hands and feet. Good circulation and a healthy lining of the arterial walls play an important role in our ability to keep our hands and feet the correct temperature. Amla works great. (44)

Apparently, amla used in clinical animal experiments improves brain cells by reducing DNA damage resulting from aging. (45) However we are not rats. Humans consume and are exposed to many more toxins and health threats, including medicines, than are lab rats.

Heart Health Checkup for Amla

Do you have thinning hair and/or acne?
Do you have acid indigestion?
Do you have hypertension?
Do you have broken capillaries or spider veins on your face or legs?
Do you have blood shot, sore red eyes? Or retinopathy?
Is your tongue red, dry cracked?
Is your memory or concentration poor from overwork?
Do you easily get angry or overemotional?

Is your urine thick, dark but without infection?
Do you suffer from severe menstrual cramps and odorous blood with clots?

Amla is a deep, effective liver and blood cleanser. If you use amla how will you be able to adjust/eliminate your heart drugs? The answer lies in prevention. If your heart tissue is rejuvenated and if blood vessels become more flexible and brain cells less damaged from stress–then we know amla is working. Those measures may be determined with medical testing as well as from our own observations of chest comfort and blood pressure. Adding amla to our diet we feel and look younger. Amla helps us to feel protected or at least cooler and look younger.

Your Daily Amla – Triphala, Amalaki tea and Chyavanprash

Amla [AKA amalaki] is one of the three fruit ingredients in the most widely used Ayurvedic formula Triphala [AKA Trifala]. Conveniently made into powder or pills, a general panacea for almost all imbalances, Triphala is excellent for detoxifying and rejuvenating the body. Amla can be taken in place of Triphala by people with excess heat in the digestive tract. It gently detoxifies the body by purifying the blood and supporting healthy, regular elimination.

Amla powder can be used to make tea or mix 1 teaspoon of dried raw amla powder with juice, yogurt or add to your favorite smoothie. I add amla powder to my recipe when making spicy, fermented lemon pickle along with turmeric, garlic, chili pepper, salt and oil. Amla is also the main ingredient in the traditional Ayurvedic semi-sweet jam called Chyavanprash. This tasty herbal paste delivers the healing benefits of amla deep into the tissues earning it the title of the perfect herb for overall cardiovascular support.

Ayurvedic Heart Support

Arjuna, guggul and amla--Can you use these great remedies the same day? Yes. They are water soluble so take them with water, juice, apple sauce or a little yogurt, but not coffee or tea which might wash the herbs out too quickly. You can also find a single remedy called Trifala Guggul [AKA Triphala Guggulu] powder or pills which combines amla and two other cleansing/balancing fruit powders along with guggul to cleanse and recondition the digestive tract, lungs, heart and blood vessels. In doing so you help protect heart action as well as the integrity and flexibility of your blood vessels.

There is a great adventure in creating good health that we too often miss by simply treating symptoms. Isn't it better, wiser, more fun to reverse aging, and improve beauty and sexuality while protecting our heart health? All that can only be done with rejuvenating herbs, not with drugs that replace the heart's functions and sedate vitality. The heart is made of flesh, blood, and air. Its electricity needs the spark of life we receive from foods and herbs.

Q & A: Mushrooms and heart health
I want to use a mushroom to improve my heart and breathing– *Cordyceps reduces fatigue and stress.* http://www.absorbyourhealth.com/product/cordyceps-mushroom-extract-40-polysaccharides-500mg-100-capsules/?ref=4041

EIGHTEEN

INFLAMMATION, OXYGEN AND "THE NEW MARTINI"

Inflammation, at the heart of so much human pain, suffering and illness, deserves special remedies that protect heart tissue and the flexibility of blood vessels. In previous chapters you have read about healing red cherries, berries and grapes that provide iron and antioxidants. Healing desert aloe vera and nopal cactus, a high fiber source of vitamin A, ease digestion while regulating blood sugar balance. Cooling, rejuvenating gotu kola and amla from India improve memory and nerves. Cooling blood-, liver- and lymph-cleansing herbs such as manjistha, covered in a later chapter, clear skin blemishes, joint aches and reduce allergies. Flaxseed oil and squid oil are sources of omega 3 that reduce cell damage. Inflammation that makes our blood vessels brittle and crack begins the deadly scenario of plaque blocking circulation. Cholesterol, required for a healthy brain and nervous system, acts as glue to fix a crack in inflamed blood vessels. The bottom line is: Cooler is better for our blood and its pathways throughout the body. Are you adding cooling foods to your diet? Aloe, amla or tart cherries? Modern medical testing is useful to chart the damaging effects of inflammation *after* it has already harmed our body and brain. But healing foods and herbs are ways to prevent organ damage before it happens. The remedies you choose will depend upon your needs, age, experience and convenience. We are not all cooks or herbalists but increasing our sensitivity to our signs of health can gradually improve life force.

Acid/Alkaline Balance

An old popular expression was that someone had "hot blood" if he were angry, antsy, or sexy. These may be very good depending on

223

circumstances. However, "heat in the blood," a TCM traditional Chinese medicine description that includes an excess acid condition, goes beyond emotional imbalance and under certain circumstances can be fatal. Inflammation may start with a stress- or dietary-related liver imbalance leading to facial flushing, headaches and dizziness. If left unchecked, chronic inflammation may lead to broken capillaries and chronic bruising. "Heat in the blood" may even become what TCM doctors call "reckless blood" when blood breaks through fragile blood vessels and leads to hemorrhage and stroke. As blood vessels become more brittle from inflammation and blood becomes more acidic, you can expect to see more enlarged and broken blood vessels in legs, chest and face. Your cardiologist may not pay attention to broken capillaries marring your legs or face, but a TCM doctor can recommend curative herbs.

So called "heat in the blood" conditions are observed by the tongue color and an excess condition in the radial pulse. The body of the tongue is dark red, red purple, or bright red, dry, coated yellow, brown or gray, or bald without coating. Not a pleasant sight. There is often bad breath from stuck bile and constipation or dietary abuse. The pulse feels unusually fast, pounding, high or irregular and excessive indicating that heat (inflammation) has entered internal organs and affects the quality or viscosity of blood and its flow. A pulse that is fast and thin may indicate chronic inflammation and weakness or chronic fatigue from long term infections or diabetes.

Poisons, infections, dehydrating fevers and illnesses such as diabetes, cancer or smoking aggravate heat markers. Long term hormone imbalance and emotional turmoil have additional symptoms specific to the person. Your physician can order laboratory tests, however the extent of inflammatory illness often does not show up immediately. It is wise to watch for little everyday signs of inflammation such as chronic thirst or hunger, acne or itchy rash, joint redness and swelling, thinning hair, infrequent thick, dark urine from reduced body fluids and a strong body odor. Does a person leave a noticeable odor, not perfume, after leaving a closed room? Body odor can smell burnt, rotten, or sour depending upon which organs are affected. A dry cough and thick mucus are signs of inflammation and dehydration affecting the sinus, throat, and lungs. Chronic excessive hunger or digestive acidity points to inflammation affecting the stomach. Inflammation in one area of the body can affect overall wellness. For example, when chronic inflammation is present, and your cholesterol is high and a small, dense size, you are more at risk for heart attack or stroke. Taking niacin to make cholesterol "fluffy" may help to make your cholesterol less harmful. However, if you reduce inflammation, you reap many additional benefits.

Kudzu

Tropical Asia has long been a source of healing anti-inflammatory foods and herbs. Most Chinese and South East Asian grandmothers add them to cooking, often not knowing why or how they work, except that their flavor and texture are traditional. Take for example kudzu [AKA kuzu, ge gen, Puerria lobata] a green vine that could quickly dominate thousands of acres in our southern United States if it weren't treated as a weed! Instead of using kudzu as a rejuvenating, beautifying, heart healthy food as Nature intended, we see little plastic bags of dried kudzu root for sale in health food stores and online. Kudzu starch is used as a thickener for sauces that is easier to use than arrowroot. It's benefits go far beyond that.

Kudzu makes the digestive tract alkaline reducing heart burn, stomach aches and irritable bowel, and brings rejuvenating moisture especially helpful for postmenopausal women or anyone who smokes. (Avoid it during pregnancy or cancer. It is a phyto-estrogen.) It lowers high blood sugar, reduces anxiety, and protects the heart and blood vessels. Asian women are famous for their esoteric beauty secrets. Beautiful Thai women drink a tea made with kudzu root native to northern Thailand to counter aging by reducing wrinkles, grey hair and vaginal dryness a result of aging and lack of sexual hormones. Youth is fresh, moist, flexible. We think of age as withered and rigid, ready to snap like a dried tree limb. The same applies to our blood vessels.

Dissolve dried white chunks of kudzu root in a little cold water to make a paste then add that to hot water or liquids while cooking to thicken sauces. It should always be cooked at least a few minutes.

Evening Primrose Oil

The night-blooming garden primrose flower is the source of evening primrose oil which acts as a blood thinner useful for reducing joint pain, headaches, and heart and blood vessel inflammation. Like tree ear mushroom, amla or serramend, an enzyme from silkworm that you will read about later, evening primrose oil can substitute for aspirin as a blood thinner. Its added benefits enhance beauty and comfort. Not an oil used in cooking, evening primrose oil is sold in health food store capsules and is an ingredient in a few expensive wrinkle creams. You should keep the oil capsules along with flaxseed oil or krill oil in the refrigerator to keep them fresh. In the United States evening primrose oil comes from the flower of the Oenothera biennis that grows wild and quickly spreads as a garden ground cover. The plant has been used as an anti-inflammatory to treat heart disease, infertility, arthritis, depression, juvenile hyperactivity ADHD, impaired immunity, as well as alcoholism and obesity.

If you take 2 grams of evening primrose oil in capsules for a couple of days you may notice that the skin around your nose, mouth or chin is lighter, shows less redness or inflammation in capillaries because evening primrose is cooling. The nose, mouth and chin color, the presence or absence of blemishes and acne there, indicate the presence of inflammation respectively in the lungs, heart and sexual area (uterus and hormone balance in women.) A temporary outbreak of acne is common for women who are overheated with acidic inflammation during PMS time. However long term acne, itchy rash, and rosacea result from chronic inflammation and acids in the blood. Rosacea triggers include alcohol, caffeine, spicy foods, topical steroid medicines and some hypertension drugs and opiate painkillers.

The seeds of evening primrose is one of the few sources of gamma linolenic acid, GLA, an essential fatty acid. Other natural sources are coconut oil and mothers' breast milk. GLA reduces inflammation because it stimulates the production of prostaglandins (PFE1) which are messenger molecules that act similar to hormones but are produced throughout the body. According to University of Maryland Medical Center, "Gamma-linolenic acid (GLA) is an omega-6 fatty acid found mostly in plant based oils such as borage seed oil, evening primrose oil, and black currant seed oil. Omega-6 fatty acids are considered essential fatty acids necessary for human health, but the body can't make them. You have to get them through food. (46.)

Early Native Americans used evening primrose for treating skin and digestive complaints, to increase female fertility, and to reduce liver toxicity. Problematic cholesterol levels and hypertension can be reduced with evening primrose oil. The mechanism appears to be the action of the prostaglandins (PGE1) on preventing blood clotting and arterial spasm. Therefore, evening primrose can be used as a blood thinner, pain relief remedy with fewer side effects compared to aspirin. (47.) Evening primrose oil stimulates fat burning in weight loss regimes, and is often recommended for treating eczema, dermatitis, psoriasis, acne and rheumatoid arthritis.

Evening Primrose Oil: Cautions and Drug-interactions

Evening primrose oil has few side effects, according to the National Center for Complementary and Alternative Medicine, but can cause temporary stomach upsets or headaches for some people. Pregnant women and those on blood thinning or epileptic medication are advised to avoid evening primrose oil. University of Maryland Medical Center warns to avoid doses of GLA greater than 3,000 mg per day because high levels may increase inflammation in the body. GLA should be avoided by people taking certain blood thinning medicines and certain drugs that treat schizophrenia. (48.)

Oxygen and You

In chapter 5 we learned that heart patients are sensitive to temperature changes and quite vulnerable when it comes to avoiding colds and flu. On cold days spent outdoors expect blood pressure to rise for a while due to narrowed blood vessels. Cold air passing through the body may increase urination or in extreme cases aggravate hypothermia.

Normally we breathe through the nose or mouth which moistens and warms the air. Then air travels through the voice box and down the windpipe which divides into two bronchi that enter the lungs. Within the lungs, the bronchi branch into thousands of small tubes the bronchioles which end in round air sacs the alveoli covered with a mesh of tiny capillaries. When air reaches them, oxygen passes through the alveoli walls into the blood in the capillaries so that oxygenated blood can travel to the heart through the pulmonary vein and its branches. The heart pumps oxygen-rich blood to organs. Certain diseases limit the transfer of oxygen from the alveoli into the blood, for example pneumonia and COPD chronic obstructive pulmonary disease. The heart and all vital organs require oxygen for the cells to work and maintain life.

Have you seen people with tubes stuck up their nose who carry their oxygen with them? Medical oxygen therapy aims to decrease shortness of breath and fatigue and may improve sleep for people with breathing disorders. For people who do not require medical intervention, there may be an easier, more holistic way to get oxygen into the body. That is to add an extra molecule of oxygen to water with food grade H202.

Hydrogen Peroxide Therapy with H202

Food grade hydrogen peroxide therapy sometimes called oxygen therapy or ozone therapy is controversial with enthusiastic advocates and enemies on both sides. Hydrogen peroxide is water with an extra molecule of oxygen. Instead of H20 (water) it is H202. You have probably used ordinary hydrogen peroxide, the everyday disinfectant stored in black plastic bottles and sold in pharmacies, for cleansing wounds. However that form contains only a trace of hydrogen peroxide along with a host of irritating chemicals and should NEVER repeat NEVER be taken internally or used as oxygen therapy. The hydrogen peroxide therapy [H202 therapy] I refer to is entirely different.

Our body creates and uses certain free radicals to destroy harmful bacteria, viruses, and fungi. In fact, the cells responsible for fighting infection and foreign invaders in the body, the white blood cells, make hydrogen peroxide and use it to oxidize invaders like a zap gun. The intense bubbling you see when hydrogen peroxide comes in contact with a bacteria-laden cut or wound is the oxygen being released and bacteria being destroyed. It turns your skin white and burns. The ability of our cells to produce hydrogen peroxide is essential for life.

228

Advocates of H202 therapy believe it is a basic requirement for good health. For example, we know that vitamin C helps fight infections by producing hydrogen peroxide, which in turn stimulates the production of prostaglandins.

On the other hand one of the greatest complaints about using hydrogen peroxide, other than the store bought variety for rinsing wounds, is that it burns as it destroys germs. Medical grade sometimes called food grade or 35% hydrogen peroxide should never, I repeat NEVER, be used undiluted. Anti-peroxide health experts somehow imagine that people may be insane enough to use it straight, undiluted and will therefore scorch their skin and internal organs.

Normally it is recommended to use one drop of food grade peroxide in an 8 ounce glass of spring or other pure water for rinsing face and hands, as mouth wash, and to whiten teeth. H202 therapy advocates recommend adding one cup of food grade peroxide to a warm bath and soaking for an hour. You absorb oxygen through your skin as well as the air you breathe.

Some H202 enthusiasts advocate adding 1 drop of food grade peroxide to an 8 ounce glass of spring water and drinking it first thing in the morning without food in order to increase oxygen in the body and thereby protect against certain diseases including cancer, arthritis, heart disease, infections and depression. New York MD, Dr. Majid Ali, recommends soaking the feet in water adding medical grade hydrogen peroxide as a treatment for gout and a number of physicians inject a solution containing H202 into a vein as an alternative cancer therapy. The therapy has been recommended for just about everything from arthritis to multiple sclerosis to diabetes to emphysema to name a few.

Do not be confused. There are a number of strengths and grades of hydrogen peroxide. (49.) However, only 35% Food Grade hydrogen peroxide is recommended for internal use and only when highly diluted. Food Grade H202 is available for individual use online. It is usually not sold in pharmacies.

If you want to try a form of oxygen therapy to improve breathing but are hesitant to use diluted peroxide you might add one drop of food grade 35% peroxide to water in a room humidifier or a glass bowl. David G. Williams in his article, "The Many Benefits of Hydrogen Peroxide, advises that "35% Food Grade H202 must be handled carefully. (50.) For example dilute it with spring water not tap water. Do not touch the Food Grade peroxide because it burns. From purchaser comments online, I have learned that frequent internal use of peroxide interferes with metal tooth fillings. Such metal amalgam should be removed to be safe from heavy metal toxins released into the blood. Is there another way safe way to increase oxygen in the body? Yes. It is to increase the germ-killing, health-building potential of the air we breathe and the water we drink.

Oregano Nature's Germ-fighter

I mentioned oregano in the chapter on fighting colds and flu. Oregano has anti-inflammatory, anti-microbial, and anti-fungal effects, and according to recent research may kill MRSA, listeria, and other pathogens. Oregano contains vitamins A, C, E, and K, as well as fiber, folate, iron, magnesium, vitamin B6, calcium, and potassium. Getting enough good clean air is a challenge for heart patients and especially if they are frequent travelers. Airplane air is notoriously challenging.

Take for example, you are on an international flight or stuck in an airport, subway or other public place. There are people from everywhere, some coughing, sneezing, others simply looking restless, feverish or worried. How can you protect and calm yourself and increase your immunity to infections in a world troubled by wars and plagues? As you inhale boost the germ-fighting potential of the air. Swallow oil of oregano capsules daily to fight infections and boost digestive power, it increases bile-flow, while eliminating inflammation and poisons. Follow the manufacturer's direction; if it irritates, then take it with cooked food. When you travel wear a face mask sprinkled with lavender and oregano essential oils. Both are antibacterial and soothing. It may also discourage unwanted chit-chat with passengers. Here is a more social use of oregano. Heart failure patients and heart patients in general are warned against the use of alcohol. Here is a recipe you might use in moderation with medical approval.

The New Martini

Oregano the digestive aid and germ fighter helps to slow cellular deterioration and the rate at which we age. (51.) Here is your new, rejuvenating Martini: Add fresh or dried organic oregano leaves to steep for up to two weeks in gin. I pour up to ¼ cup of the dried whole cooking herb or 3 heaping tablespoons of the dried power, straight from the supermarket herb jar into the liter gin bottle and keep it sealed away from heat and light in the refrigerator. The gin will turn darker from the herb as its healing power is released. An oregano Martini does more than kill germs, parasites, and boost immunity. It gives you more oxygen in a natural dietary way. You can add other herbs as needed such as mint to reduce spasm, and a sprig of rosemary to boost a weak heart and adrenal energy. When mixing the Martini add lemon juice to cleanse the liver and give the beverage added tang.

Alcohol in any form passes through the liver and is by nature heating. Steeping herbs in gin or vodka you have made a tincture with medical effects. Start with a medicinal dose of 10 drops in water and see how it feels. For sensitive people, that may be strong enough. Otherwise mix your martini, adding lemon for flavor and cleansing, and ice as usual which dilutes the alcohol.

Rosemary Fights Aging

I tried a designer Martini called "aromatherapy" at a local Killington, Vermont restaurant called The Garlic. The atmosphere is cozy and the home made pasta dishes delicious. The especially heady Martini is made with gin steeped in rosemary herb, with added lemon juice and topped off with Champagne. I ran home and added dried rosemary, an herb I have always loved, into a bottle of gin and waited a week until the color turned pale yellow. Use enough dried rosemary leaves to have about ½ inch of the herb on the bottom of a one liter bottle.

Rosemary, an evergreen in the mint family, is strong, can speed heartbeat, and has many health and anti-aging benefits that include it being a good source of iron, calcium and vitamin B6. Laboratory studies have shown rosemary to be rich in antioxidants, which play an important role in neutralizing free radicals. It has been traditionally used to improve memory and circulation. Rosemary is stimulating and heating so avoid it if you have a fever or headache or a chronic red tongue and fast pulse.. It can raise blood pressure if overused. Recent studies reported in July 2014 *Medical News Today* indicate that rosemary can improve digestion, enhance memory and concentration and protect the brain against aging. (52) That's a lot to ask of a Martini. But you get the idea. Why not make healing herbs part of a lifestyle you already enjoy?

Ginger Breathing

Raw ginger root is well known as a digestive aid and pungent herb used especially in Asian cooking. It increases sweating for some people and is recommended for a variety of health problems including nausea and travel or morning sickness in pregnant women. It clears the senses. Do not eat ginger if you have a red, dry yellow-coated or bald red tongue, stomach ulcers or digestive pain. Gingerols in raw ginger have analgesic, sedative, anti-inflammatory, and antibacterial properties. Ginger tea may also improve migraines.

For our purposes ginger root contains a good amount of potassium, manganese, copper, and magnesium. Potassium, an important component of cell and body fluids, helps control heart rate and blood pressure. But there are some cautions for heart patients. Ginger root may be contraindicated in patients with history of gallstones. Ginger root is also known to potentiate the toxicity of anti-coagulant drug warfarin [AKA Coumadin, Jantoven], resulting in severe bleeding episodes.

If you are not using warfarin and don't have any of the other cautions, cut a piece of raw ginger about the size of your thumb nail, peel it and slice it or leave it whole and chew it. If chewing it feels too hot then slice it and add hot water to make a tea. Then sit, relax, quietly, slowly breathe air warmed and fortified by ginger. Let it detoxify your gut feelings, burning off old hatreds, disappointments, and grief. Air is more than air; it marks the passage of time.

Heart Health Checkup

Do you have acne, arthritis, diabetes, allergies?
Do you frequently have low energy, low backache, weak legs?
Are you short of breath and depressed when tired?
Do you frequently travel on airplanes or other public transport?
Do you breathe from the throat up instead of from the waist down?

Adding extra oxygen to the body helps clear congestion and improves digestion, helps to fight diseases and build strength and immunity. Adrenal energy tends to lag during late afternoon to cause fatigue, aches and low vitality or depression. That is a good time to use an adrenal tonic such as rosemary tea instead of coffee.

If you feel shut in as though in a room without windows, unable to breathe deeply, or are ready to cry very easily, then look back at homeopathic pulsatilla in Chapter 3. If you are short of breath due to phlegm or chronic sinus congestion you may prefer a warm ginger tea. Warm fenugreek seed tea is recommended for asthma with excessive phlegm and wheezing. Increasing oxygen intake helps fight mental dullness and depression.

Q & A: Deep Calm Breath

I want a natural way to enhance breathing, while reducing stress and inflammation – *Inhale or apply essential oil of lavender. It is relaxing and rejuvenating.* http://www.absorby-ourhealth.com/product/lavender-essential-oil-100-pure-thera-peutic-grade-aromatherapy/?ref=4041

NINETEEN

YOUR HEART IS A MUSCLE

Heart muscle, like any muscle, needs nourishment, hydration, safe stimulation and rest. Otherwise it may become tense, flaccid, stressed, stiff or cramped. The heart rhythm may become irregular. My ECG (electrocardiogram) ST and T waves are irregular. After retesting several times I was told, "That may be just the way you are." I am an off-beat person, my rhythm is syncopated like Hungarian gypsy music. I am not surprised. My energy can become hyperthyroid fast at times: The thyroid is sensitive to emotions. Your heart may flutter for a second when falling asleep or if you become very tired, over-excited or upset. But that is normally not a cause for worry. Occasional skipped heartbeats or extra beats can result from stress, fatigue, extra caffeine or other reasons. This chapter considers those milder discomforts which may be treated at home with rest and diet. According to medical sources one-third of all arrhythmias occur in normal hearts, and rarely are cause for concern. They are not the kind of arrhythmia that makes you grab your chest, gasp for breath, sweat profusely and "see stars"—that is a case for 911 and quickly. Ordinary skipped beats are temporarily interruption of energy, the electrical charge, through the heart. We quickly recover. But we may provoke an irregular heart beat without knowing it. For example with medicines or extreme emotions.

Heart medicines and supplements are complex and sometimes hard to digest resulting in digestive discomforts, including spasm and irregular heartbeat. Do you feel discomfort when pressing ribs on your right side below the nipple, under the ribs? That is where your liver is located. It may be inflamed or enlarged. Do you have an irregular heartbeat when you feel your pulse or listen to your blood pressure cuff? Are there times when you look jaundiced, that is, have a yellow or orange cast? You may be a liverish person, especially if you feel impatient, restless, antsy. Maybe you have overeaten rich, hard to digest food that lead to an irregular heart beat, heart burn , feeling weak and dizzy or a headache. You may find relief with a dose of about 8 – 10 little Chinese patent remedy pills called Xiao Yao Wan recommended for ordinary chest pain, rib pain, indigestion, food allergies, and bloating and by the way, depression and anxiety. The Chinese call it "stuck liver Qi."

The digestive herbs in Xiao Yao Wan (Free and Easy Wanderer pills is based on this formula) are ginger, mint, bupleurum a bitter digestive herb, three blood-enhancing tonics and a diuretic fu ling [aka poria]. It works very well to ease discomforts in the digestive and emotional center and to enhance healthy circulation. Chinese herbalists recommend it for indigestion, depression, anxiety, allergies, chest and rib pain and digestion- or emotion-related irregular heartbeat. It is a convenient and easy fix.

However, there are irregular heart rhythms that become life-threatening. Our heart is a muscle after all and, therefore, subject to electrical signals. The Heart Health Checkup at the end of this chapter can help you to determine risk factors that might endanger your heart's song. But for now let's consider the most dangerous sorts of irregular beats and a few natural remedies you might use to steady your heart.

Visiting doctors is very important for heart patients especially for their regular diagnostic checkups. Sonar imaging in echocardiograms, the sorts of sensitive equipment inspired by war time, can look into and around your heart to record its actions. With state of the art testing your heart doctor can determine a physical cause of a heart irregularity, such as blocked blood vessels, and what area of the heart is involved making the heart beat irregular. It is wise to get tested if you often feel an irregular heartbeat, skipped or extra beats, and especially a heart that is struggling or galloping, or a fast heart that flutters at times of stress. Adrenal fatigue is also a big factor that most medical doctors will ignore.

There are important contributing factors to arrhythmia that you can control. They include an anti-inflammatory diet, regular gentle exercise such as walking, and stress reduction techniques such as deep breathing, yoga, meditation, or prayer what ever works for you. Herbs traditionally used in Asia for improving heart performance offer additional benefits.

Irregular heartbeat definitions: If your heartbeat is abnormally high and you are not exercising or emotionally upset, you have tachycardia. If your heart rate slows to less than 50 beats per minute, you have bradycardia. These are often temporary and can be controlled with lifestyle changes.

Atrial Fibrillation

Atrial fibrillation [AKA A-fib] is dangerous and life-threatening. It is the most common type of serious arrhythmia. A-fib occurs when the heart's upper two chambers (atria) do not contract in response to the heart's pacemaker electrical impulses but start reacting to various other electrical signals so that the atria do not forcefully contract to send blood into the ventricles to be pumped throughout the body. Then the atria "fibrillate" rapidly vibrating which can cause the heart rate to climb out of control.

With A-fib you may feel the heart quivering or not feel anything unusual except possible dizziness, weakness, shortness of breath, or flu-like symptoms. If it is temporary most people mark if off as stress and let it go. However if episodes last more than 24 hours or heart rate variance is extreme, the heart experiences considerable strain, which may lead to heart attacks or congestive heart failure. Regular occurrences of A-fib can also increase a person's risk of stroke. According to medical sources, "Because blood is not forcibly contracted into the ventricles, but flows into them by virtue of gravity, it pools in the atria and the heart ultimately pumps less blood through the body. Clots on atrial walls may break off and enter the arteries."

Contributing factors to A-fib include heart disease from a buildup of plaque or blockage in blood vessels, long term high blood pressure, and hyperthyroidism or age leading to malfunctioning of the heart's electrical conduction system. The primary goals in treating recurrent A-fib are to normalize heart rate and rhythm through various therapies and to prevent the formation of blood clots.

Most people think that irregularities like A-fib occur in older people with a history of heart disease, but it is not necessarily true. Take for example someone I will call Sam. He is just thirty. His wife is expecting their first baby. Sam, recently graduated with an advanced college degree, is working at his profession, and he is a runner who neither smokes nor drinks. You'd think he'd have perfect health. But his in-laws have moved in to help with the baby after delivery. His wife is anxious. Sam has surrendered their front room to make room for relatives and has stopped his stress-management running to be available to his family. He stopped running competitively since his heart felt uncomfortable after he gained twenty pounds eating "comfort foods" and sweets. When he tried to run his heart raced and a cardiologist put him on a heart drug that only increased his depression. He dreaded becoming addicted to medicines because his father had the same problem and took the same drugs recommended for him.

Sam felt that his heart made him old and sick. He needed a life change but couldn't very well send his family packing. I encouraged him to walk barefoot for at least half an hour instead of running daily. Walking barefoot on grass, the beach, or concrete or using grounding copper wire attached to your body or your bed sheet or computer in your home is known as grounding. As we said before, the earth has a healing electrical charge that helps us detoxify from radiation and stress. The earth is a natural source of electrons and subtle electrical fields essential for proper functioning of immune systems, circulation, synchronization of biorhythms and other physiological processes and may actually be, as nutritionist Dr. Joseph Mercola DC, wrote, "the most effective, essential, least expensive, and easiest way to attain antioxidants." Grounding may be the first, most important step a person with A-fib can take to correct their heart's underlying electrical irregularity.

To soothe his nerves I advised Sam that he play even-tempered Bach on the piano instead of his favorite Beethoven's *Appassionata*. With my dietary advice Sam slimmed his diet and waistline and added heart-regulating herbs I will cover in this chapter and he found that he no longer needed his heart medicine.

Everyday stress-related versus life-threatening arrhythmias

Skipped or extra heart beats due to stress, stimulants, drugs, alcohol, or low potassium levels can often be remedied in an otherwise healthy person with rest or diet changes. But those irregularities can also be caused by lack of oxygen, mitral valve prolapse, or aging. Most cardiologists will not prescribe drugs unless arrhythmias happen frequently and on a regular basis, and are accompanied by heart disease. However two types of arrhythmias, ventricular tachycardia and ventricular fibrillation require immediate attention (53.)

Causes of Arrhythmia

Coffee is a nervous system stimulant and caffeine acts as a diuretic that can contribute to a magnesium deficiency that may lead to arrhythmias. Electrolyte imbalances from sweating, chronic diarrhea or improper amounts of potassium, magnesium, sodium in the body are possible cause of arrhythmias.

Sugar-fib

A rather new and popular category of dietary "no-no" dubbed "excito-toxins" cause inflammation damaging to blood vessels. Sugar is a major culprit we'll cover in the following chapter. Also high on the list of excito-toxins are high GI (glycemic index) foods such as white flour and puffed or highly refined grains. Eating too much sugar in one sitting can cause a person's insulin levels to surge, which leads to electrolyte imbalance due to potassium deficiency. According to medical sources, too much chronic insulin release can cause arterial inflammation, as well as affect overall hormonal balance including adrenal response. Researchers believe that oxidative stress and inflammation underlie A-fib because these problems affect electrical activity in the heart. People with A-fib have significantly higher levels of C-reactive protein (CRP), a marker of inflammation in their blood. The test for CRP is one of the routine blood tests given to heart patients.

How can we avoid food toxins in our everyday life? The more natural, simple organic ingredients in a food or drink, the better. Are you listening junk food eaters? Avoid white flour, fried foods, refined sugar, pastry, sodas. Overeating or drinking alcohol, obesity, smoking, and excess stress aggravate heart irregularities for people who are sensitive or have an underlying problem. Chemical additives like monosodium glutamate (MSG) over-stimulate brain neurons to the point of cell death. Increase magnesium: Toxins tend to consume magnesium, an electrolyte that supports healthy heart function and structural integrity. Magnesium helps our blood vessels to relax and remain flexible so blood can pass through them. Excito-toxins play a key role in depression, obesity and degenerative brain diseases like Alzheimer's, they contribute to strokes, especially in people who are magnesium-deficient.

Street drugs and medications can cause the heart to beat irregularly. Prescription drugs like Ritalin (methyphenidate) prescribed to treat attention deficit hyperactivity disorder, tricyclic antidepressants and even birth control pills can disrupt the heart beat. Exposure to mercury from vaccines, toxic fish or dental fillings and lead from paints, batteries and some drinking water can cause oxidative stress and poison enzyme systems.

Air pollution has been shown to increase the heart's stress response which can increase risk of arrhythmia in people with pre-existing heart disease and abnormal heart rate. Avoid smoking, smokers, and places where it is allowed.

Do leg cramps indicate a heart arrhythmia? Not necessarily. Leg cramps often felt as sharp pain and spasm in the calf, often occurring at night in bed, may results from dehydration prompted by excess sweating, chronic diarrhea, or muscle fatigue, alcohol use, and an electrolyte imbalance. Usually drinking more water and gentle exercise relieves the pressure. There are at least twenty conditions associated with cramps including emotional disorders, panic attacks, hyperthyroid disorders, and lacking adequate vitamin B12.

A Heart-protective Diet

We can't live in a bubble. But how can we detoxify the body and protect against excito-toxins? Daily consume organic dark, leafy greens like chlorophyll-rich kale and spinach to help prevent arrhythmias.

Dark greens are full of magnesium required for over 300 enzymatic reactions in the body. Sources of magnesium include avocados, almonds, pumpkin seeds, and whole grains. Low potassium levels also cause arrhythmias. But bananas, oranges, figs, raisins, yogurt, whole grains and potatoes can help you get enough potassium for proper electrolyte balance. A diet high in potassium is associated with lowered risk of stroke-related death. Bananas and almonds are a good source of GABA, a natural brain chemical that slows the brain that is over-stimulated when we are anxious. A heart healthy diet includes cold-water fish and shiso leaf already discussed. Anti-inflammatory omega-3s relax the smooth muscle in blood vessel walls to keep blood pressure low and can help keep the blood thin.

Relaxation

Reducing stress any way possible goes a long way towards protecting us from sudden shocks to our nerves and our heart's electrical wiring system. Take a warm bath, get a massage, do yoga or tai chi. Call your friends, walk around the block while practicing deep breathing. The way we exercise is important. Sudden bursts of activity catch the heart off guard and can lead to palpitations. It's also important to engage in a ten minute cool down after exercising, especially when exercising your legs. I read some years ago that General Motors could not keep up with its employee medical claims and was in fact going bankrupt due to them. It seems that a large percentage of their employees were obese men who never exercised during the year and many smoked. On weekends during the season they went hunting and drinking with the boys. When these out-of-shape men shot a deer and dragged it to the car, they had a heart attack. No surprise.

Emotional Detox

Emotional stress not only causes arrhythmias, but is linked to hypertension, type II diabetes and obesity. Most of us recognize the importance of mind-body therapies like yoga, meditation and tai chi to attain a higher level of wellness. These therapies encourage slow, deep abdominal breathing, especially important for people with arrhythmias. Deep breathing increases our ability to cope with stress while reducing the likelihood of a sudden cardiac event. Some people prefer moderate exercise, playing with pets or children, gardening, playing games, or listening to relaxing music on a regular basis.

When was the last time you saw a sick or depressed person laugh– not a snide, sarcastic snicker, a nervous titter, or tight-lipped grin than might register a complaint but a comfortable, happy laugh? When was the last time you laughed out loud, had a really satisfying belly laugh? Was it a comic movie, a joke, seeing something funny happen to a friend or pet? Laughter is healing for your heart. Lee Berk, a researcher at the University of California, Irvine showed that laughter, like physical exercise, produces a high level of endorphins that reduce pain and generate a sense of well-being. In numerous experiments, he confirmed that laughter bolstered the healing potential of mind, body, and spirit, among them by lowering stress hormones, raising beneficial hormones, and boosting natural disease-killer cells and antibody levels. (54.)

Watching a movie by the Marx Brothers or Charlie Chaplin may be a good way to lighten bad news. Think of it as laugh therapy and you won't feel guilty about promoting happiness and wellness. University of Maryland cardiologist Michael Miller, MD, has shown that laughter creates healthier functioning blood vessels. Specifically, laughter appears to cause the endothelial lining of blood vessels to dilate more robustly and increase blood flow. So exercise your laughter muscles and laugh as much as you can.

Herbs for Your Heartbeat

We have covered Ayurvedic heart herbs arjuna, guggul and amla in a previous chapter. They help reduce harmful cholesterol, detox impurities and strengthen the heart muscle. As such they clear the "plumbing" of the heart system of debris. What herbs may be useful to support or regulate heart action? That concerns the "electricity" of the heart. All the herbs covered are important and have been in use a long time. But some with apply more to your situation and wellbeing. We will consider hawthorn berry, Chinese Salvia milt. (danshen) herb, and HeartCare Ayurvedic capsules. People using prescription heart medicines should read the cautions below concerning these herbs because they may augment or replace the actions of heart drugs.

Hawthorn Berry

Most of us have heard of hawthorn (*Crataegus species)* which is native to the Mediterranean including north Africa and all of Europe and central Asia, and grows wild in many areas of North America. I have friends in Vermont who make hawthorn jelly that tastes a bit like rosehips. The tree can live longer than 400 years and may bloom twice yearly depending upon weather conditions. There are many hybrids ranging from the English countryside hawthorn to China's haw fruit and beyond because hawthorn grows in most soils. Your best source is most likely your health food store capsules.

Hawthorn has been used to treat heart disease as far back as the 1st century. By the early 1800s, American doctors were using it to treat circulatory disorders and respiratory illnesses. Traditionally, the berries were used to treat irregular heartbeat, high blood pressure, chest pain, hardening of the arteries, and heart failure. Today, the leaves and flowers are used medicinally as well, and there is research that suggests hawthorn is effective in the treatment of mild to moderate heart failure. (55.)

Both animal and human studies suggest hawthorn increases coronary artery blood flow, improves circulation, and lowers blood pressure. Hawthorn has been studied in people with heart failure and a number of studies conclude that hawthorn significantly improved heart function and a person's ability to exercise following heart failure by significantly improving shortness of breath and fatigue.

1000 mgs Hawthorn of a day
keeps an ACE inhibitor away

One study reported by University of Maryland Medical Center found that hawthorn extract (900 mg/day) taken for two months was as effective as low doses of captopril in improving symptoms of heart failure. Captopril is a prescription heart medication, an ACE inhibitor, used to treat high blood pressure, congestive heart failure, kidney problems caused by diabetes, and to improve survival after a heart attack. A large study found that a standardized hawthorn supplement was effective in 952 patients with heart failure. The study compared conventional methods of treating heart failure with different medications with hawthorn alone and in addition to the drugs. After two years, the clinical symptoms of heart failure (palpitations, breathing problems, and fatigue) decreased significantly in the patients taking the hawthorn supplement. People taking hawthorn also took less medication for their condition.

Chest Pain and High Blood Pressure

Hawthorn helps combat chest pain (angina) which is caused by low blood flow to the heart. In one early study, 60 people with angina were given either 180 mg/day of hawthorn berry leaf flower extract or placebo for 3 weeks. Those who received hawthorn experienced improved blood flow to the heart and were also able to exercise for longer periods of time without suffering from chest pain. University of Maryland Medical Center reports that hawthorn extract was found to be effective for hypertension in people with type 2 diabetes who were also taking prescribed medicines. (56.) You should talk with your doctor before taking hawthorn if you have high blood pressure to make sure your heart is strong enough and not racing or galloping to keep up.

Hawthorn is available in capsules, liquid extracts and tinctures. In Chinatown you can find dried sliced hawthorn berries to add to tea. A number of slimming teas, including Chinese "The Well Known Tea" contain hawthorn since it has been popular for centuries. Hawthorn should not be given to children. Side effects are rare, but may include headache, nausea, and palpitations a feeling of a racing heart. Avoid hawthorn if pregnant. If you become dizzy, have angina, headache, or feel exhausted when using hawthorn stop taking it. Your progress should always be monitored by your doctor.

If you are currently being treated with any of the following medications, you should not use hawthorn without first talking to your health care provider: Digoxin, beta-blockers, calcium channel blockers, and phenylephine a medication that constricts blood vessels and is commonly found in nasal decongestant products. Other remedies that affect the heart may interact with hawthorn such as cat's claw, coenzyme Q10, the herbal spice fenugreek seeds, fish oil, ginger, and nitrates which are medications that increase blood flow to the heart. Taking hawthorn together with nitrates might increase the chance of dizziness or light headedness.

Danshen root (Salvia miltiorrhiza)

Danshen is a perennial herb that grows in China on sunny hillsides and the edge of streams. (57.) Its violet-blue flowers bloom in the summer and the leaves are oval, with finely serrated edges. The fruit is an oval brown nut. Danshen's roots, the medicinal part of the herb, are a vivid scarlet red. Danshen is related to our culinary herb sage. It is popularly called Chinese red sage.

Danshen thins the blood by preventing platelet and blood clotting. It also causes blood vessels to widen which can improve circulation. It is used for chest pain (angina), stroke, and heart and blood vessel problems. It has also been used for menstrual disorders, including pain stemming from poor blood flow, reducing abdominal masses, chronic liver disease (hepatitis), and anxiety or insomnia caused by rapid heartbeat and tight chest. It is also used to relieve bruising and to aid in wound healing.

Weak or herb-sensitive people may experience temporary side-effects such as upset stomach, reduced appetite, or itchy skin from using danshen so the dose should be smaller in the beginning and monitored by a health professional for best results. It may be a safe, simple alternative for people who normally use nitroglycerin or other treatments for angina.

Danshen or any herb that regulates circulation should be used with caution or avoided by pregnant women. Since danshen seems to act as a blood thinner, it should be avoided for a week or two prior to surgery. Danshen has been used to help eliminate blood clots and irregular menstruation. It has estrogenic effects and there is a warning against using it long term since it may eventually increase bleeding.

Also women with estrogen sensitivity or who have active estrogen-related cancers should avoid danshen.

An interesting additional advantage is that danshen may improve chronic fatigue. Its chemicals relax the heart muscle allowing more blood to fill the heart and be pumped to the brain. (58.) Drug/herb interactions for danshen include a warning to avoid taking it with Digoxin or blood thinners. (59.) Note: using a blood thinning remedy is not appropriate for everyone or at all times. Herbs are generally safer than medicines because they act like foods without aspirin's typical side-effects such as bleeding ulcers and a danger of increasing the risk of hemorrhage. That brings us to the use of danshen for stroke another circulation problem that has increased over time due to our sedentary lifestyle and bad habits.

Stroke Warnings

A stroke occurs when the brain does not get enough oxygen either from a blood clot blocking blood vessels or too much blood from the rupture of blood vessels leading to bleeding in the brain. The former is called ischemic stroke and the latter is hemorrhagic stroke. Both are deadly. Do not try to treat it at home but call 911. Here is how to recognize stroke symptoms:

Stroke warnings = F.A.S.T.

> Western medical people have invented a quick way for us to recognize that someone is having or has had a stroke. No need to remind you these are signs late in the game. It is better to prevent them. The abbreviation F.A.S.T. indicates typical stroke symptoms.
>
> F is for Face. Ask the person to smile. If one side of the face or mouth droops, there is a likelihood a stroke has occurred.
>
> A is for Arm. Ask the person to lift his/her arms. If one arm is weak or falls down, that side of the body may have been weakened by a stroke in the corresponding part of the brain.

S is for Speech. If the person's speech is slurred, hard to understand or if they cannot repeat a simple sentence, then you can suspect a stroke.

T is for Time. Call 911 immediately if you suspect a stroke. Like a heart attack, time is of the essence. Permanent damage may occur unless the patient is treated preferably in an accredited stroke center or hospital with trained personnel who treat stroke victims. Acupuncture is quite effective in reducing the effects of stroke such as paralysis and inability to speak or swallow.

Other subtle signs of a stroke may include a sudden unexplained severe headache, dizziness, loss of balance and vision problems.

Women and Stroke

Women can have unique symptoms for stroke compared to men. Diabetes, high blood pressure, and high cholesterol, raise the risk of stroke in both sexes. But women may have unique risks, such as migraines, pregnancy, and birth control pills. According to Western medical sources, when you add smoking to birth control pills, the risk of stroke doubles. Signs of stroke such as slurred speech, facial droop, numbness on one side occur in both genders, but in women chest tightness, a migraine with aura, or even a sudden case of hiccups can be stroke signs.

Western herbal suggestions for stroke prevention address general cholesterol-reduction and circulation enhancement. For example gingko, garlic, cayenne pepper, turmeric, green tea, hawthorn, spinach, pine bark and grapeseed extract. But we can get more specific than that. After the doctors have sent the patient home there are some things you can do to make him/her more comfortable and if used before too long, less than a year after the stroke, may improve or reverse symptoms. It depends upon the type of stroke.

Stroke Prevention/Natural Treatment: A Chinese medical approach

In China stroke [syncope] is broken down into two kinds, flaccid and tense, with two different treatments. Either may be a complication of extreme exhaustion and worry. Aging and habits are of course factors. In Shanghai I studied acupuncture and herbs in several hospitals. At a hospital specializing in neurological illness I witnessed treatments for stroke. One young woman in her early forties had to be lifted to a bed from a wheelchair for treatments. There was no energy in her arms and legs that flopped. She had had hypertension leading to paralysis, a "flaccid stroke."

A flaccid stroke may be the case for weaker or older people who tend to have a pale tongue and weak pulse or blood sugar irregularity. The person during and after this type lies still with mouth open. Muscles are loose. They lose control of their bowels. The person may be pale and chilled or unconscious. They feel cold to touch. A warming treatment of acupuncture and moxibustion (a warming treatment for acupuncture points) is used to revitalize energy and muscle tone. Apply a small dot of warming red Tiger Balm or other heating cream to the area just under the nose between the nostrils. Applying pressure there just under the nose with your finger or toothpick pointing upward toward the brain encourages oxygen to flow in that direction. Apply a dab of heating ointment to each area, the tip of the middle finger combined with the point under the nose, encourages blood to flow to extremities. In addition massage the hands and feet to warm them.

The other type of stroke is tense. That is the case of overheated people with lots of inflammation/dehydration signs like red, dry tongue, fast pulse, flushed complexion. The main difference in aspect is that the flaccid type is cold and weak with flaccid muscles, while the tense type is hot with stiff, contracted, immoveable muscles. Do not apply heat to the tense type. A cooling rub may be used in the areas under the nose, hands and feet. Either type, flaccid or tense, require immediate medical intervention and will require ongoing treatments suited to the type of stroke until the condition is improved.

Typical signs of the two types of stroke are easy to recognize if you know TCM diagnosis. The (internal cold) flaccid type looks pale, feels cold to the touch, loose and drooling. The tongue may hang out or feel too large. The person confuses their words, may lose the ability to speak or the use of one side of the body. The fingernails are white—blood is not reaching the extremities.

The (internal heat) tense type looks red/purple, a tongue that goes to one side indicating that liver inflammation has surged up to the head damaging blood vessels and affecting movement on one side. There may be bad breath and the hand on the affected side is cramped up unable to open the fingers. Physical and occupation therapy are used to reeducate muscles after a stroke. Massage and retraining the brain with a black box are used by physical therapists. And a special rowing machine is being used experimentally as well as injections of an enzyme that helps release tense muscles by Dr. Raghavan at the Rusk Rehabilitation Center of New York Langone University hospital to trick the brain into better health and arm function. The person after a stroke uses the non-affected side then the affected side so that the association is strengthened in the brain. Gradually the affected muscles are retrained.

Danshen and Stroke

In China danshen (Salvia milt) injections and an oral herbal extract are given to stroke patients in order to protect the integrity of blood vessels in ischemic stroke. Danshen injections are also given to patients to quickly reduce blockage in blood vessels from clots and cholesterol. (60.)

Risk factors for stroke and heart disease

Many of the people most at risk of developing heart disease are also at risk for stroke because their lifestyle issues are the same. Many are overweight and have a sedentary lifestyle. They smoke, drink and have inflammatory habits. They have hypertension, diabetes, a history of heart trouble sometimes with accompanying cholesterol issues. There may be a family history of stroke. Sometimes a stroke may seem to come from nowhere. But traditional Chinese doctors, as you know, notice many small but vital warning signs, changes in circulation that show up on the tongue, pulse, or other indications. An issue of *Neurology* magazine from August, 2014 describes a woman novelist aged 66 who woke up one morning unable to read what she had written the day before. An ischemic stroke had affected the part of her brain associated with the written word. She could speak and understand speech but not writing. Over a period of about six months she had to relearn to write and understand the written word. She was using medicine for A-fib but had no other symptoms and her diet was healthy. She neither smoked nor drank alcohol.

Is it a good idea to use danshen as a prevention treatment for heart disease and stroke? Very possibly. Individual cases vary however, a long history of use and recent clinical research has shown danshen's effectiveness in protecting blood vessels and circulation. (61.) Studies have shown how danshen reduces vascular and organ damage in a number of ways, including scavenging peroxides, reducing adhesions in the endothelium and leukocytes.

How to use danshen

In a sense we are all heart patients because our heart is impacted by stress, infection, and blood loss. I have used danshen as a heart-strengthening and circulation-regulating herb following non-cardiac surgery when my blood pressure dropped to a dangerous low. The powdered herb may be added to tea and Dan Shen Wan pills are recommended for chest pains resulting from poor circulation and lack of oxygen for the heart. Danshen is a heart protector. Dr. Wen Zi, a Chinese herbal doctor and Western-trained MD cardiologist, believes that as many as 80% of all heart operations could be eliminated by the use of danshen. In China, Dr. Zi has seen danshen work in a wide variety of coronary diseases. Cases of angina showed close to 90% of those tested were significantly helped and about 80% of arrhythmias were corrected or at least improved. And in many cases, mitral valve problems improved.

Danshen versus Arjuna

Danshen, commonly used in Chinese herbal medicine and arjuna well-known in Ayurveda in India, both are considered heart tonics that help regulate heart action, strengthen the heart muscle, and reduce the buildup of harmful plaque. But how do they differ and can they be used at the same time?

Danshen and an enlarged heart

Danshen appears to improve the force of heart contractions and relax the smooth muscle of the coronary arteries, improving circulation to the heart. According to Carolinas Medical Center, danshen may prevent heart damage. It helps your blood circulation by thinning the blood and helping to regulate blood pressure. When your heart has too much stress from chronic high blood pressure or long-term heart arrhythmia, you can develop cardiomyopathy, a heart disease that weakens and enlarges your heart. Cardiomyopathy can be associated with congestive heart failure, coronary artery disease and atherosclerosis, or hardening of the arteries.

What are signs of an enlarged heart?

Extreme fatigue develops with a weakened heart because blood cannot be pumped effectively to all parts of the body. Your cardiologist may examine the pulses in your feet and legs and neck along with taking your radial pulse at the wrist. If you have a strong, steady pulse in your feet and by your ankles and no swelling there from water retention it is more likely your circulation is healthy. Chest pain and an irregular heartbeat are important heart symptoms that may develop with an enlarged heart. You should check with your doctor as soon as possible.

Shortness of breath, called dyspnea, is an enlarged heart symptom associated with cardiomyopathy. The heart cannot fully empty blood out of its chambers when it pumps; blood backs up into the lungs which causes shortness of breath and cough. A person with an enlarged heart may need to sleep with his head elevated on several pillows, or even sitting up, because the dyspnea is much worse when reclining.

Arjuna bark (Terminalia arjuna)

Arjuna reduces cholesterol and strengthens heart muscle. I emailed Dr. SK Maulik in India to ask about his clinical studies on arjuna published in 2011 in *Current Pharmaceutical Technology* entitled, "Therapeutic potential of Terminalia arjuna in cardiovascular disorders." He answered that many experimental studies have reported arjuna's antioxidant, anti-ischemic, antihypertensive, and antihypertrophic effects, which have relevance to its therapeutic potential in cardiovascular diseases and clinical studies have reported its efficacy in patients with ischemic heart disease, hypertension, and heart failure. A few of the results from human clinical trials are cited here. (62.) Arjuna improves heart function by decreasing oxidative stress and lowering overall cholesterol. It reduces left ventricle swelling that is associated with a greater risk of heart failure, stroke, arrhythmias and sudden cardiac death. It may be a good treatment for heart weakness and "broken heart syndrome" because it improves the heart's ability to push blood out into the body.

Arjuna vs Danshen

Arjuna improves heart muscle function and pumping action by strengthening coronary arteries, lowering blood pressure and reducing chest pain. Danshen treats atherosclerosis (hardening of the arteries) and angina improving the force of heart contractions and relaxes the smooth muscle of the coronary arteries, improving circulation to the heart. (63) With casual observation it seems as though danshen and arjuna do the same work to improve cardiovascular conditions and reduce health risk. However the laboratory studies do not report the fact that in the herbal traditions of their origin—Chinese and Ayurvedic medicines—these herbs are most often combined with supportive herbs that improve their results.

For example, Dan Shen Wan (AKA Dan Shen Pian] pills made in China and sold in Chinese herbs shops everywhere combines danshen with medical camphor to dilate blood vessels and tienchi ginseng, a neutral heart tonic (not stimulating like red ginseng) that helps reduce cholesterol. Another example from Ayurveda is HeartCare pills that combine arjuna with other tonic herbs. The impact of the herbal *combination* is greater than any single herb.

Another caveat is *who* will be able to recommend/prescribe these herbs. According to American Botanical Counsel a Chinese pill containing Asian herbal ingredients Compound Danshen Dripping Pill [AKA Cardiotonic Pill] produced by Tianjin Tasly Pharmaceutical Co. Ltd. in China will soon enter phase III testing and could become the first Traditional Chinese Medicine (TCM) product to obtain drug approval from the US Food and Drug Administration (FDA). The pill is sold as a prescription drug in China, Vietnam, Pakistan, South Korea, India, and the United Arab Emirates and reportedly is taken by about 10 million people every year to treat angina and coronary heart diseases. In 2014, its international sales brought in over $148 million.

An FDA drug approval for Compound Danshen Dripping Pill, which could take ten years from the beginning of Phase III trials, entails "official recognition of the safety and efficacy of an herbal preparation in the conventional healthcare system," according to William Morris, PhD, president of the Academy of Oriental Medicine at Austin, Texas. "But" he added it could also be "a step backwards by Chinese herbalists who have their own methods of traditional diagnosis and many years of common use of the pill. It is not likely that Western trained physicians would consider using an herbal combination for which they have little or no experience. Doctors use what their hospitals prescribe which is what insurance companies cover.

When to use Danshen

Danshen is primarily a Qi moving herb used to get blood circulation flowing. It might have to be combined with other tonic herbs to build vitality or blood. Signs such as a purplish tongue, an irregular or "stagnant" pulse, and chest pains may best indicate the need for danshen. This will show up long before medical testing shows a heart problem. So danshen can be used as a preventive treatment to avoid heart problems. It can be combined with cleansing herbs to reduce plaque.

Danshen and tonic herbs

When heart qi is insufficient the tongue is pale with a white coating. The pulse may be deep, hollow, slow, irregular or shaking. You may lose your sense of taste or easily forget what you just said. Tonic herbs such as hawthorn and/or astragalus or digestive (anti-bloating) atractylodes may be combined in order to support heart qi at the same time as the danshen ingredient moves stuck circulation. Depending on the pallor of the complexion and tongue, severity of chest pain or poor digestion more or less tonic herbs may be used with blood-moving herbs.

As an analogy, comparing a simple herbal formula to a car: You need clean fuel (blood cleansing/thinning herbs) you need a spark (qi-moving herbs like danshen) and a powerful motor (heart muscle tonics.) Asian medicine adds another element – our emotions (herbs to harmonize emotions, encourage balance and enhance serenity. Western medical drugs for cardiovascular disease may work well for crisis intervention and protection from heart failure and attack, the traumas that can kill. However keeping blood vessels open, reducing plaque, keeping blood pressure low, in a word, the aim of heart drugs, does not accomplish the ultimate support we need for a healthy heart, which includes a calm clear mind and the joy of living. This is more possible with rejuvenating, supportive natural remedies.

Two Useful Herbal Combinations

Your acupuncturist/herbal practitioner can help you to decide about your herbs and monitor your progress with traditional diagnosis. If you aim to supplement or replace your medicines with herbs for heart health, there are also safe, effective herbal combinations you can buy online and in some herb shops. Check my suggestions for purchase in the Resource Guide. I mention only two herbal combinations here briefly, one from Ayurveda the other from Chinese medicine, and include extensive university and NIH research and other information on them, including ingredients, in the Notes at the back of this book and online at my website www.asianhealthsecrets.com/

HeartCare

Arjuna is a primary herb in this excellent Ayurvedic herbal capsule made by Himalaya Herbal Healthcare company. For sale in India it is called Abana and in the West it is called HeartCare. Clinical trials have shown the ingredients to be effective for a variety of heart wellness issues. (64.) During pregnancy avoid or use with guidance herbs that affect circulation. The recommended dose for HeartCare is three capsules 3 times daily until healthy cholesterol levels are reached and thereafter two capsules 2 or 3 times daily to maintain heart health and comfort.

Su Xiao Jiu Xin Wan [AKA Suxiao Jiuxin Wan]

In Chapter 7, I described these tiny Chinese herbal pills that melt in your mouth, cool your throat, clear your senses, and taste like medical camphor one of its main ingredients. The two ingredients are medical camphor to dilate blood vessels and ligusticum (chuan xiong) an aromatic herb that enhances heart action by facilitating blood flow and qi and reducing pain. Many TCM practitioners prescribe ligusticum to treat irregular painful menstrual periods and headaches. It is also given to patients with inflammation caused by injuries, carbuncles and boils. The effect of the Su Xiao Jiu Xin Wan pill is like natural nitroglycerin to ease chest pain and improve circulation. For simple chest pain, shortness of breath from pollution, melt 3 -4 pills under the tongue. For severe chest pain, heart attack, melt 12 – 14 pills under the tongue and call 911 immediately for an ambulance. Taken regularly 3 pills once or twice daily the pill helps regulate blood pressure. The NIH has reported this product to be very useful for reducing angina. (65.)

It is worth repeating that a heart attack is a medical emergency. Do not try to drive yourself to the hospital. DO NOT DELAY because life-threatening irregular heartbeats are the leading cause of death in the first few hours of a heart attack. Arrhythmias may be treated with medications or electrical defibrillation by the ambulance medical team. They will also give you oxygen, even if your blood oxygen levels are normal, so that your body tissues have easy access to oxygen and your heart doesn't have to work as hard. Because it is vital to increase oxygen for the heart as soon as possible, it is wise to use the the famous Chinese "heart-reliever" pill called Suxiao jiuxin wan.

Chinese Suxiao jiuxin wan (pills) for angina pectoris and heart attack: Keep the small ceramic bottle of pills at your bedside, in your wallet, or purse.

The Unavoidable Hand of Culture

Describing various common herbal treatments for heart issues covered in this book, I remark at how the role of culture plays a hand in the description, diagnosis and treatment of heart disease. The Chinese are an energetic, aggressive people who quickly establish their businesses when moving to a different country. They bring their language, diet, and customs to the new neighborhood. They seem to tirelessly work, play, travel and experience the world at large. A few years ago a magazine called *Entrepreneur* featured stories on millionaires under age thirty. The cover photo had a young, smiling kid in his twenties, black suit, thin black tie from the 1950s, and very colorful plaid socks – a newly made millionaire head of one of many startup companies that are bi-products of silicone valley. I was not at all surprised he looked Chinese.

Chinese herbal formulas for the heart aim to increase qi (energy), free the flow of qi and ease chest pain. For example Dan Shen Wan. The Chinese formula gets quick results, the worker back at work and trouble-free as soon as possible. In traditional Chinese medicine, the heart is seen as the master of our body and mind that keeps us well and emotionally balanced. Perhaps the Chinese philosophical and medical tradition that most closely resembles Ayurveda is Taoism, the middle way, a life away from the crowd.

Ayurveda the great Asian health tradition from India promotes heart health with suggestions for a vegetarian diet, gentle exercise such as yoga, meditation, and complex herbal remedies such as HeartCare. However as important as these practical measures is a lifestyle and philosophy that aim to ease tension, anxiety, aggression, and bring about our awareness of higher goals including self-understanding.

Ayurveda explains heart disease as a result of our Western drive to accomplish, succeed, and in a word acquire wealth. Ayurvedic herbal remedies such as HeartCare recommended for heart comfort reduce cholesterol the result of a rich, fat diet and sedentary lifestyle–the computer age, overweight, diabetes, and chronic aches.

In America our prescribed heart drugs, stents, and invasive surgery aim to take over the heart function, control the heart, liver and blood vessels. This manipulative approach is even embedded in the language we use to describe heart troubles. "Heart attack" attack is a war term. Under attack we use strong means to take control. "Heart failure" is practically synonymous with business failure. We are demanded to measure up, succeed or else. When that fails and we suffer a heart problem, we go to the doctor who gives us strong medicine to fix us. The underlying causes of heart disease, such stress, age, a fat diet and pollution, may be nearly the same throughout the world however how we approach heart problems, how we think about ourselves and our heart are a product of our upbringing, environment, and what we expect from ourselves.

Heart Health Checkup

Describe with a word or two how you feel about:

- Your work
- Your family
- Your love life
- Your sexual satisfaction
- Your financial security
- Your hopes and prospects for the future
- Your home and where you live
- What do you do to relax? To feel well or younger?

You can immediately instinctively feel what area of your life needs improvement. There may be no easy fix. But you can reduce physical and emotional stress by using a clean healthy diet, exercise and relaxation techniques.

Q & A: Relaxation

I want to immediately relax – *Inhale or apply uplifting essential oil of peppermint, which is calming and energizing. Therapeutic 100% pure peppermint oil helps relieve nasal congestion and improves digestion. Use between 6 to 12 drops of essential oil per ounce (30ml) of carrier oil. Diffuse essential oils by using a device specifically designed for that purpose like a lamp, candle or fan diffuser.* http://www.absorbyourhealth.com/product/peppermint-essential-oil/?ref=4041

TWENTY

REJUVENATION TONICS

Rejuvenating herbal medicines raise our level of wellness, resilience and courage. Nature's tonics affect the emotional content of our heart as well as its structure and function. Heart patients and caregivers need vitality and courage. Often our friends and family, who act like a tonic, boost our confidence and the pleasure of living a full life. They make us feel better by just being there. For a caregiver you would not choose someone who irritates or depresses you. The same goes for your choice of an herbal tonic. A tonic improves the body and gives the Spirit ease. That is why I offer a variety of choices in this chapter. Remedies described here appeal to a wide audience. Some of you may prefer a food or a time-tested herb. Be selective in your choice because the remedy can reward you in many ways.

Modern medicine that only aims to combat disease, kill germs, or stop our ability to make cholesterol—misses an important point. A tonic reduces the effects of everyday stress naturally helping us to live longer and better. Are there tonics specific to heart issues? Yes. Our ultimate goal is not only to control symptoms but to reduce damage from aging, illness and medical treatment and to regain wellness. How do you choose the right tonic? In part that depends upon your greatest need, whether fatigue, chronic pain, nervous tension, or any number of complaints. Fortunately, most traditional herbal tonics are multi-tasking adaptogens that improve our body and outlook by supporting blood, energy, and organ function. More recently science-based herbal extracts such as resveratrol from grape seed are also available. Americans have gotten used to taking supplements like candy. But how do they know the stuff is working? That's where self-observation is helpful.

When someone asks me to recommend a natural remedy because they feel weak, short of breath, or chronically tired, I look at their tongue for signs of inadequate Qi (vitality), poor circulation and/

or blood deficiency even though they may not officially register as anemic. You have made this sort of observation in the Heart Health Checkup sections. A tonic whether a food, herb, or supplement does not kill germs but it may heighten natural immunity. It gets your body to work better, with more ease and less pain and depression. Do you often feel weepy, vulnerable or have chronic complaints such as back or leg pain, or poor memory? It may be that physical issues such as shortness of breath, adrenal weakness and inadequate digestion are hampering your ability to cope. Do you sit all day for work or pleasures? You risk gaining heart-damaging belly fat, triglycerides (dense lipids in body fat) and water retention. In the long run tonics help you to reduce toxins that harm the heart.

Herbal Tonics vs. Vitamins

North America has been vitamin conscious a long time. Go into any Walgreens, CVS or Walmart and you find rows of vitamins and a few heart health products such as fish oil. If digestion is poor the healing power of vitamins and minerals can be neither absorbed nor properly used by weak organs. You burp fish oil. Concentrated natural extracts originally found in foods work much stronger and faster than herbs. They mimic drugs and you can't always combine them with medicines. We will cover several herbs and extracts you can safely use.

Tonics enjoy a long herbal tradition chosen primarily for their energetic effects upon our vital forces and not primarily for their vitamin content but for how they affect our organs, our blood production, and energy. In other words, how well the heart works depends upon our digestion, breathing, the health of heart tissue and blood vessels, and so on. Since Asian herbal formulas were born long before clinical laboratory testing was available and have a history of millennial use, their appropriate choice depends upon the herbalist's assessment of the patient's needs and our self-observations such as those included within and at the end of this chapter.

Most people, including allopathic health professionals, believe that a heart attack can come without warning. One of the aims of this book is to use simple observations to

become more sensitive to your health, your patients and loved ones. That way we get a sense of what may go wrong and how we may be able to take appropriate preventative steps in the right direction.

If you had a stomachache you might ask yourself, "What did I eat to cause this?" You would probably already know if your emotional upset was causing the digestive pain. You might even instinctively relieve the pain with self massage to improve circulation in the belly. A tonic used at the right time for the right reasons may help you to avoid such discomfort. Only you know for certain the reasons why you are hassled, what your real diet and lifestyle are, which are not necessarily what you tell health professionals. If you want some assurance you can deal with inevitable stress, aging complaints, seasonal weather changes and life's shocks, take a tonic. Let me explain very simply.

In Chinese medicine, energy and blood tonic herbals are combined in order to enhance proper blood production and support organ tissue (yin) and organ function (qi and yang.) Herbs, foods and animal ingredients are chosen along with highly valuable adaptogens such the ginsengs as longevity tonics that provide protection against illness and aging. In Ayurveda highly respected tonics are made from nourishing herbs, spices and fruits meant to be taken as daily foods and part of an overall plan to achieve wellness and spiritual awakening.

By now a number of traditional herbs have been laboratory tested and are manufactured under modern conditions by Western companies. You can find a number of these tonics in your local health stores, chain stores, and online. My Resource Guide at the back of this book and Products section at www.asianhealthsecrets.com list select recommended sources that are safe and inexpensive.

Chinese Energy Tonics [AKA Qi Tonics

Since qi (AKA vital energy] is pervasive, enabling organs to function, a qi tonic is an energy boost for the endocrine system. A qi tonic may affect the functioning of a particular organ such as a digestive herb, for example, ginger for stomach qi or a sexual tonic made from herbs that affect hormones such as testosterone for kidney/adrenal qi. However the ginsengs, considered superior tonics, accomplish an overall stimulating and rejuvenating effect. They are famous adaptogens.

Energy tonics appropriate for heart patients or anyone who needs enhanced energy without increasing inflammation might include a combination of ginsengs such as Chinese or red ginseng [AKA Panax ginseng] along with American ginseng [AKA Panax quinquefolium] which is moistening, neutral and not stimulating (or as the Chinese say "heating.") Other herbs in the formula may include Eleurthero ginseng a nerve tonic and royal jelly chosen for nutritional value. Panax ginseng, a well-known sexual tonic and energy tonic, when used alone, is inflammatory which means it can raise blood pressure for persons who are susceptible.

Studies of men over the age of 55 have shown that regular use of Panax ginseng significantly reduced all-cause mortality. (71.) Tienchi ginseng [AKA notoginseng] is a cardiovascular tonic that reduces chest pain and harmful cholesterol clumping. It can be taken alone or in combination with other ginsengs. Raw tienchi powder can be added to water as a tea or to soups during cooking. It is cooling for the entire body. It helps maintain blood vessel elasticity. It is useful for bruises, chest pains, and chronic inflammatory discomforts, including hot palms, heart palpitations, or hypertension.

Tienchi Ginseng (AKA Sanchi, notoginseng)

- Raw Tienchi Ginseng: Cooling, reduces hypertension and harmful cholesterol clumping and chest pain
- Steamed Tienchi Ginseng: Warming, increases blood production and circulation

Some people become weak and blood deficient because their vitality is low or after losing blood following an accident, childbirth, surgery, or an illness. They tend to feel chilled, wear heavy clothing, and use quilts on their beds during the entire year. More than likely, their tongue is pale and pulse slow or deep and weak. They may have low blood pressure or hypo-adrenal symptoms. They require a warming form of tienchi called Steamed Tienchi ginseng powder, which can be added to water as a tea. Tienchi, in other words, maintains healthy blood circulation but works differently depending on whether or not the powder is used raw or steamed.

How do you know you need to take ginseng? Or put another way, what can ginseng or a combination of ginsengs do for you? If you are weak and run-down, chilled, tired, sometimes short of breath, have a slow metabolism and low sexual drive and capacity, a combination of ginsengs can help you to get back on your feet. If you are taking heart medicines, you may have to avoid Panax ginseng or begin with a smaller dose if it interferes with hypertension drugs. Always monitor your blood pressure at the same time daily.

Michael, who took various heart medicines to reduce hypertension, found that when fatigued (and over medicated) his blood pressure became so low that he felt weak, dizzy and spacey or very tired so taking a ginseng combination brought his blood pressure up to a comfortable reading. When you take your blood pressure with an arm cuff, you can listen to your heartbeat. If it sounds slow, weak, hard to hear your heart muscle may also be weak. You may have slight or temporary chest pain (angina) because blood is not reaching the heart. A tonic such as ginseng or others that strengthen the heart muscle such as hawthorn or ashwagandha may be a comforting and balancing addition to your health regime. Before you add an energy tonic, check with your doctor who may want to simply lower the dosage of your heart drugs. Here is something to remember:

Do not cut the dosage of your heart drugs yourself. As one respected cardiologist explained, "Don't skip a day or take your medicine every other day. The heart does not like that."

Ashwagandha an adrenal tonic for muscles, nerves and sexuality

I have mentioned ashwagandha, an important Ayurvedic medicinal root known as Withania somnifera or Indian winter cherry, in chapters describing sleep remedies and those that enhance muscle strength and memory. The many uses of this superior herb are due to its benefits as an adaptogen and adrenal tonic. In addition, it helps reduce brain cell degeneration, stabilizes blood sugar, lowers cholesterol and has anti-inflammatory benefits. Ayurvedic doctors describes its actions as strengthening for muscles and nerves treating problems as diverse as sexual weakness to insomnia and memory problems. Scientific research papers from 2000 compiled in the *Alternative Medicine Review* and published by the NIH show that "Studies indicate ashwagandha possesses anti-inflammatory, antitumor, anti-stress, antioxidant, immuno-modulatory, hematopoietic (blood enhancing), and rejuvenating properties. It also appears to exert a positive influence on the endocrine, cardiopulmonary, and central nervous systems. Toxicity studies reveal that ashwagandha appears to be a safe compound."

Cleansing and Balancing

It is best to add a tonic to an overall wellness plan. First cleanse acids and impurities from body and mind then fortify vitality with herbal tonics. You can use both during the same day but separate them by several hours. Bitter detoxifying herbs such as dandelion are best used during morning hours because they are laxative and diuretic. The Mediterranean herb oregano and dandelion release bile. Use them regularly until body odors, dark urine, constipation, and skin blemishes are gone. Then you can fortify energy with a tonic taken during late morning or afternoon.

Backache and Poor Memory

Ashwagandha root works as an excellent immune booster that nourishes and rejuvenates the nervous system. Weak, exhausted, overworked people can add ¼ tsp. of ashwagandha powder to a cup of water or warm milk twice daily during the late morning and afternoon. If you have chronic fatigue, backache, poor memory, weak muscle strength, low sexual vitality, and lack drive, ashwagandha is very useful to reduce signs of aging. It is available in capsules and is sold as a powder in all East Indian groceries, herb shops and online. A renowned adaptogen, ashwagandha promotes rejuvenation, mental and physical health, and provides a defense against dangerous environmental factors. Research has shown that ashwagandha root extracts support healthy immune system function.

Ashwagandha helps maintain proper nourishment muscle and bone, while supporting the proper function of the adrenals and reproductive system. It is a famous sexual tonic for tired, achy, overworked intellectuals, but it has many other uses as well. Ashwagandha may be a promising alternative treatment for Alzheimer's and Parkinson's. Ashwagandha has powerful antioxidant properties that destroy free radicals implicated in aging and numerous diseases. Used by both men and women, it acts to calm the mind and promote restful sleep. It is especially beneficial in arthritis, hypertension, diabetes, and chronic stress-debility. Recent research affirms that ashwagandha also protects brain function. (72.) Other studies reveal ashwagandha's antimicrobial properties against bacteria, including Salmonella. It enhances macrophage immune cells. Ashwagandha can be considered both a vitality tonic and detoxifier. So you can stay strong with ashwagandha, your muscles, brain, nerves, heart and immune cells will be protected from stress and disease.

Tibetan Goji Berry

Because our planet has increasing environmental pollution, we use superfoods to protect longevity. The goji berry has been described as "quite possibly the most nutritionally dense food on earth." It has been praised and used in Asian medicine for centuries as a healing plant that exhibits amazing properties. Traditionally regarded as a longevity, strength building, and sexual potency food, in studies with elderly people, the goji berry, given once per day for three weeks, was reported to increase spirit, optimism, appetite, sleep, and recovery of some sexual function. Given to patients undergoing chemotherapy, the berries where shown to provide significant protection for the liver.

There are over 40 different varieties of the goji berry found throughout the world. However, the Tibetan goji berry found at gojiberry.com is noted for purity and grown wild in ancient soils free of pollutants and pesticides. The Tibetan Goji Berry should not be mistaken for the Chinese Wolfberry. The Tibetan berry is considered by experts to be the most potent goji because of the wide variety of vitamins, minerals and phytonutrients. (73.) Here, according to recent research are a few ways goji supports heart health. It protects the liver, increases metabolism and boosts immunity, aids circulation, helps regulate blood sugar and cholesterol and is rich in phytonutrients.

Add a handful to hot and cold cereals or blender drinks. Add a handful to your water bottle and eat them as you drink. I add ½ cup of Tibetan goji berries to bake in my apple pie.

Chinese Blood-enhancing Tonics

Chinese herbal blood tonics especially nourish the pancreas, liver, lung and kidney because they are understood to be part of the energy system that regulates blood and hormones. Use a cooling, moistening blood tonic when you have chronic thirst, dry mouth, a red or deep mauve tongue that is dry or has dark markings on the sides of the tongue which correspond to the liver area. You may or may not be anemic in blood tests. It is easier and more effective, with fewer side-effects, if you use an herbal combination tonic. I have included several popular ones here. For example, some blood [AKA yin] tonics are semi-sweet and moistening like rehmannia, a form of Chinese foxglove. Herbal rehmannia, either raw or cooked, has been used to treat rheumatoid arthritis, asthma, urticaria (hives), and chronic nephritis (kidney inflammation) in Chinese studies. But used alone it can cause diarrhea. It is combined with other herbs to prevent hypertension, for example in Hypertension Repressing Tablets. (74.)

Shou Wu Chih liquid tonic

All Chinese herb shops and supermarkets sell liquid tonics as well as raw herbals and pills. He shou wu [AKA fo-ti] is often used as a rejuvenation tonic in China and is especially recommended to help reverse prematurely graying hair. It tastes bland and semi-sweet. The Chinese name translated is Mr. He's black hair. The Chinese often give clues to the use of an herb by its name. Healthy blood nourishes hair, skin and nails as well as internal organs.

According to East Earth Trade Winds, eastearthtrade.com: Shou wu chih, one of the most popular liquid tonic formulas for men and women, gently increases the energy level and it tonifies, warms, and invigorates the blood, nourishes the liver and kidneys, and benefits the eyes. It is said that regular use strengthens the bones and tendons and improves sleep. Since it nourishes and relaxes long muscles it can be used at the end of the day to relax and help relieve chronic backache. I once gave a body of He Shou Wu liquid as a gift to an exhausted, hard-driving executive and he liked the taste and feel asleep, a refreshing nap, at his desk. The action of blood enhancing herbs work in part according to our needs. In other words they can correct stress, dryness, and long term exhaustion not as a quick pick-up for energy but for long term rejuvenation after burn-out.

Based on the herb Polygonum multiflorum (he shou wu, fo-ti)), it is suitable for long-term use. Take 2-3 tablespoons, up to three times a day with tea or water or in soup. It contains: Fo-ti, angelica root, rehmannia, ligusticum, Solomon seal, Angelica dahurica, cloves, Citri medica, and cardamom in distilled water base.

Astra Essence pills

Are you feeling your age? Is it getting harder to hear or see people, sleep, think clearly, or remember things? Are you sometimes dizzy and confused? Do not despair or give up by thinking, "Oh well, it is just part of aging." There are blood enhancing herbs to the rescue. They support our senses as well as reduce heart and blood vessel stress and inflammation. The Chinese have long recognized the mind-body connection. When the physical body is not well, its mental activity is impaired. Confusion, lethargy, fatigue, and irrational anger are all signs that our mind/body is out of balance. Physical symptoms such as dizziness, headaches, frequent urination, and hair loss may also occur. Complex herbal combinations help restore beauty and vitality while boosting immunity.

Astra Essence pills, made in California by Health Concerns, is a botanical tonic based on the historical wisdom of traditional Chinese medicine. This powerful blend of potent herbs can help tone the blood, restore kidney/adrenal/hormone balance, and work to vitalize mind and body. Chinese medical theory and practice link our internal organs with our senses by way of acupuncture meridians. In other words if your dry eyes hurt or you have blurry vision, the treatment from your herbalist/acupuncturist would be to nourish the liver, the source of oxygen-rich blood that nourishes the eyes, muscles and blood (moisture) that protect the eyes. You might have acupuncture done along the liver meridian, for example in the feet, to draw inflammation away from the eyes.

Blood and "essence" enhancing formulas have restorative properties for overall wellness and rejuvenation. Astra Essence is used to treat certain conditions including: mild memory loss, recovery from prolonged illness or injury and sexual problems. Each tablet of Astra Essence contains medicinal herbs like astragalus root and seed, ligustrum fruit, ho-shou-wu root, lyceum fruit, rehmannia, eucommia bark, cuscuta seed, ginseng root, tang kuei root, and cornus fruit [AKA Japanese cornelian cherry]. Notice that moistening blood tonic dried fruits are here combined with qi (energy) tonics ginseng and astragalus in order to benefit absorption and digestion of the other blood-enhancing herbal ingredients. If such qi tonics were not added, the sweet moistening blood building herbs would cause diarrhea and nausea from excess fluids.

Nourishing Mushrooms and Fungi

More and more you can find exotic mushrooms in supermarkets and gourmet shops. I have mentioned heart-healthy fungi such as the blood- thinner tree ear [AKA cloud ear] the mysterious black crinkly "paper" sliced in popular Chinese dishes such as hot and sour soup. Two other medicinal fungi deserve more than a mention. They are reishi and chaga, They are fungi because they do not have the characteristic shape and taste we expect from mushrooms such as shiitake.

Reishi [Ganoderma lucid.] is an immune-enhancing tonic recommended for cancer-prevention and as an anti-inflammatory for arthritis. Called the "immortality mushroom" it has been prized for centuries among Chinese herbalists. Often the Chinese god of immortality is depicted carrying a crooked brown staff with an irregular round top, a reishi mushroom. You can find reishi tea in many

Chinese supermarkets, reishi powder or sliced dried hard mushrooms and capsules. (75.) Regular consumption of red reishi enhances our immune system and improves blood circulation. Generally, reishi is recommended as an adaptogen, immune modulator, and a general tonic. Reishi (ganoderma) is also used to help treat anxiety, high blood pressure, hepatitis, bronchitis, insomnia, and asthma.

I sometimes cook reishi along with another famous anticancer mushroom Coriolus versicolor (AKA Turkey tail mushroom, yun zhi,). Find them online. In New York, I buy dried, sliced reishi and coriolus from Lin Sisters herb shop at 4 Bowery in Manhattan's Chinatown. The mushroom water extract is easy to make in a slow cooker, or crockpot. That is the traditional method. Fill the crockpot with water and add a handful of sliced reishi and cook at high heat for about 3 hours until it comes to a boil. Then let it slow cook for 8 hours. Allow it to cool then drain the liquid into a glass containers for the refrigerator. Drink a glass or two as you like warm or cold daily. Re-cook the same mushroom again in fresh water to save money. For busy non-cooks I recommend taking capsules recommended in the Resource Guide.

Astragalus

I have already mentioned astragalus as a major ingredient in various herbal formulas, A valuable tonic, it is often added in order to boost overall energy and enhance the function of other herbs in a rejuvenation formula. Astragalus has known anti-cancer benefits and increases our T cells, which boost immunity. T cell levels drop with stress and grief. As a general tonic, astragalus has been used in experiments to slow the aging process. (76.) You might add a handful of the sliced dried herb, that resembles a tongue depressor, to cook with soups. Its flavor is pleasantly sweet. Cut pieces and steep them in brandy for two weeks to make a delicious tincture.

From India

There are several traditional Ayurvedic tonics that are very popular for daily use. One is Geriforte (pills or herbal syrup) (77.) and the other is a semi-sweet herbal paste called Chyawanprash. Made up of many herbals and spices, they are rejuvenation and longevity tonics widely used in India and available at Indian groceries in North America and online.

Chyawanprash's formula of herbs, spices, fruits, and minerals has been in use since the 4th century B.C. This herbal jam has a brown color, a sticky consistency, and a combination of sweet, sour and spicy tastes. Dabur, Himalaya, and Zandu are some of the most popular chyawanprash brands sold in India and worldwide. Organic India also distributes this preparation. Chyawanprash contains a mixture of 49 Ayurvedic herbs. Amla [AKA Indian gooseberry] is the main ingredient of this tonic as well as ashwagandha, pueraria a female hormone supplement touted as a way to improve sexuality and breast size, pippali, a rejuvenating pepper, white sandalwood, cardamom, tulsi, brahmi a brain and nerve tonic, arjuna for the heart, Nardostachys jatamansi used for mental disorders including epilepsy, stroke, convulsion, and hysteria, anti-bacterial neem and many others. The herb extracts are combined in pasteurized safflower honey and clarified butter. It is often referred to as a fruit jam containing honey. It's very nice to take a teaspoon on an empty stomach first thing in the morning.

Modern Science-based tonic capsules

Most of us want to avoid hassle or spending wasted time and money. This gives rise to lab-tested concentrated extracts. They can be great, easy to use and offer exact dosage and assured purity. Instead of eating ten pounds of cranberry or drinking so much red wine that it reduces cholesterol but ruins your liver, you can take capsules of their heart protective phytochemicals. For example there is Longevity Power Pack made by Absorb Your Health containing three supplements Artemisinin, pterostilbene, and liposomal resveratrol. Artemisinin is a powerful antiviral derived from the Chinese herb sweet wormwood whose first recorded medicinal use was in 200 BC. Pterostilbene fights cognitive decline, high cholesterol and triglycerides and promotes longevity. Liposomal resveratrol derived from several plants including grapes has been shown to prolong lifespan and to act as an antiviral and anti-inflammatory agent. Check for their effectiveness with regular heart testing and blood tests.

Heart Health Checkup

Do you require better energy, endurance, improved performance and enhanced sexuality? Do you suffer discomforts during inclement weather or fatigue and chronic pain from excess stress? You may benefit by using adaptogens such as a combination of ginsengs such as Ginseng Complex sold by Vitamin Shoppe

Do you want a tonic that is energizing, digestive, improves appetite and mood, and makes you look and feel younger? Do you prefer an herbal paste, such as Chaywanprash taken one teaspoon at a time once or twice daily? Or pills such as Geriforte? Tastes vary.

How do you know how much of a tonic to use?

Dosage for tonics is individual but here are some suggestions. Try a tonic using the lowest recommended dose. I smell herbs to see how they may affect me before taking them. You will be surprised how you will be drawn to certain herbs and herbal traditions by instinct or Karma. If you feel fatigued after using a tonic, it may indicate that your real energy, not hype, is taking over and you actually need to rest in order to recover strength. Continue with the tonic and give yourself a few days of beauty rest. Try to get to bed on time.

If you develop a rash, chest pain, or other allergy symptoms, stop taking all herbs and allow balance to return. If taking a tonic upsets your stomach it may be that the food/herb combination you are using is too difficult to digest. Many people who are unused to using herbs and supplements try to take everything at once. It's a mistake. Unfortunately, what seems convenient to your schedule may not suit your stomach. Try taking the tonic on an empty stomach. If you feel the effects of the tonic too strongly, take it with food and a digestive herbal tea. It will take time for your body to adjust to new herbs.

Drink plenty of water and eat cleansing green and yellow vegetables to allow poisons to be flushed out by the kidneys.

Although certain herbal tonics may be famous as sexual tonics that improve libido or sexual response, for example Panax ginseng, ashwagandha, or gokshura (Tribulus terr.) which we cover later, do not expect the results to be immediate. Tonics improve organ tissue and function, but it takes time and care to alter our vitality.

Q & A: Exhaustion
I want something to heal physical, mental and emotional exhaustion. --*Adrenal strength gives us courage and prevents fatigue and an aching back. Ashwagandha improves memory, concentration, and vital energy.* http://www.absorbyourhealth. com/product/ashwagandha-auto-renew/?ref=4041

Michael's Realtime Three

Comes leaf season, a multicolored end to a Green Mountain summer of recovery. We have walked along country roads, intoxicated with the leaf bedecked trees, the array of wild flowers, bees buzzing about them. In the valley where runs the branch of a river past the village of Sherburne Letha and I have sometimes spotted beavers frolicking. It's their form of sport when they are not busy building. We have gone almost daily to the spa at the Woods in Killington to work out in the gym, swim, soak in the hot tub, sweat in the sauna, scald in the Swedish shower. This is the essential exercise component of heart healing. Follow the system that suits you at your time of life. I boxed as a young man and did yoga, for a while we did Qi Gong in a park in Chinatown. I'll let you know what's next.

My diet must be beyond healthy--revivifying--and that was made easy by Rutland's weekly farmers' market, the largest and most varied in Vermont. The fruits and vegetables are freshly picked or dug out of the rich soil by our farmer friends. Everything is seasonal: late Spring brings strawberries into July, then blueberries, next raspberries and blackberries in August, and finally, with the hint of fall, apples. Among the many veggies, I love the baby carrots in late spring, arugula and the lettuces, a little later new potatoes and peas, summer means corn and autumn pumpkins. All along Letha bakes fruit pies (graham cracker crusts, no sugar) and at leaf season pumpkin pies to satisfy my sweet craving.

Now Letha and I needed to think about packing to return to New York. Living in Manhattan's Chelsea, seeing the neighborhood grow more trendy, I'd dreaded the day our four-story apartment building (one of twins) on a quiet, school street would be bought by a so-called developer, who would gut it, refurbish the hallways and those apartments from which the company could force out tenants, and flip the buildings to hot money from China, Russia, or a Made in America tax dodger. The nightmare has happened over a period of two years of intolerable noise, dust, and a scaffold that blocked out the daylight. The workers were illegals who I chatted with in the idiomatic Spanish picked up in my travels. Busy as beavers, they were *simpatico* guys. Except that one was a spy for the developer, who hoped to evict the few remaining, rent-stabilized tenants, of which we were number one on his hit list.

The commotion from construction hadn't done my overworked heart any good, but we returned to a finished building with marble staircases, an intercom with cameras to spy on the tenants, and lousy plumbing. I wasn't worried. For a while during the Great Depression, well before I was born, my father and mother ran a luncheonette that fronted for a wire room and fed the guys in back who gambled and played the horses. There was no lottery, no off-track betting in those days. The outfit was owned by Murder Inc., who actually made their money in the rackets. But growing up I knew my father's friends who were in with the mob. I learned a few things. Then time at Harvard Law taught me a more conventional way to fight, so going up against a crooked developer, I can hit with either hand, or both.

We had a new, undisclosed landlord (that hot money) and a new managing agent we'll call Con Realty. I did some spying and found out the two buildings, bought for $4 million, had been sold for $14 million. A two-room apartment with kitchenette now goes for $3,500/month market rent. Of course, Letha and I weren't about to give up a rent-stabilized pad in Chelsea. Con Realty made its move, based on faulty info from their spy. I showed my cards: proof that the two buildings together were valued, for tax purposes, at a preposterous few hundred thousand dollars. Con, or the landlord, was cheating on the real estate taxes.. I conveyed to the company my concern as a citizen and taxpayer, and they have behaved properly, if grudgingly, ever since.

Unfortunately, it costs deep down in the heart to wage war against New York's present-day thugs. Call it stress, aggravation, or the good fight. Chelsea is a charming neighborhood with theaters, boutiques, and ethnic restaurants of all sorts at hand. I'm friendly with the people who do honest work, from the super to the shoemaker to the pharmacist. I get angry at wiseguys and cheats. That's not good for my heart, especially the blood pressure, but I believe that suppressing anger is worse than feeling it. Doctors will recommend everything from meditation to sublimation to medicine to alleviate anger. I suppose the pills and methods help, but for me justified anger is useful. Employ your strong feelings, and they become a tool that will take leave when the time is right.

PART FOUR

LOOKING AT YOU

Breathe Deep and Stretch, Wiggle Your Toes, Have No Fear:
Friends Silkworm and Caterpillar are Here

TWENTY-ONE

BREATHE AND STRETCH

The General Theological Seminary has a quiet garden near where we live in Manhattan's Chelsea neighborhood. Squirrels gather chestnuts as we walk the stone path and breathe air refreshed by grass and large trees. Though late Autumn I remove my shoes to feel wet grass under my toes. Michael, sitting on a stone bench, does yogic deep breathing. Soon he smiles and I know his breathing has worked its magic. His blood pressure is lower and he is relaxed.

Years ago in a Shanghai hospital devoted to treating neurological disease I learned a qigong technique from a traditional doctor who had taught it to hypertension patients for over forty years. He told me, "Sit with your hands on your thighs. Inhale one by one into each part of the body from your head to toes and with each exhalation, tell your body to relax. Eventually," he said, "after practicing this breathing technique for at least twenty minutes daily, people with hypertension may notice that their palms sweat as they relax and their blood pressure becomes normal."

You don't need a beautiful garden in Chelsea only a quiet, private place and a little time devoted to your health. Often throughout this book I have described breathing techniques I have adapted from qigong and yoga, natural remedies such as homeopathic gelsemium and pulsatilla used to deepen and calm our breath, and I have stressed the vital connection between our breath and our heart health and our happiness. Too often our breath is shallow, we stifle our emotions and feel the result with chest pain, nervousness, insomnia, and eventually hypertension. Let's enhance energy with oxygen while moving blocked circulation by breathing and stretching. You might use vigorous movement like fifteen minutes of brisk walking or bouncing in place to enhance blood circulation and free your mind. Your heart will find a happy home. Some people do simple yoga stretches to start the day. I lie in bed with a tube pillow on my spine to open the chest and breathe and I walk my feet moving the ankles to start blood flowing.

Here is another breath of fresh air. Monday mornings I talk with a lively radio legend show host Marie Griffiths. She calls me the "Hungarian Princess." She's the "sexy Greek." Her program, "MG Live" from Montreal on mikefm.ca, a multilingual station broadcasting programs for some sixty years, is carried on the Net and in podcasts throughout the world. We have fun discussing healing diet, herbs and natural treatments to entertain her very large audience of health seekers. Recently a radio listener asked, "What is the easiest way to bring down high blood pressure and reduce stress without using medicine?" Over half the adults in the USA have high blood pressure from age, diet, and pollution. I remembered the qigong doctor's advice and answered, "Sit quietly and breathe slowly and deeply into the abdomen allowing your breath to drop down through your legs and exhale through your feet." It sounds too simple. But it works.

However, the trick is to actually do it. There are lots of yoga and meditation centers offering deep breathing instruction. How many of us leave our work to attend a class? We sit and type or inhale car exhaust while walking or driving. Here are easy ways to incorporate a little yoga into your lifestyle.

Carry, Breathe, Walk

Weight-bearing exercise is recommended to strengthen muscles, reduce the threat of bone fractures, improve posture and enhance endurance. Why do it only at the gym? I am lucky to live around the corner from supermarket shopping. Carrying groceries home in a backpack has become my new favorite exercise. I suggest you find a post office or other pleasant stop besides a pastry shop in your neighborhood. Add deep breathing this way. Inhale through the nose while taking five steps, exhale through the mouth while taking five steps. Without stiffening any part of the body, gradually lengthen the breath for a longer count but no more than 8 or 10. Inhaling and exhaling longer deepens the breath. Of course walking in traffic congested areas is neither fun nor healthy. However, you can reduce sinus congestion and help protect against colds, flu and super-germs that colonize in the nose by cleansing with organic tea tree oil. Place a drop of tea tree oil on a Q tip moistened with water and swab out each nostril. To avoid irritation in your nose we mix the oil with water or aloe vera gel. Next is a way to soothe your brain.

Nasya oil is soothing and calming

You would expect Ayurveda, the ancient health and enlightenment science from India, to have a practical answer for stuffy nose, stiff shoulders and neck, headache tension, and hysteria. It's nasya oil literally oil for your nose. Cleanse inside the nose as part of your daily hygiene. Do you have pollen or other allergies that hamper breathing? Do you have a stuffed or runny nose and itchy eyes? Soothing nasal passages will improve them. You might cleanse, moisten and soothe sensitive tissue and ease allergic irritations by cleaning the nose. Some people use a neti pot, a small pitcher, to flush sinus passages. A neti is too dramatic for me.

If your nose is dry or cracked from harsh weather or radiator heat, use some coconut oil on a Q tip to massage inside the nose. It's a healthy fat for the brain as well as for nasal passages. If you tend to be hot tempered and irritable place organic aloe vera gel on a Q tip or your finger and wipe out the nose with this cooling, soothing and balancing plant gel.

Nasya oil lubricates dry nasal passages, delivers the benefits of the herbs directly to the nose and brain, and keeps allergens from directly irritating the nasal lining. According to Ayurveda, healthy uncongested breathing is important to ensure proper flow of prana [life force] throughout the head and body. Cleansing, balancing and soothing, nasya oil is traditionally used to improve vocal quality, strengthen vision and promote mental clarity.

Prepared nasya oils are available online and may include brahmi, calamus, skullcap and eucalyptus essential oil in carrier oils such as olive oil and sesame oil. Dropping 1 – 2 drops into each nostril at bedtime relaxes stiff neck and shoulder and improves sleep as well as deepens breathing. Then lie flat with palms up while breathing into the lower abdomen to help relax spasm pains. As you inhale imagine positive energy such as light, a happy place or pleasant memory to lull your awareness deeper as you sink into deep relaxation. When you notice painful areas such as shoulders or back, breathe into those areas to relax them.

The ingredients in the nasya oil sold online by Banyan Botanicals offer advantages for the brain and nerves. For example brahmi, a form of gotu kola, is recommended for improving memory and comprehension. Calamus root, a swamp plant used medicinally since the ancient Greeks, was a popular digestive tonic used by Native Americans and in the Middle East as an aphrodisiac. It is said to improve memory and help ease anxiety. Skullcap, as we learned earlier in the book, enhances circulation, sending oxygen to the brain to help improve mental clarity. All too often we think of the nose only when it bothers us during allergy season. Our nose and sinus passages are intimately linked to the brain, cerebral nerves and emotions. Yogic deep breathing practices not only improve breathing but enhance calm, centeredness, and satisfaction.

Exfoliate to improve complexion and breathing

We don't realize it but our skin is the largest surface area of our breathing apparatus and a defense against environmental stress and illness. The skin, lungs and large intestine are connected energetically through meridians. That means our outer surface is linked to our deep reserve of oxygen, nutrients, and ultimately our immune strength. Our skin breathes. Sweating allows the body temperature to normalize protecting us in extreme hot or cold weather. I wonder if it may even help release pent up emotions. A sauna, steam bath or exercise that causes perspiration is one of the best ways to rid the body of chemicals, pesticides, and heavy metals picked up from the environment. It is essential to allow our skin to do its work by not clogging the pores and scalp. Applying oils, creams, and cosmetics cannot assure beautiful, clear skin if our cellular nutrition remains impoverished and our blood polluted by poisons and stress. Oxygen has to be present to energize every cell and protect against fatigue and infection.

Skin brush, glove, and ginger bath

Here are ways to encourage our skin to breathe. At least once a week use a gentle skin brush or complexion glove made of a natural fiber or give yourself a vigorous "brushing" with a clean, rough facecloth to help remove dry skin and dead skin cells. Then shower or bathe as usual. In India people assure radiant skin by applying a complexion paste made with chickpeas flour, healing, anti-inflammatory turmeric powder, fenugreek powder which exfoliates (removes dead skin cells), oil and water. It smells spicy but clogs the plumbing when you wash it off. There are simpler modern ways to exfoliate, cleanse and feed your skin. For example, I dissolve papaya enzyme pills in water and apply it as a facial mask to exfoliate dry skin. Try Natural Beauty Pack by Absorb Health made with three high tech treatments, one bottle each of Matrixyl Firming and Hydrating Serum to build collagen, Vitamin C, E, and Ferulic Acid Skin Revitalizing Serum, and one jar of Retinol Skin Softening and Healing Serum. They contain no harmful parabens, sulfates, or phthalates. Matrixyl is an anti-aging, collagen building peptide. Vitamins C, E and F protect against sun damage and retinol is vitamin A to improve mottled pigmentation, fine lines and wrinkles. You absorb vitamins through your skin as well as orally.

If you have ruddy dry skin and tend to have rashes, a cooling oil will work better because retinol can be irritating. Consider a neem oil, coconut oil, black seed oil, castor oil, or bhringaraj oil rub. Mix the oil with aloe vera and briskly rub it on with your face cloth before a shower.

Cooling, detoxifying Ayurvedic Bhringaraj oil

Having a cool head of healthy hair and an unblemished complexion helps you relax, breathe deeply and be happy. Bhringaraj is known as Eclipta alba in Latin, han lien cao in Chinese and false daisy in English. A member of the sunflower family it is commonly used internally in Ayurvedic pills for treating liver disease and skin disorders, including eczema, dermatitis, hair loss and insect bites. The herb is an anti-inflammatory, antimicrobial, a detoxifying blood and liver rejuvenating treatment for reducing the ill effects of cirrhosis and has been shown to slow the progress of certain cancers. (78.)

In Indian herb shops and online you can find hair oils and massage oils that contain bhringaraj, to cool inflammation and reduce skin itching, redness, and infections. We actually absorb herbs very effectively through the skin. Since blood vessel inflammation is a key factor in the origin of heart and circulation problems it may be of benefit to apply a cooling oil regularly. You might apply the oil to skin and scalp with your hands before a bath or for a stronger treatment leave it on overnight. If the treatment feels too strong, too cooling and sedating, the oil can be applied a few drops as a scalp treatment or on the bottom of your feet for about twenty minutes then removed with warm water. This feels relaxing and calming. It deepens the breath and could start a whole new trend in family therapy. Imagine a hot argument squelched with a mutual foot massage with a cooling oil.

Heart Stretches

There are many good ways to stretch in order to enhance our flexibility and grace and to lengthen muscles. The salute to the sun is known to yoga practitioners. Affirmations can be added to the walking and breathing exercises I have already described. Although many of us do not exercise no matter how important it is, fortunately there are ways to add comfortable daily stretches to your life. Here are a few that can help free blood circulation and help you get a good night's sleep.

Lying in bed to begin or end the day

My cats love this one. They follow along watching my arm move up and down. Lie on your left side with knees together bent in a fetal position. Both your arms are extended out in front lying on the bed. As though you were an opening book, lift the right arm up and over with the palm facing up. Follow your moving arm with your head and eyes and place the outstretched arm on to the bed opposite the arm on the bed. Your arms are spread wide apart but the pelvis and legs do not move so that you have twisted at the waist. Rest looking at the right hand. Relax and lift the right arm back to the beginning position. Do that five times and then switch sides. Repeat the entire stretch several times but do not strain or move too quickly. Your arms are a leisurely relaxing book.

Passive Stretches

I love passive stretches that require no work. Lie flat on your back on a tube pillow or a soft five inch diameter rubber ball so that the tube lies along the length of your spine or the ball stretches the middle or upper back. Relax your shoulders back and down toward the bed. It may be painful for a moment as your muscles change position away from the forward crunch that's frozen in place from doing computer work. Lie there and breathe through the length of your body until you feel stretched and relaxed. It may improve your sleep as well as your breathing.

Another useful passive stretch is also a massage done with a wooden Ma Roller or a thick glass bottle. While lying flat on the bed or floor, place the wooden roller or a bell canning jar perpendicular to your neck. Placed crosswise on your neck you can then rub the hairline, tight muscles and tendons in your neck as a deep massage. You will be amazed how the neck, jaw, chest and heart are all linked by nerves. Easing muscle tightness in the neck helps the shoulders and chest to relax. You may even be able to move congested lymph in the brain to move through the neck and shoulders. You may feel pain or electrical sensations running down your arms. Eventually as muscle tension relaxes you can breathe deeper and send more healing oxygen to your heart.

Office Qigong

Working seated for long periods of time, we are advised to get up and walk around the room to increase blood circulation. I don't do it often enough, do you? It breaks my concentration while writing. But simply standing and stretching up the arms over my head helps reverse the effects of gravity on internal organs. Imagine reaching for Heaven and planting your feet in Earth. Swinging the arms gently in any direction is a good thing to do. Try it in the office and people may join in.

Rolling your shoulders in circles breaks apart upper back tension. Roll in both directions, front and back. Seated in a chair, stretch up and bend over and touch your knees, if possible your ankles, and holding that position for a few minutes breathe into your lower back muscles. It's all about sending oxygen where it needs to go.

Your Gut and Heart

If you take a complicated cocktail of medicines, if you eat a meal while tense or upset, if you spend lots of time seated or driving, you may develop chest pains unrelated to your heart. That is because the chest is part of energy flow that proceeds from your mouth through the entire digestive tract. When emotions get stuck we choke on our food, our "gut feelings" and air trapped in places that hurt. Open the passage way to smooth digestion and breathing by opening a valve that connects the small and large intestine. It is called the ileo-secal valve located about half way between your navel and your right groin. Press firmly downward towards the right groin to open the valve allowing food and air to pass from the small into the large intestine or gut. It may feel like opening a door in a dike to allow water to flow into a field. It is a deep passageway of energy known to acupuncture doctors as well. Meridians of the gallbladder, bladder, and small intestine circulate qi in the head, shoulders and back and can affect heart rhythm especially when they are troubled by stuck energy flow. "Go with the flow" has become a common place expression of comfort. We can think of it as a deep healthy river of life force.

Heart Health Checkup

Look at the palms of your hands. Are they red and do they feel warm and dry? Is one or both palms of your hand dry and lined or cracked? Those are signs of internal inflammation resulting from what Ayurvedic doctors call excess Pitta. Pitta (inflammation) can become aggravated from an overly spicy diet, alcohol, smoking, diabetes, hormone imbalance, unbalanced emotions and may be your constitution if you tend to be a hot tamale. Inflammation and dehydration interfere with breathing and stretching, heart rhythm, and underlie dangerous damage in blood vessels. You may have inflammatory arthritis or a dry cough, dry skin, bloodshot eyes and thinning hair from dehydration. Drinking lots of water is not enough to correct such dehydration. You may need to take corrective herbs for diabetes (high blood sugar) a condition that has been linked with stroke for heart patients. High blood sugar has been found to be aggravated by some heart medicines notably the statins.

A cooling diet of green vegetables, dandelion and kale, bitter melon, a few complex carbohydrates such as oatmeal (avoiding wheat and sugars) nuts, seeds, fish or krill oil, olive oil, green or white tea, and in general the cooling diet advice found in this book are helpful to correct what Chinese doctors call "internal heat" and what Ayurvedic doctors call "excess Pitta." If you are a hot tamale, eat greens, cucumber, use cooling massage oils such as bhringaraj, and laxative bitter digestive herbs to enhance bile flow until your hands become pale, soft, and supple. You will have fewer blemishes and "hot" emotions such as rage and jealousy.

Are your palms very pale, cold, moist, stiff? An Ayurvedic doctor may say your "Vata" (nerve energy and circulation) needs help. You will benefit from warm, cooked foods, root vegetables and spicy soups with garlic, flaxseed oil, and herbs to balance body, mind and nerves like ashwagandha, healthful oils such as sesame oil used in cooking and massage, certain sweet fruits such as peach, prune, sweet dark grapes, and warming, stimulating spices that enhance circulation such as cinnamon, clove, nutmeg, allspice, cardamom, ginger and pepper. So the next time you stretch to the ceiling look at your hands. The next time you breathe deeply in meditation and hold the heart mudra look at your hands.

Q & A: Happy Thoughts
I want a way to improve my meditation and relaxation without taking pill or tea. – *Inhale the fragrance of essential oil of grapefruit. Grapefruit is refreshing and calming, but it should not be eaten by people using certain heart medicines because the interaction is dangerous. Inhaling the fragrance is like waking up to a happy morning.* http://www.absorbyourhealth. com/product/grapefruit-essential-oil/?ref=4041

TWENTY-TWO

FEET, YOUR SECOND HEART

There is an old Chinese saying, "The feet are a second heart." That's difficult to understand because we stand and walk on our feet. Like our heart our feet support us and point us in the direction we walk. But there are other ways our feet keep us well. Let's consider the quality, volume and ease of your blood circulation from head to foot. The foot contains the endings of meridians passing throughout the body and internal organs. People who use reflexology recognize the connection. Look at this chart showing where energy pathways pass through us into our feet. The area closest to the toes roughly corresponds to the top areas of the body, the middle of the foot to the digestive center and the heel to the hips, lower legs, and sciatic nerve.

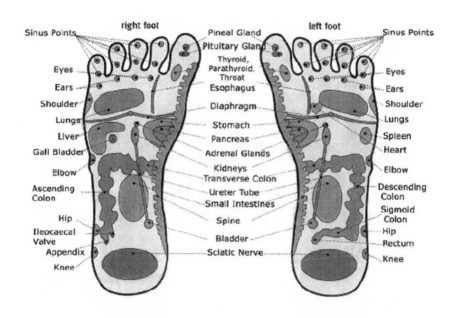

A tea kettle full of boiling water builds up steam and whistles. In our body inflammation, pain, and acidity can give us signs we are too hot and tense. Our hands and feet become red, joints swollen and painful when excess inflammation is trapped in the body. Here is an example that brings this home to heart patients.

Michael spends days at the computer writing his long, complex and highly engaging books. In addition he is often awake during the middle of the night scanning stock market results. Evenings to relax we watch classic movies on television. All this sitting makes his neck and shoulders very stiff. Lately his blood pressure is higher than usual and his temper hot. He is prone to gout and winter holiday rich foods and drink may have aggravated it.

However now what bothers Michael most is a painful swollen red area on his foot that corresponds to eyes, the mitral valve and lungs. He knows he needs more and better exercise and fewer sweets, muffins and congesting foods. He has quit his statin drugs because the muscle pain he experienced from them made walking and exercise impossible. He still needs to reduce the painful results of a sedentary lifestyle, no exercise, rich eating and overweight–pain, swelling and possible uric acid buildup in his foot. That will enhance circulation in vital heart and lung areas.

I usually give Michael a foot massage during the evening while watching television. It is an intimate bond we both enjoy. We have always been nuts about each other. We love to touch and kiss, a life-long happy lust. However, now the red hot swollen area on the bottom of his foot is painful to touch. Upping his gout medicine has not worked. He drinks very little water, mostly teas that I prepare and coffee. Using a diuretic heart drug such as Lasix or a gout medicine can cause kidney stones and increase gout if you don't drink lots of water to flush the kidneys. Laser acupuncture on the sole of the foot and foot soaks have improved circulation. Homeopathic remedies such as apis mel., homeopathic bee venom, may be used to reduce arthritic inflammation. But that is not enough to improve possible congestive heart problems.

I am not suggesting that everyone with foot pain has heart troubles. There are lots of reasons for foot pain, including injury, arthritis, overweight, and diabetes. But if the feet are the second heart, then enhancing circulation in the feet benefits the heart and circulation.

One of my favorite mentors for natural medicine and the author of over forty books, Dr. Bernard Jensen, was known to say, "Walk on pebbles at the beach, walk in beach sand and it will improve circulation in your head." Blood flows from head to feet and back again.

What does this have to do with chronic heart problems? Another term to describe congestive heart failure is left or right ventricular failure, or failure of the left or right lower pumping chambers (ventricles) of the heart. Left ventricular failure typically results from high blood pressure, decreased blood flow and oxygen delivery to the heart muscle (ischemic heart disease), or diseases of the aortic or mitral valves within the left heart. Fluid and blood may accumulate in the lungs, producing shortness of breath. Right ventricular failure may develop independently or more commonly follow or result from left ventricular failure. Causes include lung diseases (COPD), inflammation of the tissue that surrounds the heart or diseases of the valves within the right heart (tricuspid or pulmonic valvular disease). Fluid and blood may accumulate in the abdomen, legs, and feet, producing swelling (edema). Dieting alone won't reduce that sort of fluid retention. Sudden weight gain, swollen belly, ankles and feet may indicate a weak heart, valve trouble, heart failure.

Get your blood moving

If you stand or sit all day your circulation is obviously challenged. If you are overweight you are twice as likely to develop chronic heart failure symptoms as the heart becomes overstressed, tired and weaker. Does walking or exercise improve your breathing? Getting your blood moving, your heart pumping, may reduce pain and swelling due to stagnant energy and poor blood flow. In many ways regular gentle exercise such as walking, biking, swimming, dancing provides great heart health protection. Unless you have an in-house massage person, another easy way to get your body and mind back into balance is with a nice foot soak.

Foot Soaks

A lemon foot soak is cooling, refreshing and helps reduce fever and pain in red, inflamed swollen joints. Lemon contains vitamin C to boost natural immunity and help cleanse the lymph system. Add the juice from one organic lemon to at least one liter of warm spring water or filtered water and soak away your irritations and angers, melt muscle tightness and renew a sense of wellbeing. If you do not have a lemon use ¼ cup of apple cider vinegar. Apple cider vinegar is alkaline and detoxifying for the liver. Used regularly it may improve skin rashes as well as joint aches.

Oxygen kills germs and keeps us alive and well. Hydrogen peroxide contains an extra molecule of oxygen. It is H2O2 oxygen suspended in water. The usual peroxide sold in pharmacies in a black plastic bottle, which contains only about 3% H2O2 and many chemical additives, is a skin cleansing treatment for cuts but is not safe for other medicinal use.

Food Grade Hydrogen Peroxide is 35% H2O2 and extremely dangerous to handle. It turns flesh white, burning it, when it touches your skin. That white burning is from oxygen killing germs. Food Grade Hydrogen Peroxide, available online, is the only form that may be used for a foot soak. However it can NEVER be used undiluted. The safest way to use Food Grade Peroxide is to add no more than 3 tablespoon of it to 2 gallons of water and soak your feet for no more than 15 – 20 minutes. We absorb liquids readily through the porous skin of our hands and feet.

Do not soak your feet or apply the diluted food grade peroxide mixture to broken skin. The foot soak in itself may feel irritating. Your feet may tingle. This treatment is recommended as a weekly treatment for gout and may make your painful toes and swollen foot temporarily turn red as uric acid is gradually broken down by the oxygen treatment. Be sure to rinse off the hydrogen peroxide water with clear water after the treatment. It will dry your skin and can increase skin cracks. After the foot soak and clear water rinse put on clean cotton socks and slippers.

Homeopathic Calc. Fluor for circulation and tissue repair

According to homeopathic William Boericke, MD, Calc Fluor [Calcarea Fluorica. Fluoride of Lime, Fluor Spar] taken orally as directed is a powerful tissue remedy for "hard, stony glands, varicose and enlarged veins, and malnutrition of bones." If you have chronic dry cracked skin on hands and feet use homeopathic Calc. Fluor. 6x between meals to improve circulation. Calc Fluor preserves the contractile power of elastic tissue. For heart patients that means homeopathic Calc Fluor provides relief from sluggish circulation and poor elasticity of blood vessels. It has also been used to treat varicose veins, hemorrhoids, backache, and weak muscles. If you take heart medicines it is best to take homeopathic remedies separately from them and with professional guidance.

Your Feet: Your good health from the ground-up

There are many massage creams and foot rubs available in all pharmacies. There must be a lot of painful feet. Did you know that of the 206 bones in the human body over half are in the hands and feet? There are 52 in the feet and 54 are in the hands. Each foot has 26 bones, 33 joints, 107 ligaments, 19 muscles and tendons. We become tired from standing but the impact of walking can actually strengthen bones because bone, a living tissue, tends to fuse. Babies are born with 300 – 350 bones but some of their bones start to fuse as they grow up. Unfortunately, if you walked very early while your bones were soft or if your mother, while pregnant or you during childhood had poor nutrition, your bones may be irregular or your weight unevenly distributed in your feet and legs. Your leg lengths may not match which causes a strong impact when you walk and can eventually cause loss of cartilage in one or both hips and knee joints. The uneven leg length can sometimes be corrected with chiropractic adjustments or shoe inserts.

A nice soothing foot soak and foot rub can help relax tense leg muscles, increase circulation and treat specific problem areas by using reflexology. Study the foot chart provided in this chapter to see if painful areas of your feet may correspond to health problems. The point for the heart in near the center of the left foot. If you find painful areas, swollen or discolored areas on the bottom of your feet, massage the area with a firm circular motion, breathe into that area and press deeper with your fingertips then relax.

A Homeopathic Cream for Pain Relief

Homeopathic massage creams are recommended to relieve stiffness, injuries, muscle pains, bruises and sprains. One useful cream in a tube made by NatraBio is called The Rub. The ingredients are arnica recommended for bruises and sprains, aconitum for acute injury and physical trauma, belladonna for inflammation, calendula for healing, hamamelis for cuts and bruising, hypericum for pain, ruta for arthritis and strains, symphytum for bones, ligaments, and joints.

Here are acupuncture points which you may massage gently or apply a stimulating essential oil such lavender.

Acupressure on hands and feet

You can easily massage the following points I will describe for balancing heart and kidney (adrenal) energy as a routine treatment to help prevent/treat heart failure. If you have chest pains be sure to have medical tests and guidance to determine the cause.

Many years ago, one of my acupuncture teachers endocrinologist Dr. Yves Requena, MD from France said in a lecture, "Certain acupuncture treatments are recommended according to our typical imbalances that occur during seasonal changes. For example treat the liver points in the foot (liver 2 and 3 located near the large and second toe) during spring to ease circulation. However people over 40 tend to need energy and balance for their heart and kidneys in order to maintain wellness." The heart and kidney(adrenal) energies are our deepest most fundamental source of vitality. I discussed this in the chapter on heart tonics. For example, ashwagandha an herbal adrenal tonic, is also used to tone heart muscles, reduce low back pain and enhance memory.

The acupuncture points recommended by Dr. Requena are Kidney 3 (KD3) at the ankle and heart 7 (HT7) at the wrist. Acupuncturists know how to locate these points, but since you are not using needles you do not need to be so precise. You might massage the areas illustrated below at the inside of the ankle and wrist. I recommend KD3 and KD7 for kidney/adrenal stimulation and HT7 at the palm side of the wrist and the entire palm. If your hands and feet feel cold to touch your circulation is poor and you will benefit by massaging the entire hand and foot areas where many acupuncture points are located.

Kidney acupuncture meridian points in the foot

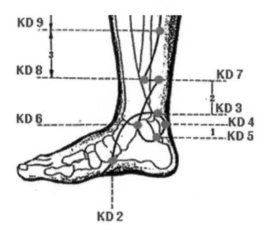

Heart acupuncture points in the hand

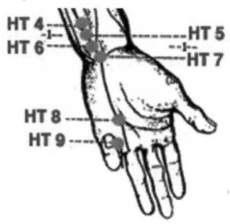

Get up and walk

I asked Michael which of my recent treatments have helped him the most to reduce his foot pain and swelling and shortness of breath, which aside from other things are both symptoms of heart failure. His answer was, "They all worked together – the food grade hydrogen peroxide foot soak, foot massage treatments, the homeopathic foot rub, and walking. If you can't walk you'll die sooner. Stopping the statin drugs enabled me to walk with much less pain and walking increased my breathing and stamina."

Heart Health Checkup

Observe the flesh of your palms and soles. Are they dry, red, cracked indicating inflammation and/or dehydration? Do your feet feel hot or burning? Is the skin rough? Do you have broken capillaries in your legs? Swollen feet or toes? You may have high cholesterol or other blockage to your circulation, arthritis or gout. Do you have an itchy rash made worse from hot weather or drinking alcohol? A cooling foot soak such as water and lemon juice may made you feel cooler, but you need to address your internal inflammation especially your bursting blood vessels.

Kudzu root [puerria] is a popular food used in Asia and a Chinese medicine. Normally it is used in cooking as a natural vegetarian thickener for sauces. However research has shown its effectiveness when used regularly for reducing inflammation, gastric acidity, and protecting blood vessels and enhancing rejuvenation by reducing wrinkles and grey hair. Some people calm anxiety and improve sleep by taking some at bedtime. It is estrogenic therefore not for everyone. Also see shatavari as a source of phytoestrogens.

Are hands and feet pale, moist and cold indicating poor circulation and a nervous condition or weakness? Are you overweight? Does walking tire you? Are you often short of breath? Do you sleep with several pillows or awaken coughing or choking?

Without changing your medical routine or omitting regular medical checkups, add some enjoyable natural health practices such as deep breathing, massage, or foot soaks and see if you feel an improvement.

Then gradually along with the cooperation of your health professionals incorporate a heart healthy exercise routine into your daily schedule. You may enjoy walking, tai chi, qi gong, swimming, or dancing. Start slowly and build your stamina gradually. Perspiring during exercise helps rid the body of pollution and heavy metals.

Q & A: Happy Feet Rub

I want a healthy pure massage cream that I can use for tired hands and feet – *Therapeutic Foot Cream has herbal ingredients such as aloe, eucalyptus, mint and honeysuckle flower to alternately heat and cool tired feet, while also including natural antioxidants to help penetrate deep and soothe dry rough skin.* http://www.absorbyourhealth.com/product/therapeutic-foot-cream/?ref=4041

TWENTY-THREE
TRADITIONAL AND TRUE

The Roman Army marched on its stomach. Each soldier was given a ration of vinegar, whole grain and a little mill with which to grind the grain to bake unleavened bread. The rest of their diet was made up from whatever foods they seized during campaigns. Vinegar as a heart healthy food is a source of potassium necessary for heart rhythm and a liver-cleanser suited to protect against inflammatory conditions. Once in New York Chinatown while Michael was getting acupuncture for chronic pain, the elderly doctor's assistant, a cheerful energetic woman said, "We Chinese believe that everyday we protect the liver by drinking one teaspoon of apple cider vinegar in water and eating one carrot." That illustrates the principle of yin and yang. A nourishing carrot, a source of vitamin A, supports liver tissue is therefore yin. The sour wine effect of vinegar is yang, stimulating liver action as a general liver tonic and blood cleanser.

Why use vinegar as a health tonic? Apple cider vinegar makes body fluids more alkaline protecting the immune system against allergies and mucus congestion in sinus cavities, throat and digestive tract. Vinegar counters fatigue. The taste is bracing, refreshing, and light. Add ½ to 1 teaspoon of apple cider vinegar to a glass of water used to rinse your mouth after brushing your teeth. Splash some on your face and scalp to relieve irritation and itching.

Drinking apple cider vinegar water is said to relieve symptoms of candida yeast infections and heartburn to enhance weight loss and to treat type 2 diabetes. Carol Johnston, PhD, directs Arizona State University's nutrition program. She has been studying apple cider vinegar for more than ten years and believes its effects on blood sugar are similar to certain medications. "Apple cider vinegar's anti-glycemic effect is very well documented." She explains that the vinegar blocks some of the digestion of starch. "It doesn't block the starch 100%, but it definitely prevents at least some of that starch from being digested and raising your blood sugar," Johnston told webmd.com.

Simple and true

Unfiltered, unpasteurized apple cider vinegar is the best kind to use as a source of vitamins and minerals because it is unrefined and contains much of the natural richness and health benefits of organic apples. It tastes invigorating. Remember the 2011 dietary study published in the *British Medical Journal (BMJ)*: An apple a day keeps the statins away. Start the day with 1 tablespoon of unfiltered, unpasteurized organic apple cider vinegar in a glass of water. The dosage recommended for easing arthritic pain and stiffness is three such glasses of water daily. The same amount may apply to heart patients and may as an added benefit help curb a sweet tooth, depression and fatigue. Start with a dose that works for you and increase gradually. For weight loss, drink the vinegar water between meals so that it does not dilute the stomach's digestive juices. If you take medicine for high blood sugar, have regular checkups and adjust your dose of vinegar accordingly. You may be able to reduce your medication.

Improve your walking with chicken's feet

Here is another old Chinese food remedy, also popular in the Caribbean, for arthritis that helps to support cartilage and ease joint pain. Why bother about a joint remedy in a heart book? The more you walk the better it is for your heart! Your circulation will flow from head to feet and back to feet again. You will benefit from endorphins released during movement, enhanced breathing, and a boost for your mood and circulation. How can you get more cartilage? The natural cushion between our joints, our cartilage, thins with age and wear and tear from loose ligaments, poor posture, bad habits, and stress. You can help delay age-related cartilage loss by eating cartilage-rich foods. For example, add a packet of unflavored gelatin to water or juice daily. Drink it so it goes to your joints.

Chicken Feet Soup

My Hungarian grandmother, Erzibet cooked pig's knuckles long enough to make a natural gelatin. I slow cook in a crockpot at low heat for 10 hours soup bones from organic beef, chicken, egg and shrimp shells, adding onion, garlic, green herbs, and chaga mushroom with a tablespoon of apple cider vinegar to make a tasty soup stock. The glucosamine comes out of the bones and shells into the broth. No need to buy expensive, hard to digest arthritis supplements.

Braised chicken's feet are a popular Chinese dish. Chicken feet are sold raw, cut and cleaned in some butcher shops. Here is quick recipe for chicken feet soup followed by my own version using chicken bone left-overs. Chicken feet can smell and taste rather bitter and the oil from them is heavy. But if you are game here is what to do. Makes two quarts in a slow cooker.

Ingredients
- 4 – 6 organic chicken feet, each about 5 inches long
- 2 cups sliced vegetables including carrots, onions, sweet potato, celery and optional okra.
- 1 large clove of garlic, herbal seasonings such as oregano, parsley, thyme, rosemary, sliced fresh ginger, turmeric and pepper
- 1 sliced apple
- water to make 2 quarts.

First scrub the chicken feet with a food brush and water then soak the feet in water adding some apple cider vinegar for about 15 minutes and rinse them. Some people cut off the sharp nail tips off with a kitchen scissor. But they contains the most glucosamine. You are ready to assemble the soup ingredients. If you want to improve flavor and digestibility use brewed tea instead of water and simmer this at low heat for up to six hours until it is well cooked. Skim off the fat after it cools in the refrigerator. You might use this as a soup stock discarding the chicken and vegetables. Here is my frugal housewife's recipe for Mulligatawny Soup using leftover chicken bones as a stock.

Letha's Mulligatawny

This is a favorite soup in our house–rich, spicy, and full of protein from yellow lentils. It features the bitter healing properties of turmeric and tangy flavor of sweet curry. People in India who use turmeric daily have a very low incidence of Alzheimer's disease. Turmeric has anti-cancer, digestive, and anti-inflammatory effects that protect delicate blood vessels making turmeric root and powder an all round healing food. You can add turmeric to coffee, soups, apple sauce or just about everything. Color cooked whole grains, breads and pasta with its bright yellow hue.

Another ingredient revered for over 2,000 years throughout Asia and the Middle East is black cumin seeds (nigella sativa) which was found in King Tut's tomb apparently to cure his headaches, digestive troubles and increase immunity after death. According to modern medical sources other uses for black cumin seeds and oil include lowering blood pressure and cholesterol and as a cancer treatment. This recipe makes at least one quart of soup.

Ingredients
- Leftover chicken bones and cartilage from an organic roast chicken
- 1 cup yellow lentils or split chickpeas (chana dal) soaked in water overnight
- 1 ½ to 2 cups chopped vegetables including onion, carrot, celery, garlic
- 1 Granny Smith apple or other organic apple cut into 4 pieces
- ½ tsp cardamom powder, ½ tsp turmeric powder, ½ tsp ginger powder, ½ tsp cumin powder, black pepper and paprika to taste, 1 bay leaf, ½ tsp black cumin seeds (nigella sativa)
- 1 – 2 tsp sweet curry powder to taste

Soaking the legumes overnight reduces acids that hamper digestion and cause gas. Bring the soaked lentils to a boil, turn off the heat and move the pot over the stove. Add 1 tsp baking powder to the hot cooking liquid which makes it bubble up to a foam. That releases gas into the air. After it foams for a moment thoroughly rinse the lentils in clean water and replace the water for cooking until the lentils are done.

In a separate pot cook the vegetables, apple, herbs and spices, and chicken bones for about 30 minutes until the vegetables are soft. Correct the seasoning and strain the ingredients preserving only the liquid which becomes your soup stock. Combine the seasoned stock with the soft lentils and simmer them an additional 15 minutes to blend the flavors. You may want to blend the ingredients to make a smooth soup or leave the lentils soft. Serve it hot with garlic toast.

What's the point of eating gelatin or a soup stock made with chicken feet or bones, pigs knuckles or horses hoofs? It is not only the cartilage but a natural source of inexpensive, non-shellfish glucosamine that you get from them. Glucosamine does not increase cholesterol levels however, some research suggests that glucosamine might increase insulin levels and affect blood pressure. To be cautious, if you take glucosamine sulfate pills and have high cholesterol or hypertension, monitor your cholesterol levels closely. The bone soup stocks won't bother you.

Friends that Crawl and Squirm

Daily foods and herbs may detoxify the body and build vitality but heart health sometimes calls for stronger, unusual medicines. I first began research on medicinal leech therapy to treat chronic pain and enhance circulation to avoid surgery for carpal tunnel syndrome. It works! To my surprise, on the Internet I found clinics abroad that successfully treat heart disease using the current Ayurvedic and Eastern European health practice of placing live medicinal leeches on the skin to remove toxic lymph fluid and support any number of other health benefits without the aid of surgery or drugs. Leech saliva is an anti-inflammatory blood thinner. In addition, an American herb company Health Concerns makes a capsule containing an enzyme that silkworms produce in order to dissolved their cocoon—a marvelous natural blood thinner. Make friends with creatures used for medicines. They live on bushes, under leaves and rocks. Nature has provided answers to our worst health problems if we respect the earth, learn its wonders, know where to look for them and how to use them.

Friend Leech

Herophilos (335-280 BC) the Greek physician known as the first anatomist and Hippocrates of Cos (460BC-370BC) the father of medicine both used leech therapy for blood letting to balance the body's "humours." During the 1800's the demand for medicinal leeches in Europe was into the millions annually and American barber shops and pharmacies used leeches to remove black eyes and bruises. The practice became less popular with the advent of antibiotic drugs, but is still used in traditional Ayurvedic medicine as a blood cleansing treatment. Today the American medical establishment considers the leech a "medical device" used in hospitals mainly by plastic surgeons in order to speed healing and reduce bruising following surgery.

My search for medicinal leech therapy sent me to Silesian Holistic Center in Greenpoint, Brooklyn a working-class Polish neighborhood in New York that I grew to appreciate for shops selling poppy seed coffee cake and pickled cabbage. Andrew Plucinski, a large, friendly, rosy-cheeked man whose apartment serves as a clinic, is expert in leech therapy. His skis stand near the entry when he is not zipping down a slope in Switzerland. He professionally studied medicinal leech therapy in Poland after leech therapy saved his leg from amputation.

Patients I have seen visiting Andrew's clinic include people who come to cure everything from tooth and sinus infections, headaches, depression, arthritis, and heart disease. One four year old little girl had several leech treatments to help reattach her fingertip that was accidently cut off. Andrew says he does not treat disease but that leech therapy enhances wellness when body systems are under-functioning. He follows an elaborate treatment protocol dating from the 18th century placing leeches on the skin over major organs in order to bring about rejuvenation by detoxifying and tonifying organ systems.

Aside from the "ick" factor that discourages most people from trying the treatment, it works wonders. Leech saliva is a blood thinner, anti-bacterial, and lymph cleansing natural remedy. It supports over 400 healing enzymatic actions the body needs in order to work well. For heart patients, the treatment helps reduce cholesterol and swelling from lymph fluid retention, a natural pain-killer without drugs. It can improve movement by reducing pain throughout the body, improve breathing, and reduce blood vessel congestion resulting from cholesterol and environmental poisons. In addition the treatment releases endorphins, those feel-good chemicals that are also increased by exercise and acupuncture.

I have used leeches for organ and lymph cleansing and to completely eliminate carpal tunnel syndrome after I had been threatened with surgery. The effects felt relaxing and somehow strengthening to be connected to earth energy. I applied medicinal leeches several times to help cleanse Michael's liver and around his heart to help control cholesterol blockage. He tolerated it nobly, although releasing toxins to be eliminated by the liver gives some people a temporary headache. It made him testy. I doubt that it will catch on to become popular.

Herbal Lymph Cleansers

What herbal lymph cleansing treatments exist? Ayurveda uses cooling deep-cleansing Manjistha (Rubia cordifolia) root a perennial climber that is best known as a lymph mover and blood purifier. It is sold as capsules or powder online. According to Ayurveda, the lymph and blood are the first tissues to become congested when the body is not detoxifying properly, and subsequently have a domino effect throughout the body unless addressed properly and early. The astringent red powder can be added to tea, applesauce or yogurt to assure radiant clear skin, improved breathing, enhanced circulation and lymph detoxification.

Silkworm Enzyme: A Blood-thinner

Silkworms are the larva of a moth (Bombyx mori) native to Asia that spins a cocoon of fine, strong, lustrous fiber that is the source of commercial silk. Silkworm cultivation began 5000 years ago in China. During the eleventh century European traders stole several silkworm eggs and seeds of the mulberry tree (the leaves are a silkworm's preferred food) and began rearing silkworms in Europe. Today, silk is cultivated in Japan, China, Spain, France, and Italy, although artificial fibers have replaced silk in much of the textile industry.

There is an enzyme in the silk worm's gut serratiopeptidase that is extremely valuable for heart patients. Silkworms used it to dissolve their cocoons before flying off as moths into the sunset. We use it to help dissolve blood clots, fibroids, and reduce chronic pain and swelling and protect against hardening of arteries. According to medical sources, Serrapeptase is used for painful conditions including back pain, osteoarthritis, rheumatoid arthritis, osteoporosis, fibromyalgia, carpel tunnel syndrome, migraine headache, and tension headache. It is also used for reducing swelling after surgery, swelling of a vein with the formation of a blood clot (thrombophlebitis.) Some people use serrapeptase for heart disease and atherosclerosis.

Serramend

One capsule of Serramend made by Health Concerns contains 10 milligrams of serratiopeptidase. Since serratiopeptidase plays a role in dissolving blood clots in the arteries, Serramend works to maintain healthy blood circulation as well as overall cardiovascular function. By the same token this supplement may relieve symptoms of inflammatory venous disease such as varicose veins or leg cramps.

The recommended dose is 1 – 2 capsules three times daily. Each 180-capsule bottle of Health Concerns' Serramend should last for up to two months at the standard serving size. As far as drug interactions, serrapeptase may decrease blood clotting. (79.)

Cordyceps: A Qi Tonic

Continuing with worm-like creatures for heart health, we have cordyceps a Chinese tonic par excellence. Although Cordyceps sinensis is often described as an herb in TCM, according to New York University Langone Medical Center, it's actually a combination of a parasitic fungus and the larvae of a moth (a caterpillar). The fungus attacks the caterpillar and destroys it from within. The remaining shell of the caterpillar along with the fungus are dried and sold as cordyceps. Sold in Chinese herb shops, the dried fungus resembles small brown dried worms and has a mild semi-sweet flavor when cooked in soups.

I recommend you buy it in capsules from outlets such as Vitamin Shoppe to insure quality and ease of use. If you prefer you can pour the capsule contents into soups or take them as directed. Many people have used cordyceps as an energy tonic and it is especially useful when recovering from illness, exhaustion and recovery from the weakening effects of antibiotic treatment.

Research suggests that cordyceps improves energy making the utilization of oxygen more efficient. That accounts for the overall physical enhancement, the added endurance, and the anti-fatigue effects seen in using a cordyceps supplement. A study quoted by the National Institutes of Health (*Journal of Ayurveda Integrative Medicine*, 2011 Jan-Mar. reports:

> The major chemical constituent is cordycepic acid with other amino acids, vitamins and minerals. Many studies in vitro and in vivo support C. Sinensis having diverse biological activities and pharmacological potential. Its effects on renal and hepatic function and immuno-modulatory-related antitumor activities are most promising.

Cordyceps alleviates symptoms of respiratory illnesses including chronic bronchitis and asthma. Cordyceps improves heart function. Numerous studies have demonstrated the benefits of cordyceps on heart rhythm disturbances, including cardiac arrhythmias and chronic heart failure. (80.)

Excellent studies demonstrate that cordyceps helps to lower total cholesterol by 10 to 21% and triglycerides by 9 to 26%. At the same time it helps to increase HDL-cholesterol ("good cholesterol") by 27 to 30%. In addition cordyceps improves blood cells, promotes DNA repair, and protects the liver, reducing hepatitis and cirrhosis, chronic kidney diseases, and tumor size in cancer patients. Research showed chronic kidney diseases improvement of 51% after one month with cordyceps supplement. Other studies show that cordyceps improves the immune system by increasing NK natural cancer-killing cells, reduces fatigue and signs of aging. Patients reported a reduction of fatigue 92%, of feeling cold 89%, in dizziness 83%, after taking cordyceps for 30 days. Patients with respiratory/breathing problems felt physically stronger and some were able to jog for 600 ft. (*Applied*

Traditional Chinese Medicine 1993) You can learn about the successful use of cordyceps for improving sexual problems in a later chapter.

Heart Health Checkup

Do you often feel dizzy and weak? Have you had hepatitis or other liver disease such mononucleosis? Do you catch colds easily or feel weak and depressed during inclement weather? Has worry and grief weakened you? Do you huff and puff walking up stairs?

Try adding some cordyceps to your chicken soup or use capsules to improve your breathing and energy. Your recovery time after exercise or injury may improve. When energy improves your mood may lighten, your muscles and joints may feel nourished and bones stronger. You will be more able to move about freely enjoying the good life of social activities, dancing, sports and sex.

Do you bruise easily? Are you taking a blood thinning medicine? Does it irritate your stomach or give you other side-effects? Do you have black bowel movements or fresh blood in the stool indicating an ulcer? Do you have stomach or abdominal pains that go away when you eat? You may want to change your blood thinner to something safer than aspirin.

Q & A: Memory Tonic

I want an herb that strengthens the heart and improves memory and mood naturally. -- *Rhodiola Rosea extract used for centuries in Siberia and Asia fights and increases oxygen uptake. It increases ability to manage emotional stress and improves mood. It has positive effects on binge eating, cardiac health, and helps normalize serotonin levels.* http://www.absorby-ourhealth.com/product/rhodiola-rosea-extract-101-500mg-100-capsules-endurance-support/?ref=4041

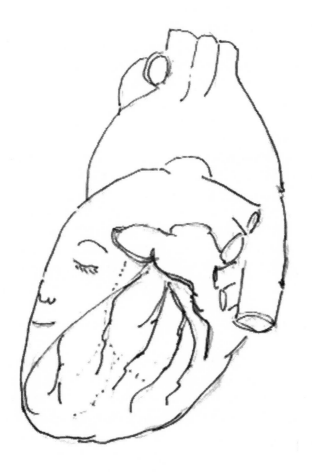

Be sure to get enough sleep

TWENTY-FOUR
CAREGIVER SURVIVAL KIT

After the doctors and hospital staff have released your patient and you are back home to the daily routine of care-giving, you and your loved one will begin to assure health. It will take all your courage and love. You, the caregiver, will need some of the healing foods and energizing herbs that I have described in this book for yourself when you ache from fatigue and suffer from anxiety, depression or frustrations. You may need a quick answer, not a pep talk or a recipe. The lastest issue of AARP magazine reports that 40 percent of the caregivers in America are men. Many of them, I suspect are new to the job and lack kitchen skills. Many are millennials. In the words of one man caregiver, "You feel so alone when its up to you to make a call and you don't know what you are supposed to do." This books gives you easy to recognize symptoms to observe daily by which you can measure progress in your healing routine. It should not substitute for the doctor, who will be called when needed, but together you and your patient can develop a comfortable rhythm in your health routine, and peace of mind.

Keeping things simple makes life easier. Care-giving can help you to organize. You might have to rely on list-making of things to do, medicines to take, or important phone numbers such as doctors, dentists, hired home nursing professionals, and financial information. But more than likely you need to find a comfortable work/rest rhythm that takes care of your patient's daily needs and offers you opportunities to regroup. If you are on your own living with your loved-one and acting as primary caregiver, at least keep track of medical appointments, important test results, current medications and heart doctor contact information.

Learn to recognize your patient's obvious signs of heart disease. There are clear, but often ignored symptoms. This book helps you to cover that territory and gives the assurance that you are on top of things. The things to watch for are not always dramatic: It may be fatigue and weakness especially swollen face, hands and feet signaling a heart problem. A sudden edema or weight gain of even a few pounds may indicate a diet too high in sodium. If it continues after adjusting diet, it is a signal to call the nurse or cardiologist. Does he/she breathe or walk with difficulty? Also possible signs of edema or congestive heart issues. Does he/she seem absent minded, for example, walk out of a store without paying? Or awaken un-refreshed by a night's sleep? These may be heart-related. Does he/she complain about digestion, headache, appear to have a jaundiced complexion or rash? It may be a reaction to diet or medications. That may be the liver complaining about medicines. If after using the natural home remedies I detail in this book fail to achieve a desired result, check with your heart specialist for advice. Is the one you care for careless about appearance or hygiene? Have they lost weight or experienced a change in mood or appetite, often signs of depression? Subtle yet effective flower essence remedies for emotional balance are covered in the chapter "A Woman's Heart." The calming, centering remedies are meant for you the caregiver as much as the patient.

Monitoring Devices

Do you work outside the home or live away from your heart patient? As Baby Boomers become seniors telecommunications companies have invented clever devices to monitor health when the caregiver is not present. According to Telecare Aware (www.telecareaware.com) people can use body sensors that measure vital signs, like heart rate and blood pressure. Cell phones can also serve a role in telecare in a variety of ways, for example by storing and transmitting vital signs, providing reminders when a measurement or medication is due, or (in phones with a global positioning device or GPS) serving as a tracking device if a person wanders away. If you feel such technology could be helpful for your loved one, a geriatric-care manager or doctor may be a resource for finding an appropriate system.

Your Feelings

On the other end of the spectrum is emotional monitoring of your own reactions. No one has invented a device for that yet. Someday Apple will invent a phone that you look into and it registers a level of emotion from 1 – 10. But for now, you have to observe yourself over time. Realize that caring for someone almost always involves caregiver frustration and guilt feelings. You may wonder, "Did I do enough? I should not feel bored, tired, out of sorts – but I do. I could slap my patient for doing this or that. I hate interference from annoying relatives or friends. I always had communication problems with my parent or partner, now it's worse. I wish this job were over. I need a break… I am getting sick from this…" The list goes on. Don't sweat it. Expect some frustrations, some rewards, and move on. Find peace and grace by creating breathing space and forgiveness for yourself. Actress Hattie McDaniel, the first black actress to win an Academy Award for her great performance as Mammy in *Gone With the Wind*, had a nice quotation about herself. "I do my best and God does the rest."

The Loving Home

The best medicine you can find is, of course, knowing that your loved one is getting better. Sharing the caring is important. Reading this book together with your patient or in a reading group may bring you closer and give you confidence that improvement is not only possible but within your grasp. Take time to breathe and stretch together, give yourself and your patient a massage and foot bath using pleasing scented oils for relaxation. Citrus essential oils lift mood and energy. Add 5 drops of an essential oil to a carrier oil such as jojoba or coconut oil and apply for an invigorating gentle massage. Essential oil of lemon relieves fatigue and sluggishness, often symptoms of a stagnant liver. Lemon also helps sharpen the memory, resolve respiratory problems, fight infection, and soothe a migraine. Lemon oil is antibacterial, antiviral, and antiseptic.

Like other citrus oils, grapefruit benefits digestion, relieves anxiety, and cleans the air. Grapefruit is particularly suited for easing the tension and mood swings of hormonal imbalance, such as PMS and menopause. Grapefruit essential oil stimulates the lymphatic system, and can help relieve water retention, and cellulite. Don't confuse grapefruit essential oil with grapefruit seed extract which is a very bitter antiviral and antifungal. Studies have shown that drinking grapefruit juice contains chemicals that can significantly interfere with the function of more than 85 pharmaceuticals. But essential oil of grapefruit does not contain these problematic compounds so you can enjoy the healing uplifting aroma without concern. Applying citrus oils can make your skin photosensitive so avoid use when spending time in the sun. I enjoy adding essential oils a mild soap and water as a floor wash for my wood floors. All these tricks for feeling better will help you both.

Here is a valuable tonic pill from the TCM tradition. It is named Aspiration for its far-reaching benefits. It can improve your spirit and ready you for the day's challenges and enable a peaceful night's sleep.

Aspiration

We aspire for a better life, with comfort and security, with the blessings of love and sharing. Aspiration polygala far-reaching herbal supplement is the name of an herbal pill remedy made by Health Concerns that is available in health food stores and online. I recommend it as a safe natural treatment for depression because the herbal combination wisely avoids side-effects. It is safe for heart patients who prefer natural treatment. It is recommended to prevent and treat depression, anxiety and their inevitable negative effects upon our digestion and vitality. To aspire for a better life we need our digestion to work properly. The digestive center is also our emotional center where we process foods and ideas. Our blood sugar and our comfort during digestion and proper elimination affect thoughts and feelings. Have you noticed how you sometimes get fed up, can't stomach something, or feel full of it? That's your digestion letting you know that you have reached your limit. Our expressions never lie.

One of the main herbs in Aspiration is polygala (yuan zhi) which has a mystical element in its history. It was used by Taoist monks who drank a tea of polygala, a bitter twig, and during sleep had visions.

There have been times when my mind was unsettled and I was unable to sleep. I chewed a couple of small bitter/sweet polygala twigs and asked myself for a dream to clarify my feelings or resolve a problem then I drifted off to sleep. Native Americans traditionally used the herb as an expectorant to treat cough and bronchitis. Polygala is used for a variety of purposes, including calming the spirit. Polygala is considered a powerful tonic herb that some say can help develop the mind and aid in creative thinking.

Polygala root is 1% methyl salicylate. The active ingredient in polygala root is a mix of triterpeonid saponins which have been studied for their benefits to the body which include calming anxiety, acting as an expectorant for people with asthma. It stimulates organs including the uterus, therefore, avoid its use during pregnancy.

Ancient beliefs held that polygala root especially improved the energy flow between the kidney and heart. If this energy connection becomes blocked, there is a loss of connection between sexual energy, i.e., our vitality and our emotions. Where does our energy most often get stuck? In our negative emotions, in our troubled digestion and labored breathing—in our center. The Taoists believed that polygala increases happiness and mental clarity. This brings us back to the caregiver. When we are split apart by the painful concern we feel in our heart for the welfare of our loved one and our lack of courage resulting from exhaustion or high emotions, we have an impasse. The connection between heart and adrenal energy is blocked so that we cannot grasp the reality of our situation. We become stuck in fear, depression, or denial.

What are the possible symptoms of these emotional troubles? Insomnia, anxiety, poor digestion with bloating and junk food addictions. Stuck liver qi gives us pain in the ribs and chest, burping, constipation, a jaundiced complexion, PMS, irritability, insomnia, troubled dreams, and difficulty staying in focus. Is your schedule too demanding to allow regular meals? Have simple, nutritious snacks--chia pudding, a boiled egg, raw celery and carrots, nuts, tea—throughout the day. If you lack courage and stamina, add a balancing tonic such as Aspiration polygala far-reaching herbal supplement.

Our digestive center is also our emotional center where we process foods and feelings.

Emergency Care-giving

Once while I was in acupuncture school during the 1980s in New York, I flew home to Albuquerque because Mother was in fragile health. She had symptoms that I feared could lead to a stroke. At her house I stayed wide awake that night in a panic pacing the floor worrying whether or not I, a student, should treat her with acupuncture. Finally I took a dose of homeopathic aconite 30C a remedy for panic, sudden high fever and severe headaches, which settled my nerves and I slept through the night. The following day I did give her a treatment and she did fine and lived 34 more years.

There are times when care-giving can be emergency care. Homeopathic remedies work quickly and well in such situations and the container of white pills can fit into your pocket. Do not mix them with medicines, foods, or beverages. I have mentioned a few useful homeopathic remedies already. You might keep them on hand. Check with a homeopathic expert whether you can use them for yourself and for your patient if your patient already uses heart drugs.

- Homeopathic Gelsemium for exhaustion, anxiety, lack of courage
- Homeopathic Pulsatilla for weeping, whining, shortness of breath with thick phlegm
- Homeopathic Cactus grandiflorus for chest pain, palpitations and arm numbness
- Homeopathic Ignatia amara for grief, anxiety, heartbreak; indecision, oversensitive and changeable moods, fear, timidity, brooding

Extend Your Horizon

How can you give yourself a break and prevent your worries from driving you nuts? Start something new and fun. I began taking a course in Mandarin Chinese and calligraphy. Sometimes late at night after everyone is asleep, I escape into a Chinese world of pleasure. You may want to take up a sport or dancing—any way you can get your body and mind free from your normal routine works well to prevent the blues. Routine dulls the mind. Doing something new and relaxing opens up new channels of communication, memory and pleasure in your brain. You and your loved-one patient may enjoy reading together or painting. Shared pleasure is always healing.

I leave the last word to my "patient" Michael who wrote this short update:

> Finally, it's spring in New York and I'm some distance from what I call my heart failure attack. It came on me with the suddenness and danger of a heart attack, though with more of a strangling feeling than acute pain. That's gone and I'm eager to walk around our neighborhood and return to the gym at the local Y. Letha and I have started doing a light version of Qigong. Still, most of my waking time is desk bound. Fortunately, I do have allies both in the prescribed meds and the supplements and herbal remedies I take daily with some precision. I am fortunate to have a loving caregiver who is also expert in Asian and alternative medicines. She knows much more about my friends, the herbs and supplements, derived from the earth and sea, grown on trees and bushes or spun off by tiny creatures. In a not very forgiving world, our hearts need all the help they can get.

Heart Health Checkup

What time of day do you feel most tired or emotionally upset? Noticing consistent periods of discomfort can help you to determine your best healing approach and remedies for comfort. Is it morning especially if you have an upset stomach or headache? Consider digestive and liver remedies. Do you wake up with pain? Consider remedies for joint (arthritis) or heart failure. Is it evening when you were most often with loved ones? Is it bedtime? Consider tonics and natural treatments for depression.

To be more specific, refer to The Traditional Chinese Meridian Clock in the following chapter to see what organ systems may be involved. It is likely that your energy will lag during mid-morning and mid-afternoon, especially if you skip breakfast. Mid-morning fatigue may point to heart weakness and mid-afternoon fatigue or 5PM wipeout results from weak adrenal energy. A tonic that addresses both heart and adrenal vitality such as ashwagandha or an herbal combination including them would be helpful. You will be surprised how effectively fatigue can be reduced by breathing and stretching, a walk around the block, a brisk shower, or a quick pickup nap.

Do you brood about your work load of care-giving? Consider engaging friends, relatives and neighbors to mutually run errands or otherwise become involved with sharing chores.

Do you feel your worries and time spent in care-giving are aging you and are too heavy a burden? Consider getting a pickup massage, body relaxing treatment, a haircut, facial, pedicure or other such treatment to change your outlook. Supplements such as Mood Enhancer Power Pack by Absorb Health can support courage and mood. http://www.absorbyourhealth.com/product/mood-enhancer-power-pack/?ref=4041

Spend time with new friends without discussing problems. Walk barefoot on the beach or in the grass to ground your energy. No beach? Then walk barefoot on a wood or stone or concrete floor.

Is your care-giving work putting your health at risk? Protect your health, mood and longevity with a combination of supplements such as Longevity Power Pack by Absorb Health. It contains Artemisinin, pterostilbene, and liposomal resveratrol. Artemisin is antiviral, pterostilbene and resveratrol fight cognitive decline and regulate cholesterol to protect the heart. http://www.absorbyourhealth.com/product/longevity-power-pack/?ref=4041

Here are wise thoughts that you might keep in mind:
- A smile is the beginning of love. Mother Theresa
- Being loved gives you strength, loving deeply gives you courage. Lao Tzu.
- The first requirement of love is to listen. German theologian Paul Tillich
- You as much as anyone deserve your love and affection. Buddha
- There are two means of refuge from the miseries of life: music and cats. --Albert Schweitzer

Part Five will help you to bring together self-observations from throughout the book so that you can craft an individual heart health routine for yourself and your loved ones.

Q & A: Anxiety, ADHD, Pain
I want something to help me to relax, take one day at a time and sleep better – *Kava and valerian, though excellent sedatives, should not be combined with alcohol or sedative drugs. One simple way to relieve anxiety, PMS, and ADHD is to use GABA a chemical that is made in the brain. It promotes lean muscle growth, burns fat, stabilizes blood pressures and relieves pain.* http://www.absorbyourhealth.com/product/gaba-3/?ref=4041

Michael's Realtime Four

Winter in the city, it's bitter cold out, and the snow left lying around in the streets looks more like grey concrete. It will melt someday or be washed away by April showers, which seem distant. I'm on a regimen of heart meds initially prescribed by my cardiologist in Vermont and seconded by my cardiologist in New York, Dr. Berdoff. Last visit, the latter gave me an "A" after the usual range of tests that included an Echocardiogram, where (thanks to Doppler ultrasound) you can see your heart bumping around on a screen. My ejection fraction (heart muscle pumping blood outward) was close to normal, and so was my diastolic function (the heart relaxing). My blood pressure remains under control (120 over 70 range), I breathe okay, Letha and I walk around Chelsea, both wearing layers of winter clothes, enjoying the neighborhood and its characters. The cardiologist seemed a bit surprised by my test results, though pleased.

Nearly all folks with heart disease, whether heart failure, post heart attack, or other, are on an accepted regimen of prescribed medications, six, eight or ten drugs is not uncommon. It's considered essential to control cholesterol, keep the arteries open, and the blood pressure down. Yet about half the patients become impatient and quit taking their meds. Why? Popping a series of pills two or three times a day can be wearing, especially if you're at work, traveling, or painting a masterpiece. You may fall victim to false confidence--"I'm okay so why should I bother?" If you don't have drug insurance, there's considerable expense. And the side effects of the drugs are a variable but crucial factor. Short term reactions to taking several drugs at a time are obvious—I get briefly dizzy and lightheaded--but what about long term side effects? Drug interactions? Your doctor may be too pressed for time to talk about the downside of drugs, but you can find out about the dangers in Letha's *Heart To Heart*.

To date, I have been prescribed eight medicinal drugs for the heart, remarkably small pills, taken regularly. Letha recommended and I am successfully taking natural substitutes for five of them. I never took nitrostat, the medical version of nitroglycerin, for an emergency. Instead, before exercise, I let three tiny pills of Suxiao Jiuxin Wan dissolve in my mouth. Tastes pleasant, and the medicinal camphor plus an herbal ingredient quickly smoothes my breathing and increases my ability to walk, work out, or even make love. Good for the Chinese!

Letha recommended, and I am using, natural substitutes for another two meds. I quit taking the most effective, and dangerous, statin, Crestor, because it caused over-all fatigue and specifically muscle pain and weakness in my legs, making it difficult to walk. Exercise is essential to keep the heart muscle pumping, so no matter what positive effect the drug induces, it's a no-go for me. I walk along the city streets, I eschew elevators and walk up flights of stairs, and there's the treadmill and other aerobic machines at the gym. Exercising and taking statin drugs simultaneously is a prescription for pain that may cause you to leave off one or the other.

Generally, the approach of cardiac drugs is negative, they prevent you from getting sicker. Statins, for example, persuade the liver not to make cholesterol, widely believed to block our arteries and *cause* heart attacks. While it is now proposed to prescribe statins more widely, including for people with only a slight risk of heart disease, the role of cholesterol is controversial. As British vascular surgeon Dr. Haroun Gajraj states, "High cholesterol has been a scapegoat for too long. Yes, it may be an indicator of heart disease but there is no evidence of a causal link." Instead, he recommends exercise (I don't do enough), weight loss (I need to), and omega 3 supplements, especially squid oil.

Cholesterol is a complicated substance made by every cell in your body, but especially your liver. Your body makes vitamin D and sex hormones from cholesterol. Your brain and nervous system depend on it. So does your digestive system. The total cholesterol number you get from testing is not predictive, and the idea of "good" and "bad" cholesterol, the hero and the villain, is too simple. Think of the cholesterol found in plaque in your troubled arteries as you would police cars at an auto accident--proof of trouble but not the cause. It's inflammation of the arterial wall that triggers the crack-up.

Statins do tend to reduce inflammation. I regularly drink what I call "Tummy tea," which Letha has described as Chinese Pu Erh tea, and I take natural statins in capsule form as found in Red Yeast Rice, easily available purchased in your health food store. Both have been used in Traditional Chinese Medicine (and Japan) at least since the Tang Dynasty (800 AD) to invigorate the body, aid in digestion, and revitalize the blood. I have felt no unwanted side effects. The FDA has on occasion attacked Red Yeast Rice products, though not because of unwarranted claims. Rather, containing lovastatin, the products do have beneficial results and therefore, says the FDA, they must be classified as a drug that needs regulation. So if it works, ban it--that's twisted bureaucratic logic. I will let the history of medical practice in half the human race, and my personal experience, determine what I ingest.

I also take capsules containing a Bergamot orange extract from a variety of the Seville orange tree that is cultivated along the coast in southern Italy. It has a number of benefits in support of cardiovascular health, which have been studied, such as producing a more flaky and less cloggy cholesterol in the blood vessels. Here is the sort of result I demand from swallowing pills: My blood sugar was way too high, one cardiologist insisting I had diabetes. Instead of taking the prescribed medicine, I resorted to cinnamon added to coffee and that product of the sunny Mediterranean, Bergamot. My blood sugar now tests normal, and I have not given up an occasional cookie!

Another replacement I have made is to drop the blood thinner aspirin because it interferes with my digestion, which is a common complaint. Instead, I take Serramend, a Health Concerns product that contains an enzyme made by the silkworm to help dissolve its cocoon when it emerges to become a caterpillar and ultimately a beautiful moth. A blood thinner, Serramend also helps relieve carpal tunnel syndrome without surgery or side effects. That's a blessing for a writer or those who work consistently with their hands. Since writing this I have added capsules of odorless aged garlic and find it to be a strong, effective blood thinner.

That's the idea: Keep the blood in your arteries flowing freely. Keep your options open.

PART FIVE

YOUR LOVING HEART

Health, Happiness and Sex

TWENTY-FIVE

A WOMAN'S HEART

It has been four years since Michael was first hospitalized with acute heart failure. I had sensed it coming a long time, had treated him with laser acupuncture for various discomforts, had urged him to lose weight, use a valuable energy tonic ashwagandha and eat fewer sweets. However, determined to put his work first, he sat at his computer days and nights. Despite my growing agitation, he insisted upon having his medical checkups follow a set schedule while ignoring his discomforts. His hospitalization was a rude awakening. Our human heart is finely tuned, it has no sympathy for mistakes as it shapes our destiny.

As caregivers we are faced with our illness that comes from worried watching. I began to write this book while Michael was recovering from what he called his "attack of heart failure." To relieve stress, I spent sleepless nights in denial chatting with friends on social networks while never referring to his illness. I barked at anyone who provoked Michael's temper. I became a mother tiger! His ex-wife, surprised about his condition, added to his concerns. When she visited us in Vermont only one week after his release from the hospital, she expected him to drive her around as usual for her vacation outings! I blew up and cried. The strong man who always got her out of jams, who had protected her pension, and catered to her whims was sick. She insisted, he yelled, she sulked, I contemplated murder. Every caregiver runs interference for their patient. You have to juggle everybody for the sake of your patient when you would rather scream. It takes a toll. This chapter may help you to deal with your own challenging physical and emotional reactions. You may be a "hot reactor" or suffer a slow death of depression. I learned from experience there is no denying feelings by pushing them down your throat.

Thanks to our love, his heart medicines, and herbs and Michael's willpower, his condition improved rapidly. I urged Michael to add natural supplements, described in this book, that worked well to improve his energy, circulation, cholesterol, and morale. I finally stopped holding my breath when his heart tests began to significantly improve. My panic left as his healthy facial color returned and he looked his handsome self. I felt more collected and safe, but predictably, with some emotional relief my body jumped into psychosomatic symptoms. Has that ever happened to you? The big problem is somewhat resolved so that you can relax but your body still knows it's not over. Unable to sleep, my blood pressure soared and my heart and hot head pounded. It was the leftover hard-wired response, the hyper-thyroid, hyper-adrenal "fight or flight syndrome" when I no longer needed it. Typical of a caregiver: Fighting his battle mentally and emotionally along with him, often times more upset than he was, I came through the war intact while my body remained battle-ready. There is a recognized medical term for this. Not only emotional Hungarians are affected.

Are You a Hot Reactor?

A "hot reactor" is someone whose heart signs such as pulse jump rapidly during a stressful situation, including a heart stress test. What can you do to manage your over-the-top physical and emotional reactions? A hot reactor may develop liverish symptoms including headache, surging hypertension, anxious mental chatter, hysteria, and rage.

People today are insulted if you call them hysterical. Hysteria is a 19th century medical term. A number of homeopathic remedies discovered during that time use the word hysteria as a symptom. But have we changed so much over time? Women traditionally were expected to stay home and care for children and parents. Today, it is common for women to work and many do not marry. Back when women were considered "the gentler sex," they may easily have developed an aching back, stiff jaw, irregular heartbeat or chest pains that we now recognize as heart symptoms. Emotional upset was called hysteria not bi-polar depression, ADHD or any number of newly named maladies. Women are still the essential caregivers, now many men as well, although the words used to describe our watchful worrying or emotional outbursts have changed.

How to Cool Emotions

When frustrated we may feel sad, angry, aggressive, and/or dizzy or develop a headache, a tight jaw, abdominal cramps, muscle spasms, liver pain, a jaundiced complexion or violent behavior. Our desires have hit the wall. Since life does not go according to plans, symptoms resembling fire surging upward in us may become chronic. We are a hot head.

Bitter Herbs: Cool and Balance Inflammation

We think of many herbs as liver cleansers or "spring tonics" because they reduce headache and jaundice, for example dandelion used as salad or dandelion root as a tea or a very bitter herb Coptis sinensis. Coptis [AKA golden thread] grows wild in northern woods in north America and Canada and is traditionally used as a spring tonic to reduce headaches, fevers, nosebleed and bleeding gums and testy behavior. Some research points to its use for menopausal hot flashes. It comes in pills. in Chinatown called huang lian. Use the herbal huang lian pills for no more than a few days. It works if your tongue is bright dark, red and you feel heat rushing to your head. You will feel cooler. Overuse may slow the thyroid or make you feel chilled or weak. Use it as needed.

Verbena [vervain] tea

Some milder tasting bitter herbs and extracts cool the liver nicely such as dandelion or skullcap, but they are not as agreeable as a soothing tea to serve to an angry or anxious person. However lemon verbena has a refreshing flavor. Verbena contains caffeic acid derivatives, flavonoids and iridoide monoterpenes which help to relax neck and shoulders. Verbena provides calming effects to the brain to help control anger. You may drink a warm cup of vervain along with your heart patient. It cools a tense moment. You may want to drink 2 to 3 cups of vervain tea daily for a couple of weeks to reduce frustration or frequent migraines. Another way to use it is as a tincture.

Depending on the person, chronic frustration may be a combination of fear, anxiety, and repressed rage so that you can't sit still and feel calm and safe. Such emotions knot up the mind and body. Cooling, bitter-tasting herbs can be used to cool the hot aspects of troubling emotions.

Sarpagandha [Indian snake root, *Rauwolfia serpentina* root]

When you are ready to hit the wall from rage or hypertension rauwolfia is a very bitter Ayurvedic herb that has been used for over 4,000 years in Asia. It became known in north America during the 1940s as a treatment for hypertension in people who tend to be irritable, strong and muscular--not weak, timid, or depressed. It works in small doses for "hot reactors." You can find rauwolfia capsules in your health food store and online. In India, where it is called sarpagandha, the herb is used to treat what they call "insanity and hysteria," also hypertension and itchy rash. It is strongly anti-inflammatory and is, therefore, not advised for women who are or who plan to become pregnant. Online find capsules and liquid extracts of this mind-mellowing herb: The capsules are easier to swallow than the extremely bitter tincture. Follow directions as needed. When feeling upset and hot headed you might add up to 5 drops of the liquid extract to water. It lowers blood pressure fast and I suspect it reduces a hyper-adrenal imbalance. It makes you feel mellow not driven or anxious.

The constituent in rauwolfia that helps lower high blood pressure is reserpine, an alkaloid substance with powerful sedative effect found in the root. This herb is occasionally useful for people who become hyper-adrenal "hot reactors" and insomniac when stressed. Do you speed up instead of slowing down when tired and upset? Does your tongue become sharp and mental focus a bit too keen? Rauwolfia helps stop the hot reactions resulting from adrenal hormones. Heart patients should use it with care and with the supervision of a professional. It may increase the action of a beta blocker heart drug. For helping to control hypertension the Mayo Clinic recommends this dosage for rauwolfia: Adults—50 to 200 milligrams (mg) a day taken as a single dose or divided into two doses.

This chapter can show you how to cool mind- and spirit-damaging inflammation, how to cool your hot reactor. However, the following herb helps to quiet your nerves, ease anxiety and improve back and leg aches and sleep.

Valerian, grounding and calming

Valerian root smells like a wet forest and rich soil musty from autumn leaves. It is bitter-sweet, dank, earthy. In the chapter on insomnia I warned against using strong sedatives for heart patients. However for the harried, otherwise healthy, caregiver given to intense emotions and hyper-adrenal insomnia, valerian can be very soothing. According to the University of Maryland Medical Center, scientists believe that valerian root increases the concentration of GABA in the brain. (GABA is a neurotransmitter, a molecule the cells in the brain and nervous system use to communicate with each other. GABA capsules have a calming effect on the nervous system to reduce physical symptoms of anxiety and has also been found to increase Human Growth Hormone release.)

Because of its calming effect, valerian can help lower blood pressure, in particular when related to stress. It acts as a nervous system sedative. However, I do not recommend it for overweight, sedentary heart failure patients. Some new cardiologists recommend taking valerian along with grape seed extract to control hypertension. Avoid combining valerian with sedatives or alcohol. It relaxes the uterus muscles and should be avoided by pregnant and nursing women. This trick may help you to decide whether or not valerian is for you. Smell it. If the aroma is relaxing and pleasant, you might try 500 mgs in capsules or take it as a tea. The recommended dose for reducing hypertension is 500 mgs once or twice daily.

Difficult situations and self-doubts

Sometimes going for a walk or calling a friend works to refresh your "milk of human kindness." Other times you may need targeted support for wellbeing. The best natural treatment for dealing with a pain-in-the-neck situation depends on your particular reaction to it. That's where your self-observations come in handy. The following sensitive remedies may be just the thing you need.

Bach Flower Remedies

Bach Flower remedies are subtle so you may need to use one or more throughout the day. They are aimed to bring about emotional balance so they work on a different level than an herb or food. They are not digested the same way as an herb. In a sense we incorporate the positive energy of the plant when using the remedy. See the list of emotional responses that are treatable with the Bach Flower remedies. (82.)

Each of the 38 flower remedies discovered by Dr Bach is directed at a particular characteristic or emotional state. It is very difficult to be objective because we tend to be over-critical or over-generous about our emotions. So think about how you typically react in your particular stressful situation without making a judgment. If you choose the wrong remedy, it will do no harm but will not alleviate your stress. Answer this question: How do you feel when you are with that person? How do you feel about that person or situation? How do you react? If you don't have a clue, there is a company in California that has prepared a questionnaire to help you choose your best Bach Flower Remed(ies) at this web address: http://feelbach.com/qti.asp You can look up the remedy for more information in the note (82.) at the back of the book.

I found that treating my tendency to be impatient helped me to deal with tense family encounters. The Bach Flower remedy Beech is recommended to "help you to be more tolerant and see the positive in others despite their imperfections." A few drops under the tongue as directed takes some of the heat out of hot reactor situations. You may need something stronger than Beech such as Bach Flower remedy Holly recommended to help overcome your pains of rage and hatred. It is liver-cooling. There are about four hundred varieties of holly. Mao Dung Qing (holly) a capsule is used as a Chinese herb to improve heart action and reduce cholesterol, but its use is limited to one week because over time it can become toxic. However, Holly, the Bach Flower remedy recommended for strong negative emotions, feels calming, may improve sleep and temporarily lower high blood pressure. It is not toxic. Calm is not the opposite of hate: Love is, compassion is. That process of understanding and acceptance may be helped along with Bach's Holly by giving us a moment of peace in order to examine our motives and develop emotional strength.

You may require a remedy to help overcome feelings of hopelessness, self-blame or self-pity as described by Dr. Bach. If you can alleviate your caregiver stress as much as possible you can remain free to help yourself and your patient. At times the burden of care-giving may feel like a heavy weight to bear. As days and weeks wear on, many who care for others fall into addictions, dark moods, and exhaustion. Do you lose yourself in daydreams, or gorge yourself with cookies or ice cream? After a twelve hour shift of nursing work do you fall into bed unable to move? Do you gain weight just thinking about snacks? Do you consume comfort foods to quell stress? Are they rich, sweet and satisfying? The price to pay is added fat and low vitality which adds up to heart trouble.

Here is something we never realize: We hold negative emotions in our fat. Belly fat has been called a stress fat because it is different from fat in other areas of the body. Stress hormones increase belly fat. Each cell contains water. The number of fat cells in our body does not alter when we lose excess weight, however excess lymph and fluids containing toxins may be reduced so that the size of each fat cell decreases. Your waistline and mood can improve with an energizing treatment such as radio frequency slimming treatments that reduce triglycerides and ,therefore, protect your heart. Each time I give a middle slimming treatment using my radio frequency and cavitation machine to one of my overweight health/beauty clients, they feel energized and positive from enhanced circulation. The slimming results are noticeable over time. Also see my book *Feed Your Tiger* for health-supporting slimming herbs, supplements and recipes. Remember: The larger the waistline the shorter the lifeline.

Honor a Goddess

Saraswati churna is an Ayurvedic herbal powder named after the Indian goddess of culture, learning, beauty and art. She plays the veena, a lovely, graceful string instrument, and near her sits a pure white swan. Saraswati herbal powder (churna) is the perfect remedy for the mopey feeling that comes on drowsy gray days of rain, a heavy, achy feeling that comes with edema and depression. The ingredients ginger and pepper warm the dietary source of intelligence and memory–our middle, our digestion. Ashwagandha is added to enhance adrenal energy and courage. Calamus root is added to calm nerve pain and nervous irritability. The powder, available in Indian herbs shops and online, is soothing, grounding, warming, energizing the higher intelligence.

Ayurvedic doctors recognize the effects of humid weather, rich foods that are sweet and heavy, and low vitality leading to overweight, sinus and breathing congestion and depression. They call it Kapha. Excess Kapha leads to body fat, fibroid masses, congestion, confusion, low spirits. The pepper and ginger in Saraswati churna warm and dry Kapha and revitalize digestion. Add up to ½ tsp of Saraswati churna to green tea. If you are sensitive to herbs, add a pinch to your tea, apple sauce or yogurt. Used over time it is said to improve intelligence and memory as it reconditions the nervous system.

Distract Anxiety/Depression

Faced with a mental demon one practical approach is to distract it. Put your energy and attention elsewhere. You might gong your Tibetan singing bowl which is made of seven metals and emits a lovely ethereal tone when struck. You might take a shower and wash your hair. I know a world famous beauty stylist, Gad Cohen, who recommends regularly cutting hair because he says we store emotions in our hair. A nice cooling rinse or hair oil can temper a bad mood. I once asked a class I was teaching what suggestions students had for improving mood. One woman replied, "When I am obsessing about something I ask myself, 'Who is thinking?' or I ask myself, 'What is my next thought?'"

Another way to change a bad mood is to laugh at a comic movie or television program–good medicine for your patient and you. From comedy royalty, Lucille Ball, we have this advice, "One of the things I learned the hard way was that it doesn't pay to get discouraged.

Keeping busy and making optimism a way of life can restore your faith in yourself."

Heart Health Check-up

What time of day are you most tired or feel out of sorts? Four thousand years ago, Chinese herbal doctors realized that since Qi energy circulates throughout the body in a predictable manner, acupuncture meridians and associated organs are full or empty of Qi energy, call it vitality, at given times of day and night. If you consulted a traditionally trained Chinese doctor and complained of symptoms that repeated at regular times the doctor would realize that certain organ systems were involved and would choose treatments suited to heal that energetic system. For example, do you feel tired and down-hearted at one of these times?

The Traditional Chinese Meridian Clock

Mid-morning around 10AM to 1PM – Heart energy, circulation and emotional balance

From 1 – 2PM in afternoon – small intestine, ability to think and decide clearly, digest properly

From 3 – 5PM in afternoon – Bladder energy, urinary health, bones

From 5 – 7 PM Kidney/adrenal vitality and longevity, endurance, memory, vitality, courage, back pain, sexual and hormonal health

From 9 – 11 PM at night – pericardium, chest pain, circulation, internal balance and body temperature control

From 11PM to 3AM – Liver and gallbladder health, nerves, muscles, vision

From 3 AM to 7AM – Lungs/large intestine, breathing, elimination

From 7Am to 9AM - Stomach and spleen/pancreas, digestion, assimilation

Knowing when organ systems are most active enables you to maximize your physical activities and diet. You are healthiest when the circulation of energy within your body is harmonious, so planning meals and rest around key organ activity can help balance energy from the inside out more effectively. For example, the liver is most active between 1 and 3 AM. It is when your body is detoxifying, eliminating what it no longer needs, and refreshing your supply of blood while you are most likely sleeping. It is not a good time to eat rich foods and alcohol. Kidneys do their most intensive reconditioning work from 5 to7 PM so it's best to have a light dinner including greens and avoid foods that are high in fat, sugar and salt. This will help lessen the burden on health during peak activity.

Are you very tired, do you grab a stimulant in that time frame (5 to 7PM?) That indicates your adrenal vitality is weak and you may benefit from rejuvenation herbs aimed at enhancing endurance. For example ashwagandha. See the chapter on tonics. Are you wide awake working or fretting at 2 or 3AM? Your liver, blood, muscles, and vision, need rejuvenating herbal support to avoid inflammation and exhaustion. Why is it that most heart attacks occur during early morning? Our adrenal energy is lacking and we are burdened with water retention from lying asleep all night. Taking steps for prevention can save you.

Q & A: Mood and Concentration

I want to improve my energy, mood and concentration. *An amino acid found in green tea, L-theanine has been found to increase relaxation and improve mood without causing sedation. It reduces cortisol, the stress hormone, and improves attention span in people with mild cognitive impairment. No time for tea? Take L-theanine in a pill* http://www.absorby-ourhealth.com/product/l-theanine-200mg-100-capsules-relaxation-support/?ref=4041

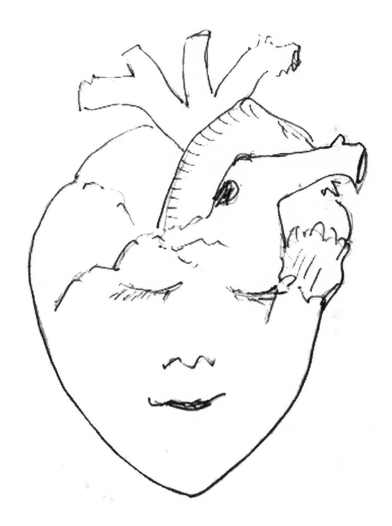

Lub-dub, Lub-dub, my Lub!

TWENTY-SIX

YOUR HEART AND SEX

You or your lover has a chronic heart condition or has had a heart incident resulting in a doctor or hospital visit. When is it safe to resume sexual activity? Most medical authorities advise that sex can resume when you feel strong enough and that is often within a few weeks of a heart attack. But sexual activity is not only sex. There are also kissing, hugging and affectionate words that we hope never stop. An affectionate smile, a gentle touch are glue that holds lovers together and abates fear. I am sure our loving sexual life kept Michael alive and active to age 80. We were never "buddies" or "pals" but had a very strong attraction. That spark of desire for the lover, your other half, brings a vital craving for life, love and wellness. Sex is a good measure of a loving relationship. It counts for more than most of us realize because sexual energy measures survival Qi. For men low sexual energy, the inability to achieve erection, has been linked to chronic heart failure. Blood is not flowing where needed either because it is blocked somewhere in congested blood vessels or because the heart is not strong enough.

The term erectile dysfunction is coldly scientific and impotence sounds pejorative. The outdated term formerly used for women, frigidity, is absurd. Physically or emotionally exhausted women may feel vulnerable, irritable or sleepy, not frozen. Let's get our head out of the laboratory refrigerator. Sexuality is an energy like everything else. It flows through meridians, is dependent upon nutrition, emotional comfort and fitness.

Unfortunately, quite a number of medicines are known to reduce libido and sexual capacity such as anti-depressant drugs, drugs for diabetes, hair loss, prostate issues, and heart troubles. The drugs may include serotonin reuptake inhibitors, tricyclic antidepressants, birth control pills, Proscar used for prostate swelling, Propecia used for male hair loss, antihistamines, medical marijuana, and anti-seizure drugs. Certain opioid pain-killers such as Vicodin, OxyContin, and Percocet lower testosterone.

Beta blockers especially damage sexuality. Tens of millions of Americans use beta blockers such as propranolol and metoprolol to benefit their heart to the detriment of t their sex life. In some cases, even eye drops containing the beta blocker Timolol, used to treat glaucoma, can decrease libido. Benzodiazepines, anti-anxiety drugs like Xanax, lower sex drive. Fortunately, you can add the following natural foods and herbal sexual tonics in most cases with no fear of discomfort. As an added benefit the remedy may ease anxiety.

Libido and the Heart

How important is libido anyway? Old school psychoanalysts described libido as the energy of the sexual drive as a component of our life instinct. Although we do not follow narrow prescriptions for sexual normality laid down by Freud, it is significant to see, from a psychoanalytic perspective, the role of sexual desire for self-preservation. Traditional Chinese medicine goes much further. It places sexual desire and capacity in the sphere of the Water Element comprised energetically of the kidney and adrenal energy and hormone-balance and their meridians. The emotional correlative is courage.

Life force and longevity, according to early Chinese doctor/ philosophers, is inherited, finite and measured as *jing*. *Jing* has been called "the essence of life" and "original Qi" our inherited vitality. Imagine someone with reduced *jing*—aged sooner than their years: stooped from bone deformity, with bleeding gum disease and loose teeth, thinning hair, scattered thinking, low intelligence, chronic inflammation, urinary incontinence, and long term irritability or low enthusiasm from depression. How did she get that way?

According to the Chinese, our *Jing* is endangered by illness, age, drugs, and excess sexual activity that leaves vitality exhausted. Then health problems result from premature aging and hormonal imbalance. So TCM gives us not only the causes but some possible results of sexual exhaustion. No wonder *jing* tonics make up an important part of Chinese medicine most often combining herbs to restore blood, qi energy, and hormone balance. Placenta, considered a potent *jing* restorative, has problems. Whose placenta was it? Human or sheep? And from where? You can order online sheep placenta capsules from the United States or New Zealand. It is rich in rejuvenating nutrients and is estrogenic which poses problems for certain cancers. Some *jing* restorative remedies include qi tonics such as cordyceps, astragalus, codonopsis, eucommia, cornus combined with blood tonics such as rehmannia and asparagus. The Qi tonics restore immunity and testosterone for drive and endurance, the blood tonics protect organ tissue and restore hormones and moisture for skin, hair and sexual fluids. In a word they rejuvenate.

Sex and Life Force

Why in a heart health book should I address sexual vitality? Because sexuality is part of life, love and longevity. Energetically speaking when we increase adrenal (sexual) energy we also support heart health. Western scientists agree there is a vital connection between the adrenal cortex and brain that supports circulation and maintains life. Recent studies have shown that men who have adequate testosterone have less heart disease. That said, there is another reason why sexual tonics have been used for centuries. Holistic medicine recognizes the interdependence of hormones, muscle strength, heart action and circulation. It all works together. Desire is not floating above the body in a castle, it motivates action.

How can we enhance libido and sexual capacity without raising blood pressure? Minerals are important for heart health especially calcium, zinc, boron, selenium and magnesium among others. Magnesium stands out as a shining star because it helps us utilize calcium and it dilates arteries, therefore, lowering blood pressure. In this chapter we find valuable herbal sexual tonics that are safe for most people such as maca and damiana providing natural sexual hormones for men and women. Several other popular sexual remedies covered later in the chapter require either special care or should not be combined with medicines.

Maca a safe hormone balancer

Maca is a yam from Peru that is available in powdered form and capsules in health food stores and online. In the high mountains it is eaten as a daily food. A sexual tonic, it is a hormone regulator used to increase libido and fertility. If you need more estrogen or testosterone because of age or other factors, by taking maca your body will make more of what you need. Adults over age 40 tend to have reduced sexual hormones. Maca brings us back up to a health quotient we need and the hormone is not synthetic. It is made by your body.

Maca has been used to increase muscle strength, libido, and endurance. Maca belongs to the radish family and has been called "Peruvian ginseng." There are no serious known side effects of maca, but like any other supplement it should not be taken in too large amounts. When you first start using maca, it's best to begin by taking smaller amounts and building up; even ½ teaspoon of the powder daily is a good place to start. Later 1 teaspoon to 1 tablespoon of the powder is an average daily dose added to smoothies or soups. Don't add it to very hot, boiling liquids because that stops its actions. Rotating a few days on and a few days off is often recommended. Taking too much at a time could throw your hormones into high gear with resulting side-effects. Increasing testosterone my raise blood pressure. If you experience this, you should take less or wean yourself off completely.

Maca's overall benefits include a source of valuable nutrients, for example the B vitamins, C, and E. It provides plenty of calcium, potassium, zinc, iron, magnesium, phosphorous and amino acids. Maca may relieve menopausal issues. It alleviates cramps, body pain, anxiety, mood swings, and depression. If you are pregnant or lactating you should avoid taking maca. Within days of using maca your energy level and stamina may increase. Athletes take maca for peak performance. If you find yourself tired most of the time, experiment with maca to see if it helps. Maca supplies iron and helps restore red blood cells, which aids anemia and cardiovascular diseases. When used in conjunction with a wise diet and good workout regime you will notice an increase in muscle mass.

Foods used for endurance by people living in harsh weather conditions and high mountains have been used to build stamina for those of us living with city stress. For example chia seeds and maca.

If you are overcome with anxiety, stress, depression or mood swings, maca may help alleviate these symptoms. Some people have reported an increase in mental energy and focus, but that may be due to maca's high nutrition and hormone balancing effects. Be very cautious if you have a cancer related to hormones like testicular and ovarian cancer, among others. If you have liver issues or high blood pressure you should consult your doctor before using maca.

Damiana

Turnera diffusa, sometimes called Turnera aphrodisiaca, is a shrub native to the southwestern United States, Central America, Mexico, South America, and the Caribbean. Some people use it to reduce anxiety and increase circulation in the sexual area. It can act as an aphrodisiac for some people. Medical sources list its uses as a treatment for headache, bedwetting, depression, nervous stomach and constipation; for prevention and treatment of sexual problems; boosting and maintaining mental and physical stamina; and as an aphrodisiac. Damiana contains chemicals that may affect the brain and nervous system.

Damiana is useful for every day anxiety, depression, low energy and diabetes. Damiana might decrease blood sugar. Medical sources warn that taking damiana along with diabetes medications might cause blood sugar to drop too low. Monitor your blood sugar closely. The dose of your diabetes medication may need to be adjusted. This is a good thing. Maya Indians used damiana to treat asthma, dizziness, vertigo, and as a body cleanser. In Mexico it is used primarily to treat female problems as an excellent restorative for the reproductive organs. For women with menopause it controls hot flashes. It is known to raise the sperm count in men. With regular use the effects become stronger increasing potency for men and regulating hormones for women.

In case you want to make a damiana liquor, mix 30 grams (1 oz. or two heaping tablespoons) of dried damiana herb with 1/2 liter of vodka and let this soak for 5 days to two weeks. Sift this and let the alcohol drenched leaves soak another 5 days in 125 ml (1/2 cup) of mineral water. Strain out the herbal liquid and filter it. Heat the water extract until just under the boiling-point and mix it with 1/2 of raw honey. Mix the alcohol extract and the water extract in a bottle and keep for a month. The mix will sink down and the liquid will become clear. Pour the liquid carefully in a clean bottle. For the best results take up to 1 glass in the evening at least two hours after dinner.

A sorter version is to do only the first step, which is to steep the dried herb in vodka to make an alcohol extract. In that case the dose is only 5 -10 drops added to water.

Note: Damiana (Turnera diffusa) raises happy brain chemicals while relaxing muscles on the prostate. Don't combine it with alpha-blocking drugs like Remeron (mirtazapine), Hytrin (terazosin) or Flomax, or Cardura (doxazosin).

Sexual Tonics: Side-effects, Drug Interactions

This is a warning: If you are taking heart medicines the following sexual stimulant herbs may have interactions that you and your health provider need to be aware of. Some sexual stimulants raise blood pressure or interfere with the action of heart drugs. Herbs that increase testosterone may result in headache, acne or fibroids in women. They should be avoided completely by men at risk of prostate cancer.

Yohimbe dilates arteries so it increases blood flow, but it may raise blood pressure to dangerous levels or cause an erection that lasts for hours. It should not be mixed with alcohol or anti-depressant medications and it may increase high anxiety or negative emotions or suicidal tendencies.

L-Arginine an amino acid helps create nitric oxide which improves blood flow to the heart and nether regions in both men and women. But you need to take massive doses of more than 8 grams to have any effects. Important: L-Arginine is not recommended to be combined with many commonly prescribed heart medicines.

Tribulus terrestris (known as gokshura in India) a desert weed, boosts testosterone so it sparks desire and improves performance in the bedroom and gym. Gokshura supports a healthy urino-genital system, protecting the kidney and prostate for men and tones the uterus for women. It protects and feeds the nervous system and is an all around good sexual tonic as well as a diuretic.

Eleuthero, Panax or Korean ginsengs relax muscles in the penis like Viagra does, and ease fatigue in both men and women. Raw Tienchi ginseng (notoginseng) and steamed tienchi are heart tonics. The raw form thins the blood so be careful with anticoagulants (ie warfarin, Plavix, ginger, ginkgo, aspirin, etc).

Saw Palmetto (Serenoa repens) relieves prostate symptoms such as weak stream, night urges to urinate and may improve libido.

DHEA, sometimes called The 'fountain of youth' supplement, may boost sex drive in men and women, and ease erectile problems, but too much may make the body stop making its own DHEA. Many experts recommend that people over 40 can safely take about 50 mgs daily not more.

Horny Goat Weed (Epimedium, known as yin yang huo in TCM (Chinese: 淫羊藿) has been used to get farm animals aroused encouraging reproduction. It increases testosterone and is used in TCM combined with other herbs to reduce chronic pain caused by age and cold weather.

Herbal Combinations for enhanced sexuality

Is there an easily available over-the-counter sexual tonic that is safe and effective? Here are several. The choice depends on your qi and blood. If you most often feel chilled, weak and have a pale tongue, if you avoid cold weather and raw foods, if, as a man over 40, you are too soft around the waistline, or have enlarged breasts, baring illness, you may benefit from additional testosterone.

One remedy that provides testosterone herbs is not a snake although it is called Python or Python Extra available at Vitamin Shoppe. Recommended to improve male sexual performance, the pills come with a warning. (83.) for inflammatory side effects such as rapid heart beat, dizziness and blurry vision. They may be due to increased testosterone, dehydration, and hormonal changes. Python includes eleuthero and Korean red ginseng, a trace of guarana extract (caffeine) and 500mg of tribulus. You can tell right away if the herbal combination does not agree with you. You may feel a headache or leg muscle pain. Sometimes reducing the dose is enough to correct this.

Some user reviews recommend taking one pill daily or alternating one day on one day off to get used to ease the positive effects.

Python Extra pills is the same formula as Python but has an additional heart herb 200 mg of Rhodiola [AKA arctic root.] If you are taking heart medicines and have been forbidden by your doctor to use herbal stimulants such as hawthorn, it would be wise to avoid rhodiola and, therefore, Python Extra. TCM uses rhodiola, (called hong jing tien,) for weak heart muscles and reduced circulation. Regular use is thought to improve intelligence and memory. That makes sense when you consider the role of blood circulation for brain function. Hong jing tien wine is a popular home made herbal liquor enjoyed during cold weather after dinner in China. I make my own by steeping the dried herb, which resembled tree bark, in vodka. It tastes pleasantly sweet and feels warming in cold weather. Unlike Python, heart tonic rhodiola can easily be used by men and women.

Sexual Rejuvenation Treatments

Although testosterone replacement therapy is available, it is expensive and can have serious detrimental side effects. Many men have instead looked to natural, herbal therapies. Eurycoma longifolia jack, also known as Malaysian ginseng or tongkat ali, is an herb native to the Malaysian rain forests. Like many other exotic plants, tongkat ali is popular in traditional medicine its primary use being to promote healthy libido and normal hormone levels in men. Its popular name in Thai "Ali's cane" conjures up a pleasant image. It is said to be an effective sexual tonic that increases sperm mobility but does not raise blood pressure. Another popular stimulating sexual tonic that supports testosterone is called PriMale. Please see the Resource Guide at the back of the book for links.

Testosterone herbs are rejuvenating when we need testosterone. Otherwise, the following herbs offer great additional benefits. The following sexual rejuvenation herbs help to rejuvenate sexual tissue damaged by age, dehydration from illness, diet or lifestyle, or early menopause.

Ashwagandha

Ayurvedic doctors value ashwagandha and shatavari for men's and women's sexuality. Ashwagandha is an excellent adrenal tonic for muscle strength, vigor and memory I mentioned in an earlier chapter. A researcher Dr. Prashanti writes about ashwagandha, "Because Ashwagandha is androgenic it naturally supports the vigorous strength that is one of the many facets of masculinity. And because it is one of the best herbs to re-build the strength and capacity of nerves, while being one of the strongest of the anti-stress adaptogens, it can profoundly support a stable calm whose foundation goes to your very cells." (84.)

Shatavari

Shatavari, a wild asparagus from India, is considered a woman's herb for rejuvenating sexuality by increasing female hormones and natural fluids to protect a fragile, sensitive vagina challenged by age, illness, or surgery. It has also found its way into numerous male sexuality formulas. Like ashwagandha, in men, it can increase testosterone, semen count, seminal fructose content, erection indexes, and much more. Shatavari is imbued with phytoecdysteroids that can mimic hormones and sapogenins to ease aging discomforts. Shatavari and ashwagandha support sexual arousal and ability in men and women. Men can use twice the amount of ashwagandha and women twice the amount of shatavari. There are so many sexual tonics to choose from that you may enjoy experimenting to see which work best. Let your heart doctor know that you are supplementing hormones and sexual energy n case they may interfere with our medicines. Some of the best hospitals, as well as independent researchers, are studying sexual tonics as a source of supportive heart treatments. In addition, I have noticed that using ashwagandha and shatavari together supports the strength of muscles, nerves and bones for enhanced physical endurance and may even help prevent osteoporosis.

An Unexpected Problem

You or your sexual partner with a heart condition have plenty of health issues to observe and medicines to take without worrying about sexual comfort. You are not likely to hear from the doctor or media about deflating sexual side-effects of heart drugs. The doctor's business is to prevent the patient from dying. Consequently, heart doctors pay little attention to a patient's sex life and less attention to the discomforts experienced by the patient's sexual partner. That means *you* if you are the wife/husband care-giver. You can easily develop a terrible yeast infection with painful vaginal sores or worse just from having sex with your heart patient who is taking a ton load of medicines or who eats lots of sugar.

What is the answer? Your heart patient lover most likely already has drug side-effects such as dizziness, memory loss, muscle aches, or diabetes without thinking about what happens to you in bed. And you certainly don't want to compromise your lover's health with a yeast infection. The sexual health certainly affects a loving relationship.

Candida yeast home cures

A yeast infection can develop for an otherwise healthy person after using birth control pills, antibiotics, after stress and surgery and after having sex with someone who has candida a yeast infection. Yeast symptoms may include uncomfortable abdominal bloating and digestive problems, hormone irregularities, a vaginal discharge that is thick white or yellow or odorous and in advanced or systemic cases vaginal sores, pain with sex, infertility or in rare cases death. Candida in the mouth, called thrush, is a common problem with people taking heavy doses of antibiotics such as HIV patients. The yeast is always present and can overtake the body when healthy gut bacteria is compromised.

A simple method for sexual comfort and protection against developing vaginal yeast sores is my yogurt method. Before sex insert with a clean finger ¼ teaspoon of plain yogurt into the vagina. It feels cooling, moistening and supports your healthy bacteria so that yeast cannot grow. If you do develop a yeast infection use this method for three nights in a row wearing a protective pad to catch the discharge.

Another useful approach is to use a homeopathic candida pill and suppository as directed to kill the yeast. For example, Yeast Gard homeopathic pills and vaginal suppositories made for Lake Consumer Products Inc. As the yeast is dying off you may experience temporary headache, cramps, or other slight discomforts. You may experience strong sugar cravings, your body's attempt to keep the yeast growth intact.

While we are discussing sexual matters, how about the issue of sexual satisfaction? It is a heart to heart topic. A heart patient may be too scared by his/her condition to try for sexual satisfaction beyond hugging and kissing. You as caregiver may be distracted by anxiety over your lover's health so that your satisfaction flies out the window. You may feel frustrated loving an "invalid." Your love has matured over time and brought changes in tempo and needs. Try to find comfort in all the affectionate things you do for each other, the kind words and warm caresses you share. You might satisfy a sexual itch with a personal method. Each orgasm a woman achieves increases her natural estrogen production which saves our bones, joints, muscle tone and mood. Take the pressure to perform out of sex. Enjoy the healing warmth of loving affection without stress.

Heart Health Checkup

When was the last time you really wanted to have sex?
Does your mind wander or are you distracted by outside events during sex?
Do you feel tired or refreshed after sex?
Are you frightened by your heart patient spouse's condition?
Do you spend time hugging, kisses, and otherwise preparing for sex?
Do you take care of your appearance and sex appeal?
Do you or your partner need help to develop libido or sexual stamina?

A general tonic combination such as ashwagandha and shatavari not only supports hormones, endurance and sexual moisture, such herbs also calm nervous tension and gradually build overall vitality.

If you or your partner plan to use a natural sexual tonic such as those described in this chapter, discuss with your heart specialist if you are ready for sex and if there are any limitations. Happiness, comfort and compatibility are the beginning and end of sexual love.

Q & A: Sexual Tonics

I want a male sexual tonic that is safe for my heart. -- *An Ayuverdic herb that has traditionally been used for enhancing male sexual health, Tribulus Terrestris displays a wide range of health benefits. It increases androgen receptor density in the brain, which may be responsible for its effects on libido. A component of tribulus, tribulosin, appears to be potently cardioprotective, and Tribulus Terrestris has also shown the ability to protect the liver and kidneys from oxidative damage.* http://www.absorbyourhealth.com/product/tribulus-terrestris-40-saponins-500mg-100-capsules-hormonal-support/?ref=4041

I want a rejuvenation tonic that protects the prostate and is rejuvenating for men and women. *Fo- Ti is a libido enhancer and longevity promoter. It is very high in zinc, which is essential for proper sexual functioning.* http://www.absorbyourhealth.com/product/fo-ti-ho-shou-wu-500mg-100-capsules-powerful-51-extract-anti-aging-sexual-health-supplement/?ref=4041

TWENTY-SEVEN

YOUR HEART-SAVING ROUTINE

This chapter does not substitute for medical testing or regular checkups with your doctor. However it will help you to organize your and your patient's self-observations gleaned from Heart Health Checkups in this book in the effort to avoid illness and mend common heart conditions. It includes several sections. The Symptoms Key contains typical heart-related discomforts, their associated health problems and possible treatment options. Another section contains possible additions and substitutions for certain medical drugs pertaining to heart health. There is a section covering diets, teas, and herbs and a section for body treatments that apply to your heart issues. Finally there is a checklist of remedies to keep at your bedside, in your desk, car and pocket. This chapter enlarges your possibilities for the care of yourself and loved ones. It is, at least, a good beginning step toward creating educated independence and vibrant health.

The Symptoms Key

Symptom(s)	Possible Problems	Possible Solutions	See Chapter(s)
Swollen face, hands, ankles; Shortness of breath	Drug allergy, Edema due to sodium in diet, heart failure	Reduce daily sodium intake; Diuretic tea; Get medical checkup	Chapter 2, Part Two

Chest pain in center of chest or arms: Abdominal pain: Jaw or shoulder pain	Emotional upset; Indigestion, Heart disease -- Important: If severe. lasting chest/arm pain get medical help immediately	For prevention: Reduce caffeine, alcohol; Breathe & stretch; Digestive herbs, teas; Treatments for circulation; A homeopathic remedy for emotional balance; Detoxification, Reduce LDL cholesterol and inflammation	Chapters 1-3, 7, 14, 17 – 24
Fatigue, weakness	Poor diet; Depression; Aging	Improve diet; Exercise; Herbal tonics	Chapters 1, 3, 10, 11, Part Three, Chapters 21 – 24
Fever, aches, nasal congestion, sore throat, weakness, chills from respiratory infection	Colds and Flu	Bed rest; Herbal teas; Antibiotic herbs for sore throat, fever, respiratory infection, phlegm; (follow-up with Serramend and herbs for asthma	Chapters 1, 5, 6, 8, 21, 23
Low sexual energy and drive	Diabetes, Heart medicines, Weakness, Aging, Fear of heart troubles	Alternative treatments for blood sugar and heart disease; Herbal tonics to slow aging; Sexual tonics for hormone balance; Stress reduction meditation, yoga, tai chi, massage	Special Alert: What doctors don't tell you; Chapters 1, 10, 17, 22, 26

Super-germ infections (MRSA etc)	Poor hygiene, Exposure during dental work, hospitalization, public places	Insist on cleanliness at home, office and hospital; Carry hand wipes; Colloidal silver and herbs to build immunity	Chapters 1, 6, 16
Aching legs, swollen veins, numbness, broken capillaries, varicose veins; poor circulation, vision impairment, retina damage	Unhealthy fats, congesting foods, inflammatory diet; Diabetes, PAD, Plaque build-up; Liver-inflammation; Hypertension; Lack of exercise	Support stockings; Herbs for diabetes, circulation; Anti-inflammatory liver-cleansing herbs, lymph cleansing	Chapters 1, 2, 4, 8-19, 22, 23
Headaches, allergies, bad temper	Liver congestion; Medications; Food allergies, Frustration, Fatigue	Check for dietary pain-triggers; Liver-cleansing herbs and green foods and teas; Calming treatments	Chapters 1, 3, 8, 12, 13, 19, 21, 22
Care-giver burnout	Overwork, Worry; Poor scheduling; Overuse of stimulants; Guilt, frustration, anger, depression	Create escape times and activities; Herbal tonics; Detoxify negative emotions with diet, herbs, Exercise, Body treatments, Sleep	Chapters, 1, 3, 5, 7, 10-13, 19-27

That should give you a general idea of helpful chapters in this book that you can use for study and for future reference. Now for a more detailed look at individual needs, go back to the ending of each chapter to see how you answered my questions in the **Heart Health Checkup**. If you are the caregiver, answer the questions for your patient. Have you tried some of the suggestions that I offered in response to your observations? Have you noticed any change in symptoms, feelings, discomforts since using those recommended treatments? If you haven't tried the suggestions yet, it is a good time to start.

I summarize the **Heart Health Checkup** observations in this section to help you identify your most pressing heart problems (and those of your patient) so that you are better able to follow-up with health professionals and try natural treatments.

Summary of Heart Health Checkup Observations

1. Page 44: The first chapter offers ways to protect heart health daily. This Heart Health Checkup HHC concerns breathing and the importance of oxygen for heart health.
2. Page 57: You observed your tongue each morning before brushing your teeth. This is a simple way to observe if your digestion and energy are serving you well.
3. Page 72: You observed your urine in the morning. Tongue and urine diagnosis can indicate how well digestion and circulation are working to enhance energy and mood. You observed the pattern of emotions that are typical/predictable for you during the day and evening.
4. Page 84: You observed your sleep patterns and how they affect energy and immunity. Chapter 5 concerns our immunity against extreme temperatures, detailing heart-safe remedies for colds and flu and insomnia.
5. Page 97: You observed the music of your heartbeat, its rhythm, intensity and quality. That music changes with fatigue, emotional upset and other factors. If you become a friend to your heart, you can anticipate its actions wisely.

6. Page 109: You observe your typical hygienic habits in regard to infections, common germs, and especially super-germs. Also special considerations for stents and a pacemaker.
7. Page 118: You observe the usual color, temperature, and skin quality of your hands as a method to observe chronic stress, dehydration, fever, weakness, and locate acupuncture points that could save your life in an emergency.
8. Page 139: You observe your tea-drinking habits after a chapter on the many benefits of Camilla sinensis and herbal teas.
9. Page 145: You observe your sugar-intake habits and hidden sugars.
10. Page 154: You note the red foods you enjoy to prevent heart disease.
11. Page 161: You observe your consumption of heart healthy fish
12. Page 170: You observe your shopping habits and reputable sources of foods.
13. Page 176: You observe you inflammatory health problems from arthritic pain, allergies, and rashes to mental cloudiness and poor memory.
14. and 15. Pages 190, 198: These two chapters deal with cholesterol and side-effects from commonly recommended heart drugs. You observe discomforts associated with heart drugs such as muscle pain and stiffness, reduced mental concentration and memory, diabetes, reduced sexual vitality and resulting depression.
16. Page 207: You observe possible symptoms and the weakening effects of intestinal parasites, common household toxic materials, radiation, lead poisoning etc.
17. Pages 213, 217, 220: With separate Heart Health Checkups within this chapter you observe symptoms indicating possible uses for arjuna, punarnava, guggul, amla and trifala. They are balancing Ayurvedic remedies that improve among other things heart weakness, water retention, common signs of aging, and poor digestion/absorption of nutrients.
18. Page 232: You observe your breath capacity, stamina, clarity, vitality and immunity made possible by adequate oxygen intake.
19. Page 256: In this chapter covering important remedies for preventing/treating heart attack and stroke, you observe your life as it is now including your work, relationships and stress levels.

20. Page 270: You observe your issues addressed by herbal tonics and decide which sort of tonic would work better for you.
21. Page 284: You observe your hands for signs of inflammation, dehydration, or weak circulation in order to evaluate your progress in using diet.
22. Page 293: You observe your hands and feet to help chose the best remedies to address inflammation and weakness affecting the entire body.
23. Page 304: You observe the effects of your blood thinning medicines, bruises, circulation, and energy.
24. Page 312: You observe the times of day and night that you have certain symptoms that correspond to energy systems, meridians, and your internal clock.
25. Page 329 The Meridian Clock
26. Page 342: You observe your vitality, attitudes and habits as a caregiver. We begin to put together your self-observations and/or observations of your patient in order to reach a global picture of where to start to rebuild health and wellness, how to proceed and markers for your progress.

I recommend reading this entire book taking notes that apply to you. If you don't cook, give a copy of the book to someone you love, someone who cooks for you or with whom to go out to restaurants. For non-cooks I have described many herbal remedies and supplements that are easily found in health shops and online. My website www. asianhealthsecrets.com has a section "Products" that contains an ongoing updated list with links for many of the modern natural supplements described in the book.

Now that you have reviewed "The Symptoms Key" and your "Heart Health Checkup" self observations at the end of chapters and the above observations summary, at this point you should answer the following three questions about yourself (or your patient).

1. My main heart health problem is ------------------. I will begin to work on one major problem at a time for example:
   ◦   I am over weight
   ◦   I am diabetic
   ◦   I have swollen hands, feet, ankles, spare tire

- ◦ I suffer too much stress
- ◦ I have frequent headaches, jaw pain, stiff shoulders, chest pains, irregular heartbeat, hypertension (get a heart checkup from a qualified doctor then reread Parts One, Three, Four)
- ◦ I am often emotionally upset
- ◦ I need sexual energy and/or better libido
- ◦ I don't have time to exercise
- ◦ I am at high risk of coronary heart disease
- ◦ I want to get off my medications

2. Do I need to improve my health and wellness as a caregiver, a heart patient, or both?

Caregivers often break down, fried from stress, fatigue, depression, anxiety, worry, grief or other problems. As a caregiver you need to protect yourself as well as your patient, family members and loved ones. The entire book will be helpful especially Parts One, Four, and Five. If you cook for yourself or patient you need to be aware of suggested foods, herbs, and tonics in Parts Two and Three. Reduce emotional wear and tear, learn to organize your healing routine, and find practical help in Part Five.)

3. What are the most valuable lessons I have learned from this book? For example, what suggestions for maintaining natural health and wellness can I easily put into operation? What new material gleaned from this book requires my further study and practice?

Possible Additions/Substitutes for Medical Drugs

Never stop taking a medical drug without discussing it with your heart doctor. Your body is used to medicines and strongly react to changes in medicines and dosage. The following suggestions should be used with your doctor's cooperation. I strongly recommend keeping current with medical heart and blood testing in order to evaluate your progress.

Most heart doctors even alternative cardiologists are unfamiliar with many natural remedies either by their training, legal restrictions, insurance coverage limitations, by choice or habit. Many Americans especially tend to be doubtful about world research (non-American research). See the Special Alert at the beginning of this book. For example, doctors attached to hospitals must follow hospital policy determined in part by insurance coverage regardless of quality patient care and safety concerns. The bottom line is don't expect your physician to welcome with open arms a natural or dietary approach to heart disease. They will need to be convinced that you are on the right tract by your having personal evidenced-based proof, including improvements in standard heart and blood tests. Do not be discouraged. It took a long time to make you sick and will take time to get you well.

While being monitored for heart health with regular checkups, discuss with your doctor the following possible drug modifications/ substitutes. If your physician is up to date with current heart research he/she may already know about these supplements.

Heart Drug/Herb Interactions

When it comes to coronary heart disease, most cardiologists agree upon a similar combination of widely used heart drugs and that using the prescribed drug protocol saves lives. For the most part even well-informed doctors are aware of the same heart studies and will agree upon a similar treatment whether or not it completely applies to you. The main goal of many heart drugs is to protect the heart muscle (myocardium) from reduced oxygen supply (ischemia) that can result from blockages in coronary arteries. In the best of all possible worlds, heart drugs may be used to increase our activity level without provoking symptoms such as chest pain, shortness of breath, dizziness, fatigue, poor memory and compromised sexual capacity.

Certain medicines slow and stabilize the heart rate and energize heart action. They may lower cholesterol, regulate blood pressure, increase the force of heart muscle contraction, or remove excess fluid from the lungs and lower blood pressure. Based on testing, your cardiologist may prescribe drugs most needed in your particular case, but medical advice based on meta-analysis of large groups may not apply. For example, the blood thinner Coumadin (warfarin) is sometimes prescribed to prevent blood clots in people with atrial fibrillation whether or not you consume foods such as garlic another blood thinner. Low-dose beta blockers have been prescribed to help reduce the risk of arrhythmias and sudden cardiac death even though certain anti-arrhythmic drugs can cause sudden death from arrhythmia.

Possible Natural Substitutes for Heart Medicines

Alternative cardiologists recommend natural substitutes for certain heart drugs along with lifestyle advice such as found in this book that are aimed to improve heart health. Never stop taking any heart medication without your doctor's explicit consent. Stopping them is like giving yourself whiplash. However, when used with nutritional supplements, cardiac drugs may offer heart-protecting benefits with less severe side effects and often at lower doses. If you hope to avoid all prescribed heart medications, follow the health advice in this book and consider using one or more of the following drug substitutes to avoid symptoms. Always follow-up with regular medical testing. The following is standard medical information from numerous medical sources. My additions are "Note" where they apply.

ACE Inhibitors

ACE (angiotensin-converting enzyme) inhibitors (Capoten, Altace, Enalapril, Vasotec, Lotensin, Monopril, etc.) lower blood pressure by inhibiting the body's production of specific enzymes that cause arteries to constrict. The arteries relax and the heart's job becomes easier. Side effects include moderate to severe cough, dizziness, headache, fatigue, bone marrow depression, and liver damage. Other side effects are weakness and rash.

Possible Alternatives to ACE Inhibitors

- Hawthorn berry—500 mg 2–3 times per day—increases blood flow in smaller vessels, acting much like ACE inhibitors, as it decreases blood pressure. It also helps to regulate heartbeat, promote circulation in the heart, and strengthen the heart's pumping power. Another option is grapeseed extract at 300 mg/day. Wild garlic also has ACE inhibiting activities.

Note: A secondary use for hawthorn in TCM is to remove masses from the colon, therefore using it may temporarily increase cramps or bowel movements. A useful combination to support the heart and general immune health during stressful times is to combine hawthorn with grape seed extract or resveratrol. If taking hawthorn increases insomnia, a feverish feeling or that the heart is pulsing in your head, your hypertension may be the result of a hyper-adrenal or hyperthyroid response. Then you should consider another herbal treatment that regulates heart action without over-stimulating the heart such as danshen or arjuna especially if your LDL cholesterol is high.

- Calcium, magnesium—400 mg magnesium, 1,000 mg calcium. Note: Magnesium also helps to relax tense muscles and stiff blood vessels and thereby moderate blood pressure. It can also increase bowel movements and help reduce bloat.
- Coenzyme Q10—60–90 mg of water-soluble CoQ10 daily, in divided doses.
- Fish oil—2–4 grams per day.
- Note: for people who prefer not to use animal products, oils beneficial for the heart include flaxseed oil and hemp seed oil.
- L-arginine—2–7 grams per day, taken at bedtime. L-arginine relaxes the muscles in coronary arteries, increases immune response, and lowers blood pressure. Research has shown that L-arginine can retard the development of heart disease, including hardening of the arteries (atherosclerosis), the most serious form of heart disease.

Note: You should not take L-arginine supplements if you are currently on an ACE inhibitor or a diuretic because a deadly interaction can occur. If you are taking an ACE inhibitor, you should avoid licorice for the same reason. Some authors recommend L-arginine as a sexual tonic, however research has shown that a very large amount over 8 grams is necessary to increase libido.

Calcium-channel Blockers

Calcium-channel blockers (Isoptin, Calan, Verelan, Norvasc, Procardia) are prescribed to lower heart rate, contractility, and blood pressure. Like nitrates and beta blockers, they may improve blood flow and improve vascular tone through narrowed vessels. Some calcium-channel blockers encourage smooth-muscle relaxation in the inner lining of blood vessels, preventing spasms and helping them dilate. Side effects include ankle swelling, constipation, fatigue, and headache.

According to medical sources, there is considerable controversy regarding an increase in mortality in patients treated with short-acting calcium-channel blockers. Check with your physician to make sure you are on long-acting, second- or third-generation calcium-channel blockers. Be careful when you combine calcium- channel blockers with digoxin for treatment of congestive heart failure and atrial fibrillation. Some of the calcium-channel blockers can increase the digoxin in blood to dangerous levels. This can cause nausea, vomiting, loss of appetite, or "heart block," a serious condition whereby your heart rate can slow dangerously. Check with your physician.

Alternatives to Calcium-channel Blockers

Several alternative cardiologists recommend taking magnesium (400 mg), potassium (500–1,000 mg), and calcium (500–1,000 mg) because these minerals help normalize mineral balance. Do not take these minerals if you have kidney problems. You must talk to your physician. Do not reduce or stop taking your anti-arrhythmic drug without your doctor's consent and guidance. If you cannot tolerate calcium-channel blockers, ask your doctor about beta blockers.

Note: If you experience chest pain due to reduced blood flow to the heart, shortness of breath, and hypertension, consider using Suxiao Jiuxin wan on a regular basis to help ease these symptoms. In China, Suxiao Jiuxin wan is often used in conjunction with beta blockers, calcium channel blockers and nitrates (nitroglycerin.) Before beginning on a regimen of this Chinese herbal medicine recommended for angina, check with your doctor. An appropriate dose may substitute for nitroglycerin pills in order to ease pain and improve circulation.

Note: When taking cardiac drugs, especially calcium-channel blockers, you should avoid grapefruit and grapefruit juice. Studies have shown that grapefruit can cause levels of these drugs to increase in the blood, which may be dangerous to your health.

Digoxin

Digoxin (digitalis) is used to control the heart rate in patients with atrial fibrillation, and will also assist the force of heart muscle contraction, especially in patients with congestive heart failure. By improving the heart's pumping ability, digoxin can help clear the body of excess lung fluid. Side effects include nausea, vomiting, diarrhea, blurred vision, headaches, and psychosis if abnormally high blood levels arise.

Note: Many people cannot tolerate digoxin even in small doses.

Alternatives to Digoxin

- Hawthorn berry is often used as a substitute for digitalis in Europe and has therapeutic benefits for a wide range of heart conditions. It can be taken as a tea or in tincture, tablet, or capsule form, all of which can be found in health food stores.

Note: Do not use hawthorn berry with digoxin because of their similar effects on the heart.

Diuretics

If you have a history of heart attack, congestive heart failure, or high blood pressure, you may be prescribed diuretics such as indapamide (Lozol) or furosemide (Lasix) which lower blood pressure indirectly by reducing salt from the body and increasing urine output, which clears excess fluid from the body and lungs. Side effects include dehydration, and loss of electrolytes, most significantly potassium and magnesium, a mineral that's absolutely essential for healthy heart function. Dr. Stephen Sinatra, MD strongly advises, that if you take diuretics, especially Lasix or Bumex, it's imperative that you supplement with magnesium (400–600 mg/day) and potassium (99 mg three times/day.)

Alternatives to Diuretics

According to most cardiologists there are no alternatives to standard, conventional diuretics if you have diagnosed heart failure. For people with mild water retention, alternatives include:

- Take uva ursi extract, 100–200 mg daily.
- For diabetes and water retention consider using cornsilk tea which lowers high blood sugar as well as acting as a diuretic.
- Take punarnava herb daily, adding ¼ tsp. of the powder to a little yogurt or apple sauce. A useful combination for heart failure is equal amounts of arjuna with punarnava herbs. However this should be closely monitored by your health provider.
- Wu Ling San water balance pills, useful for congestive heart failure and edema

Beta Blockers

Beta blockers are considered among the safest of all cardiac drugs. Scandinavian research shows that low-dose beta blockers actually interfere with the adrenaline response typical of a failing heart. This reduces the risk of arrhythmia and sudden death. Many doctors prescribe them for high blood pressure, congestive heart failure, and atrial fibrillation even though they have side effects (impotence, fatigue, dizziness, depression, and wheezing) and can deplete Coenzyme Q10, a key energy-generating nutrient. You can easily counter the loss of CoQ10 by taking 60–90 mg of water-soluble CoQ10 daily.

Alternatives to Beta Blockers

Note: You may find that taking the herbal tonic that best suits your needs can not only regulate but also support heart health. For example ashwagandha, considered a tonic for weakened adrenal vitality also supports heart action and immunity. Long term use of a natural tonic has so many benefits that it cannot compare with a heart drug. You may have to gradually adjust the dosage of heart medication when adding tonics such as arjuna, ashwagandha, danshen or others. They provide a natural heart and energy support system but they take a long time to work.

Blood Thinning Drugs and Herbs

If you take Coumadin (warfarin), limit your intake of supplemental vitamin E to no more than 200 IU/day. More than that amount of vitamin E may cause your blood to thin too much. Taking aspirin with Coumadin (warfarin) could cause overly thin blood. While taking ginkgo can prevent blood clotting, it does not give the maximum anti-clotting support that Coumadin will. Coumadin prevents excessive clot formation in the chambers of the heart and helps prevent stroke. Ginkgo is not an alternative if you have atrial fibrillation.

Alternatives to Blood Thinners

NOTE: Serramend (serrapeptase) an effective blood thinner that reduces excess fibrin, may substitute for blood thinners. Serramend has an anti-inflammatory effect, dissolves necrotic tissue (blood clots), arterial plaques, thin lung secretions, may reduce fibrinolytic activity. It treats chronic lung, ear, nose and throat disorders, sinusitis, sprains, edema, postoperative inflammation, carpal tunnel syndrome, breast engorgement, (fibrocystic breast disease) venous inflammatory disease, asthma, cardiovascular disease, inflammatory pain conditions, leg ulcers, and chronic headaches. It digests scar tissue and speeds the healing response. But, like tree ear mushroom, the dosage of Serramend is individual.

Statins

Statin drugs are controversial due to serious side effects and the debate over whether statins can prevent heart attack and stroke. They include lovastatin (Mevacor), pravastatin (Pravachol), simvastatin (Zocor), ator-vastatin (Lipitor), and fluvastatin (Lescol). They can produce phenomenal reductions in a patient's cholesterol level. According to some experts, that is not the best reason to use them. Statins may reduce inflammation for patients with a history of heart disease, previous coronary events, diabetes, or inflammatory markers such as high levels of C-reactive protein or high coronary calcium scores, but it is debatable whether they should not be prescribed in the absence of these factors solely on the basis of high cholesterol levels.

Muscle pain and weakness, flu-like symptoms, and generalized soreness are extremely common among statin users. Other side-effects may include liver dysfunction with elevated liver enzymes, problems of the nervous system, including a condition called peripheral neuropathy, and total global amnesia, which means forgetting where and who you are for a few minutes to several hours. If cholesterol LDL levels get too low, they interfere with neurotransmitter mechanisms in the brain. Another severe side effect is diastolic dysfunction and/or congestive heart failure, an outcome that was written up in the *American Journal of Cardiology*.

If you take a statin drug, make sure you take a minimum of 100–250 mg of hydrosoluble CoQ10 a day to offset the drug's depleting effect on this important enzyme.

Alternatives to Statin Drugs for Lowering Cholesterol

Note: It is wise and safe to reduce excess harmful cholesterol before it clogs blood vessels by following a heart health routine including exercise, appropriate herbs, and heart healthy foods including omega oils such as flaxseed, hemp seed, extra virgin olive, and coconut oils. A Mediterranean/Asian diet that is rich in fiber, healthy fats from olive oil and omega-3s from fish and fish oil, garlic and onions—two potent cholesterol-busters—and fresh fruits and vegetables. Soluble fiber (grapefruit, pears, and apples) helps soak up cholesterol while insoluble fiber (baked beans and oat bran) cleanses the colon, preventing rapid absorption of cholesterol.

Recommended supplements to reduce cholesterol and augment or replace statins include:

- Niacin raises HDL "good" cholesterol and lowers LDL "bad" cholesterol along with fibrinogen and Lp(a) levels, now recognized as risk factors for heart disease. Low doses in the range of 100–300 mg three times daily are often effective without side effects of flushing, heartburn, or gout attacks.
- Tocotrienols. Vitamin E compounds that possess powerful antioxidant qualities act much like statin drugs, minus the side effects, by interfering with the liver's ability to produce cholesterol. As little as 10–60 mg per day can have a positive effect. If you take regular vitamin E, look for mixed tocopherols and take no more than 400 IU per day. Vitamin E will help inhibit the oxidation of LDL "bad" cholesterol. To take full advantage of all that vitamin E has to offer, you need a combination of its two major classes: tocopherols—alpha, beta, delta, gamma—and tocotrienols (also alpha, beta, delta, and gamma forms). According to alternative cardiologists it is unwise to purchase the synthetic version, *dl*-alpha-tocopherol because it's ineffective. Gamma tocopherol is more expensive than the alpha variety, which is a reason many supplement manufacturers don't include it. Recent studies indicate that the four tocotrienols are the best combination of vitamin E biochemistry. Look for vitamin E supplements available containing full-spectrum (alpha, beta, delta, and gamma) tocotrienols as well as gamma tocopherol. More than 400 IU per day is unnecessary and may cause problems. Also vitamin E is fat soluble, so take it with food.
- Ground flaxseed is a perfect food for cholesterol control, containing essential fatty acids, high-quality protein, vitamins, precious phytonutrients, and lignans, as well as soluble fiber and insoluble fiber, all of which promote healthy cholesterol. Flaxseed is also high in linolenic acid, vital for healthy heart function.
- Soy isoflavones (including genistein and daidzein) are phytoestrogens that prevent oxidized LDL and subsequent buildup of artery-clogging plaque. (Soy can help ease menopausal symptoms and may reduce the risk of hormonal-dependent cancers such as breast cancer in women and prostate cancer in men.) Best sources are non-GMO soy milk,

soybeans, and tofu. Supplements are also available. Note: See my Resource Guide for safe sources of soy products. Soy grown in the United States is nearly exclusively genetically modified and banned in parts of the world.

- Oats. Research shows that beta glucan, a water-soluble fiber in oatmeal, oat bran, and oats, helps lower cholesterol. It's an established fact that heart patients who eat two ounces of oat bran daily for six weeks can expect up to a 10-percent reduction in their cholesterol.

- Pantethine, a component of vitamin B5 or pantothenic acid, promotes healthy cholesterol and triglyceride levels. Pantethine has no side effects and works especially well in diabetics, so it may be worth the expense. The usual dose is 300 mg, three times a day.

- Oligomeric proanthocyanidins (OPCs) are very powerful nutrients found in most fruits and vegetables; they're particularly abundant in grapeseeds and pine bark. They're also readily absorbed into the bloodstream, which means their benefits are felt almost immediately throughout the body. OPCs are incredible free-radical scavengers that help control the oxidation of LDL cholesterol. I recommend taking 150–300 mg of grapeseed extract or 100 mg of Pycnogenol (pine bark extract) daily.

- Note: PuErh tea is a natural source of lovastatin that has been used for generations to improve digestion of fat foods. Hung cha (red tea) refers to both PuErh and black teas both helpful for preventing heart disease.

Note; Arjuna has dose-related cholesterol-lowering capacity. Check the label for dosage.

Note: Red yeast rice (Monascus purpureus) is another supplement that has become popular lately in American health food stores and major stores. Chinese cooks have used it for centuries as a soup additive. The dose is important.

Mayo Clinic advises the following dosage for red yeast rice (RYR) supplements and for Chinese red yeast rice products:

Adults (18 years and older) Red yeast rice (RYR) should be taken with food. A dose of 1,200 milligrams of red yeast powder in the form of capsules has been taken by mouth twice daily with food. In Asia, the average consumption of naturally occurring RYR is 14-55 grams daily.

To treat coronary heart disease, 1,200-2,400 milligrams of Xuezhikang (an extract of cholestin that reduces cardiovascular events in type 2 diabetes patients with coronary heart disease) has been taken by mouth daily for 2-12 weeks. Xuezhikang has also been taken by mouth at doses of 0.3-0.6 grams twice daily for 4-4.5 years on average (range: 0.5-7 years). Xuezhikang has been taken by mouth at a dose of 1,200 milligrams daily for 12 weeks to 24 months.

To treat diabetes, two capsules of 300 milligrams of Monascus extract have been taken by mouth for eight weeks.

To treat high cholesterol, 1,200-2,400 milligrams of Cholestin® has been taken by mouth 1-2 times daily for up to 12 weeks. Doses of 600-1,800 milligrams RYR have been taken by mouth up to three times daily for 8-24 weeks. Two capsules of 300 milligrams of RYR product have been taken by mouth daily for 1-3 cycles of eight weeks each. Doses of 600-3,600 milligrams of Xuezhikang/RYR have been taken by mouth 1-2 times daily for up to one year. A dose of 2-4 capsules of Xuezhikang has been taken by mouth twice daily for 8-12 weeks. A dose of five capsules of 0.5 grams of Xuezhikang has been taken by mouth twice daily for two months. Doses of 0.6-3.6 grams of RYR extract have been taken by mouth daily for four weeks to 4.5 years. Doses of 0.6-1.2 grams of Monascus purpureus rice preparation have been taken by mouth 1-2 times daily for eight weeks to one year, with dose adjustment depending on cholesterol levels and tolerance. Five Zhitai capsules have been taken by mouth twice daily (for a dose of five grams daily) for two months. Three Zhibituo tablets (0.35 grams each) have been taken by mouth three times daily for a total of 3.15 grams daily. One to two capsules of Xuezhikang have been taken by mouth

2-3 times daily for up to 24 weeks. Four capsules of RYR (Hy-poCol®, Wearnes Biotech & Medicals Pte, Singapore) have been taken by mouth daily for 16 weeks.

To treat fatty liver, 0.6 grams of RYR have been taken by mouth twice daily for 12 weeks. There is no proven safe or effective dose for RYR in children.

Nitroglycerin substitute for chest pains

Note: Su Xiao Jiu Xin Wan (Suxiao Jiuxin Wan) has been proven more effective for reducing chest pain (angina) than nitroglycerin. This small Chinese pill that is melted under your tongue contains a form of medicated camphor to dilate blood vessels and herbs to enhance heart action in order to ease chest discomforts and gradually reduce cholesterol and other symptoms.

A Natural Heart Health Checklist

Are you taking Serramend, garlic, and/or cloud ear mushroom as a blood thinner? How about red yeast rice, oat bran, vitamin E, nuts, flaxseed and Pu Erh tea instead of a statin? How about hawthorn and grapeseed extract instead of an ACE inhibitor? Is your cholesterol "fluffy"? the safer large size that causes less risk of stroke? Niacin has been recommended to fluff up cholesterol and reduce LDL cholesterol.

What are your preferred regular Exercise, Body Treatments, and Stress-reduction Techniques from this book or other sources?

What heart healthy supplements do you keep at home by your bed, in your pocket, in your car or desk at work?

Have you become more aware of discovering and maintaining your heart wellness possibilities? Tests can give you numbers to compare, directions to take, but only you know how well your heart feels. Your heart health personalized program will open new doors, new relationships, new vitality and hope for you. Poor health is a prison. Open the door. Life is a gift: Open it.

Heart to Heart Conclusion from Michael

It's summer and Letha and I are once again in the mountains of Vermont. The condo, on two levels, a loft, and a back porch, is spacious and airy, very much a station in the surrounding intense greenery. For a city boy, it takes some adjusting to the blue sky and fleecy clouds and views through the trees across to a green-clad junior mountain. Our two cats are deliriously happy, running up and down a spiral staircase that leads to the loft. They don't squabble over food, and Mrs. Tiger is fascinated by the birds on our back porch. She has been known to charge when a bird gets too close, once taking out the screen door. Mr. Fluff, when he is not admiring himself in the ample mirrors, demands to be petted, purring away. It's contentment in the country!

This summer is a challenge for me. The bitter '2014 –'15 winter in New York was tough, and working long hours to finish a lengthy book kept me mostly deskbound. We had a tussle with our building management--the landlord is hot money from some disreputable place--which I disposed of with my usual Brooklyn-born tactics. Letha, aside from her writing, radio and personal appearances, has a job keeping me going. So when I had my annual heart exam, which includes an echocardiogram, at Dartmouth Hospital in July and the results were not great, I wasn't surprised. Total cholesterol was up, ejection fraction down. The former doesn't worry me because it takes a more sophisticated test to determine the quality and health implications of cholesterol. However, I still need to exercise more and to lose weight . . . don't we all?

As the summer progresses I feel stronger, my heart at ease. I confess I'm still off and on about exercise, but there are several things about the Green Mountains that act as an elixir. First, the fresh air. I do yoga breathing daily on our back porch, which faces the mountains with a ring of flowers below. The only sounds are the low, incessant hum of the insect world broken by occasional chirps of birds. We put out birdseed and have attracted mainly flycatchers, small, black and white with a sprightly tail, larger, swift blue jays, and lately a gorgeous yellow flicker, a type of woodpecker. Out front we get an occasional bunch of crows and a mated pair of ravens. Driving or walking along back roads we have spotted stunning wild turkeys, a family of curious raccoons, a stealthy fox, and even a fisher cat. Very sleek, this weasel will kill smaller species not only to eat but for pleasure.

It's vital to feel close to animal life, to feel the primal in us. Nature is our best medicine. So is fun.

Towards the end of the summer we are going to the World's Fair. That is, the fair held annually since 1867 at Tunbridge, Vermont in a valley between verdant mountains. In the old days it was known as "a drunkard's reunion" where the boys would drink and watch soft-porn shows. Nowadays the fair is family fun with a grandstand for musical entertainment (mainly country), a large midway of stands selling every sort of junk food, a Ferris wheel, a beautiful, old-fashioned merry-go-round, and farm animal shows and contests. Letha and I head for the goat show. Goats are handsome, intelligent, inquisitive, and mischievous. We drink their milk, eat their healthy cheese, and neither eat nor wear any part of them. At the fair, the goats, or rather their handlers, compete for best in each category. It is the young handlers, bright boys and girls no more than ten years old, who manage their goat's appearance and posture. It's they who deserve the prizes.

But surprise! The shed housing prize chickens, especially roosters, has captivated me. With their bright red combs atop their arrogant heads, glistening feathers ranging from orange to white to blue, their cock-a doodle-doo's and cock o' the walk attitude, the roosters on display are acting as Nature made them. They guard their pretty hens, crow when they feel like it, and fight any other rooster who tries to barge in. The rooster is a symbol of hope and grace in many religions, especially Christianity. Among other symbols, the cock became a weather vane on church steeples in many lands. I favor a citation from the Talmud, the Jewish book of wisdom: "We learn modesty from cats, honest toil from ants, chastity from doves and gallantry from cocks."

Soon, it will be goodbye to the hills with their dappled, early autumn leaves. Goodbye to our good-natured friends at the farmer's market with their abundant, beautiful pumpkins, squashes, peppers, and apples. Once again we shall enter the ring to perform, promote, strive. Whether in the country or city, life is an adventure. Living is what your heart is about. So listen to your heart as it works and rests. Open a dialogue with your best friend.

ACKNOWLEDGEMENTS

I thank Michael Foster for sharing his insights, feelings and experiences with you and his love and devotion to me. His healing and this book could not have been possible without his generosity, wisdom and the strength of our love.

Many physicians and alternative health experts have participated in our improved health, wellbeing and offered the detailed medical and natural health information found here. Among them are Dr. Robert Fafalak, MD., Dr. Russell Berdoff, MD, the cardiac medical and intensive care staff at NY Beth Israel, Dr. Bradley Grossman, D.C., Dr. Erik Steiner MD., Kareem Fahmy, LMT, Dr. Lili Wu, L.Ac. in New York, Dr. Patrick Cooley D.C., in Vermont, Dr. Eric Hadady D.C., in New Mexico, and in New Hampshire Dr. Alan Kono and Dr. James Devries.

Care-giving is a demanding job. We have been fortunate to have received much appreciated help from dear friends, including Katie McFadden in Vermont and Arnold and Judy Hererra in New York. Our families have helped sustain us in times of emotional and financial drought. I especially thank Barbara Foster for her support. I have been encouraged and helped by Christopher Phillips, CCH, RSHom (NA), Mallie Bowman, Ira (Salima) Swain, Anna Magenta, Jan Pedis, Qigong master Sharon Smith, Mieko Ikegame and Takao Shibata, Gad Cohen, Jean-Claude van Italie, and my friends at Pan-Pacific South East Asian Women's Association in New York, Dr. Orest Pelechaty in New Jersey, my brother Eric and sister Michelle in New Mexico, Bob Warner in California and C. Lynn Brooks in Texas. At times Mother has been a beacon of light in a foggy storm of troubles. I have remembered her poise and courage.

From the great healing traditions of Asia I am inedited to my mentors H.H. the Dalai Lama of Tibet, Sogyal Rinpoche, Dr. Vasant Lad in Albuquerque, Dr. Yeshi Dhonden in India, Dr. Thubten Lekshe of Tanaduk Botanical Research Institute in Orcas Island, Dr. Chao in Shanghai College of Traditional Chinese Medicine, and Susan Lin of Lin Sister Herbs in New York Chinatown.

A book can become a reality that impacts public awareness only when given the opportunity by talented Media professionals. I am lucky to know some. A big shout of thanks and *des bises* to radio show host Marie Griffiths in Montreal and the staff at 105.1mikefm. ca. In New York, I thank Kathy Davis at WBAI radio, Damaris Ojeda of Jnana Wellness Center and ARE Edgar Cayce NYC center. Many thanks also for the publishing efforts and hand-holding by Nick Caya and his staff at Word-2-Kindle.

NOTES

1. The connection between cancer and heart trouble.

   From a sample of 3,005,734 patients who received a diagnosis of a heart attack for the first time and had no prior history of cancer, the cancer incidence was nearly double in survivors of heart attack compared with the background population. During the first six months following a heart attack data showed a high risk of cancer. After six months patients remained at a 10 percent increased risk for cancer overall, a 50 percent increased risk for lung cancer and a 30 percent increased risk for bladder cancer when compared with the general population. Researchers lead by Morten Winther Malmborg, research fellow, at Gentofte Hospital, Copenhagen, suggested that the higher incense of cancers were due to smoking, alcohol use, obesity, physical inactivity and unhealthy eating—all shared risk factors for both heart attack and these types of cancers.

2. Guilinggao reduces heart cell death: quoted in PubMed. Guilinggao [AKA herbal jello, grass jelly] has antioxidants that reduce heart tissue stress apoptosis (that's heart cell death)! http://www.ncbi. nlm.nih.gov/pubmed/23467630

3. Information on electromagnetic (EMI) causes of illness and ways to protect yourself can be found at http://www.emfcenter.com/ emffaqs.htm#B1.%20What%20are%20Electromagnetic%20 Fields%20%28EMFs%29

4. Statin drugs and type 2 diabetes. April, 2015. A study published in the journal *Diabetologia* finds the use of statins - drugs commonly used to lower cholesterol - may significantly increase the risk of type 2 diabetes, and that this risk remains even after accounting for confounding factors, including age, smoking status and body mass index.http://www.medicalnewstoday.com/articles/292672. php

5. Men who skip breakfast are 15 percent more likely to gain a substantial amount of weight and 21 percent more likely to develop type 2 diabetes, earlier studies have reported. Researchers analyzed data culled from a 16-year study of nearly 27,000 male health professionals that tracked their eating habits and overall health from 1992 to 2008. During the study period, 1,572 of the men developed heart disease. The study also found a 55 percent increased risk of heart disease in men who regularly indulge in late-night snacking. From a July, 2013 report published in the medical journal *Circulation*.

6. Here are the main health benefits from organic chicken eggs, real eggs not egg substitutes or chemically engineered eggs:

   a. An egg a day may prevent macular degeneration. Carotenoid contains lutein and zeaxanthin, both help lower the risk of developing cataracts.

   b. One egg contains 6 grams of high-quality protein and all nine essential amino acids.

   c. According to a Harvard School of Public Health study, there is no significant link between egg consumption and heart disease. In fact, according to one study, regular consumption of eggs may help prevent blood clots, strokes and heart attacks.

   d. One egg yolk has about 300 micrograms of choline, a nutrient that helps regulate the brain, nervous system and cardiovascular system.

   e. One egg contains just 5 grams of fat and only 1.5 grams of that is saturated fat. New research shows that moderate consumption of eggs does not have a negative impact on cholesterol. In fact, recent studies have shown that regular consumption of two eggs per day may improve lipid profile. Research suggests saturated fat--butter, *hydrogenated* oils and lard--raises cholesterol. Eggs are one of the only foods that contain naturally occurring vitamin D.

7. Side-effects of common coronary heart disease medicines from rxlist.com: Each type of coronary heart disease medication has different side effects. Heart drugs and common side-effects:

- Antiplatelet drugs can cause diarrhea, rash, or itching, abdominal pain, headache, chest pain, muscle aches, and dizziness.
- Anticoagulants (blood thinning drugs) side effects are bleeding and necrosis (gangrene) of the skin.
- Angiotensin converting enzyme (ACE) inhibitors side effects include cough, elevated blood potassium levels, low blood pressure, dizziness, headache, drowsiness, weakness, abnormal taste, and rash.
- Vasodilators may cause lightheadedness or dizziness, increased or irregular heart rate, or headache.
- Calcium channel blocker side effects include constipation, nausea, headache, rash, edema (water retention) low blood pressure, drowsiness, and dizziness.
- Anti-arrhythmics (that affect heart rhythm) may cause dizziness, blurred vision, anorexia, unusual taste in the mouth, fatigue, nausea and vomiting.

NOTE: Most commonly prescribed heart drugs have ED erectile dysfunction as a side effect but ED may not be listed in product information as a common side effect for them. According to WebMD: http://www.webmd.com/erectile-dysfunction/guide/drugs-linked-erectile-dysfunction

The connection between statin therapy and erectile dysfunction has been controversial ever since Italian clinical researchers reported ED and lower testosterone in patients taking statins (Journal of Sexual Medicine, April 2010). Scientists have confirmed in laboratory studies that statins inhibit testosterone production (Reproductive Toxicology, online Jan. 21, 2014). This contributes to ED, especially in older men.

8. Bacopa and the brain: Animals treated with bacosides from bacopa extract had increased protective antioxidant activity in many parts of the brain, including the hippocampus the brain's memory

center. Bacopa increased GABA and glutamine neurotransmitter levels associated with calming effects. In human studies, bacopa resulted in faster information processing, increased learning rates, improved memory retention and reduced testing anxiety within 12 weeks.

9. Tranquil Mind sold by Banyan Botanicals ingredients: One 500 mg tablet contains vegetarian ingredients: Bhringaraj leaf (Eclipta alba), skullcap herb (Scutellaria lateriflora), passionflower (Passiflora incarnata), guduchi herb (Tinospora cordifolia), chamomile flower (Matricaria recutita), brahmi leaf (Hydrocotyle asiatica), ashwagandha root (Withania somnifera), vidari kanda root (Ipomomea digitata), fennel seed (Foeniculum vulgare), and pippali fruit (Piper longum.) Interestingly, the first herb eclipta, which is supportive of liver health, is most often recommended for prevention of hair loss and complexion problems. Imagine supporting healthy hair growth and liver health as you sleep. Ashwagandha helps calm the mind and improves memory as it enhances muscle strength, which is useful for the heart as are the digestive herbs fennel and pippali a pepper.

10. Safety issues with using liquid silver. The estimated amount of silver accumulation over a one-year period that is required to produce argyria is 1 to 5 grams, which is very large compared to the 50 mcg typically recommended and consumed by people using over the counter colloidal silver products. Using the most conservative figure, 1,000 mg (1 gram) of silver corresponds to the silver content in 100 liters of 10 parts per million colloidal silver.

11. Salmonella and E.coli germs on menus, a study published in the *Journal of Environmental Health*, http://www.ncbi.nlm.nih.gov/pubmed/23505769

12. Fifteen clinical trials involving 1,776 people were reported for suxiao jiuxin wan at pubmed http://www.ncbi.nlm.nih.gov/pubmed/18254051.

13. According to the manufacturer other uses for Suxiao jiuxin wan include:

- Dilates coronary arteries, improves blood flow to heart muscles, lowers oxygen consumption of heart muscles
- Improves blood flow to the brain and limbs, lowers resistance of the peripheral blood vessels
- Antibiotic effect
- Anti-coagulation of platelets
- Helps resist effects of lack of vitamin E

14. L-theanine in tea modulates aspects of human brain function. Electroencephalograph (EEG) studies show that L-theanine significantly increases activity in the alpha frequency band. In other words tea relaxes our mind without inducing drowsiness. This effect was been established with the equivalent of about two cups of black tea (approximately 40mg L-theanine). The data indicates that L-theanine, at realistic dietary levels, has a significant effect on mental alertness or arousal.

15. Tart cherry research: The University of Michigan research group published findings in the Journal of Medicinal Food which suggest tart cherries help to control weight and prevent metabolic syndrome, including high blood pressure, high cholesterol, and the risk for type 2 diabetes and heart disease.

16. Research has shown jiaogulan tea to be useful for treatment of poor appetite, cough and chronic bronchitis, ongoing stomach pain (chronic gastritis), pain and swelling (inflammation), ulcers, constipation, stress, gallstones, obesity, cancer, diabetes, trouble sleeping (insomnia), backache, and pain. From that collection of symptoms I gather that the herb is a liver and gallbladder cleanser, bitter tonic, and adaptogen.

17. The Tibetan lycium berry 'Goji' has been used since ancient times in the Tibetan culture as a food because of its neutral energetic nature (neither cold or hot nature) and used in traditional medicines for the same reason because it can be utilized in a broad spectrum

of Tibetan medical formulas. (You can find an introduction to and valuable resources for the complex, highly sophisticated and useful aspects of Tibetan medicine available to us in the West at gojiberry. com's sister website tibetandoctors.com presented by Amchi (Dr.) Thubten Lekshe. He was born in the United States in 1953 as Bradley Dobos, In 1968 he began botanical training in many systems, including studies with herbalist Dr. John Christopher, and an impressive list of renown Masters of Tibetan Medicine, including Dr. Yeshe Donden, and Dr. Tenzing Choedrak.)

Here in brief are several benefits of Tibetan goji berries. Evidence shows that its nutrients improve cell communication and have antioxidant as well as anti-inflammatory properties. These substances have been shown to increase mitochondrial function and detoxification. It has also been shown that nutrient dense foods such as Goji berries are far superior to supplementation with isolated nutrients contained in juices, capsules or tablets.

Goji berries are naturally rich in antioxidant carotenoids, vitamin A, and Zeaxanthin. They contain B-complex vitamins, Vitamin C, and important polysaccharides. These special little berries contain more protein than whole wheat (they are 10% protein) and supply 18 different amino acids including all 8 essential amino acids. In addition, Goji berries are loaded with many phytonutrients.

The Goji berry – Lycium Tibeticum/Chinensis variety is used in Tibetan Medicine to bring (neutral) tonic and immune-building strength to herbal formulas without increasing inflammation. Whereas, Chinese lycium fruit (AKA wolfberry) is considered hot, acrid and not suitable for problems in which inflammation is prominent, or where weak spleen and weak digestion (diarrhea, bloating, indigestion, bleeding and bruising conditions, water retention, etc) are evident. In Chinese medicine lycium fruit is used only in combination with other herbs to harmonize the formula, and it has never traditionally been used as a single food source

18. Bitter melon contains gurmarin, a polypeptide shown in experimental studies to achieve a positive sugar regulating effect by suppressing the neural response to sweet taste stimuli. In other

words it reduces the sweet taste in the mouth and sweet craving. It has long been used in India as a home remedy for diabetes mellitus.

19. Stevia and your heart:

Research done by the Department of Environmental Studies, Alexandria University in Egypt shows that low levels of stevia appeared to increase HDL "good cholesterol" in male rats. Another mouse study reported by Department of Cardiovascular Diseases and Leuven Food Science and Nutrition Research Centre in Belgium showed that stevia improved "insulin signaling and antioxidant defense...leading to inhibition of atherosclerotic plaque development and inducing plaque stabilization." In other words, it seemed to help prevent heart disease.

Stevia is apparently also helpful for human high blood pressure. The Department of Medicine, Taipei Medical University in Taiwan reported a study of 174 adults with mild hypertension showing that stevioside not only improved their blood pressure compared to the placebo group, but had no significant side effects.

How much stevia?

Sugar amount	Equivalent Stevia powdered extract	Equivalent Stevia liquid concentrate
1 cup	1 teaspoon	1 teaspoon
1 tablespoon	¼ teaspoon	6 to 9 drops
1 teaspoon	A pinch to 1/16 teaspoon	2 to 4 drops

20. About quinoa: About 25% of quinoa's fatty acids come in the form of oleic acid, a heart-healthy monounsaturated fat, and about 8% are alpha-linolenic acid or ALA—the omega-3 fatty acid and a form of vitamin E commonly associated with decreased risk of inflammation-related disease. Quinoa is also a good source of folate, copper, and phosphorus in contrast to whole wheat. It has twice the amount of calcium as whole wheat.

21. A 2013 study in the British Medical Journal BMJ highlights the often overlooked fact that 'everyday' soluble drugs such as painkillers, contain high levels of salt (sodium) which may cause health problems if taken on a long-term basis. For example, the study points out, if you take the maximum recommended dosage of soluble paracetamol per day for an adult this would exceed the daily recommended salt / sodium intake of 6g, roughly equivalent to a teaspoon. High sodium intake, on a long-term basis, is known to increase blood pressure, which in turn, can increase the risk of cardiovascular diseases such as heart attack and stroke. The study was carried out by researchers from Ninewells Hospital and Medical School, Dundee and UCL School of Pharmacy, London.

22. Journal of Agricultural and Food Chemistry, 2014 Aug
Capsaicinoids but not their analogue capsinoids lower plasma cholesterol and possess beneficial vascular activity.

23. Tart Cherries: Michigan State researchers found that tart cherries contain the highest concentrations of anthocyanins 1 and 2, which help block the cyclooxygenase enzymes (COX-1 and COX-2) that are sources of inflammation targeted by over-the-counter pain killers like aspirin and acetaminophen.

Tart cherries exceed sweet cherries in the anthocyanin/phenol, delivering more than twice as many per 100 grams. They also score very high on a lab test that measures how many free radicals a food can neutralize. Damage done to cells, tissues and organs by free radicals is a key factor not only in cardiovascular disease, but also in virtually every chronic, degenerative disease, not to mention, aging.

A 2012 study published in the *European Journal of Nutrition School of Life Sciences*, Northumbria University, Newcastle upon Tyne in the UK concluded that consumption of a tart cherry juice concentrate "provides an increase in exogenous melatonin that is beneficial in improving sleep duration and quality in healthy men and women and might be of benefit in managing disturbed sleep."

24. About grapes: Resveratrol inhibits angiotensin II, a hormone secreted in response to high blood pressure and heart failure.

Angiotensin II causes the heart muscle to stiffen, reducing its ability to pump blood efficiently. If red grapes are so healthy, and they are used to make red wine, why is alcohol harmful for heart failure patients? I wondered about this when I heard the director of a respected heart failure clinic say, "Alcohol is poison for heart failure patients." Alcohol is inflammatory and can be fattening. Alcohol can weaken muscles including the heart. That is why drinking alcohol may feel temporarily relaxing but threatens heart failure patients who may not even have elevated cholesterol, only a weak or "stiff" heart.

25. About cayenne: The report was part of the 243rd National Meeting and Exposition of the American Chemical Society (ACS), held in San Diego the week of March 26, 2012. A study focused on capsaicin and its fiery-hot relatives, a piquant family of substances termed "capsaicinoids." The stuff that gives cayenne, jalapenos, habaneros and other chili peppers their heat. Past research suggested that spicing food with chilies can lower blood pressure, reduce blood cholesterol and ease the tendency for dangerous blood clots to form. The research was focused on how hot substances in chilies work in improving heart health. According to Zhen-Yu Chen, Ph.D., who presented the study, "We now have a clearer and more detailed portrait of their innermost effects on genes and other mechanisms that influence cholesterol and the health of blood vessels."

Capsaicin and a close chemical relative lower cholesterol levels by reducing accumulation of cholesterol in the body and increasing its breakdown and excretion in the feces. They also block action of a gene that makes arteries contract, restricting the flow of blood to the heart and other organs. The blocking action allows more blood to flow through blood vessels. But the study, according to Chen certainly "does not recommend that people start consuming chilies to an excess. . . Capsaicinoids also blocked the activity of a gene that produces cyclooxygenase-2, a substance that makes the muscles around blood vessels constrict. By blocking it, muscles can relax and widen, allowing more blood to flow.

26. In a February, 2014 article in *the Guardian*, cardiologist Dr. Aseem Malhotra, MD is quoted saying, "The overwhelming majority of people in the low risk category are not going to benefit [from statins.] Real world data [as opposed to clinical trials] tells us that one in five people will suffer a side-effect that is unacceptable."

27. Blood test scores considered healthy by alternative cardiologists:

   Total cholesterol: 180–250 mg/dL
   Total HDL cholesterol: 40–120 mg/dL for women; 35–120 mg/dL for men
   HDL cholesterol subtypes: Greater than 25 mg/dL for HDL2; greater than 15 mg/dL for HDL3. Total LDL cholesterol: 80–140 mg/dL
   LDL cholesterol subtype Lp(a): less than 30 mg/dL for a standard blood test; less than 10 mg/dL for a VAP test
   Total triglycerides: 50–100 mg/dL
   Triglycerides subtype VLDL3: less than 10 mg/dL

28. According to Medicine.net examples of beta blockers include:

   • acebutolol (Sectral)
   • atenolol (Tenormin)
   • betaxolol (Kerlone)
   • betaxolol (Betoptic S)
   • bisoprolol fumarate (Zebeta)
   • carteolol (Cartrol, discontinued)
   • carvedilol (Coreg)
   • esmolol (Brevibloc)
   • labetalol (Trandate [Normodyne - discontinued])
   • metoprolol (Lopressor, Toprol XL)
   • nadolol (Corgard)
   • nebivolol (Bystolic)
   • penbutolol (Levatol)
   • pindolol (Visken, discontinued)
   • propranolol (Hemangeol, Inderal LA Inderal XL, InnoPran XL)
   • sotalol (Betapace, Sorine)

- timolol (Blocadren, discontinued)
- timolol ophthalmic solution (Timoptic, Betimol, Istalol)

29. In June 2009 a study entitled, "Low serum cholesterol and external-cause mortality: Potential implications for research and surveillance" was published in the *Journal of Psychiatric Research*. The study followed 4,500 American veterans for fifteen years and found that men with low total cholesterol and depression were seven times more likely to die prematurely from unnatural causes such as suicide and accidents than the other men in the study.

For many years, scientific studies have linked low cholesterol to depression and impulsive behaviors, including suicide and violence. To name only two: A 1993 study reported, "Among men aged 70 years and older, categorically defined depression was three times more common in the group with low total plasma cholesterol...than in those with higher concentrations..." And a Swedish study of 300 healthy women, aged 31 to 65, concluded that women in the lowest cholesterol group-the bottom ten percentile-suffered from significantly more depressive symptoms than the others in the study.

30. In a research paper published by MIT entitled "APOE-4: The Clue to Why Low Fat Diet and Statins may Cause Alzheimer's" Dr. Stephanie Seneff has this conclusion: "It was found that Alzheimer's patients have only 1/6 of the concentration of free fatty acids in the cerebrospinal fluid compared to individuals without Alzheimer's. In parallel, it is becoming very clear that cholesterol is pervasive in the brain, and that it plays a critical role both in nerve transport in the synapse and in maintaining the health of the myelin sheath coating nerve fibers. An extremely high-fat (ketogenic) diet has been found to improve cognitive ability in Alzheimer's patients."

Dr. Seneff is associated with the Weston A. Price Foundation, a non-profit organization formed to share the research of Dr. Weston Price "whose studies of isolated non-industrialized peoples established the parameters of human health and determined the optimum characteristics of human diets." According to that Foundation, Dr. Price's research "demonstrated that humans achieve perfect physical form and perfect health generation after generation only when they consume nutrient-dense whole foods and the vital fat-soluble activators found exclusively in animal fats." Now that's confusing!

31. The body makes ATP also recycles eighty to ninety percent of it in the mitochondria, the cells' energy battery, then releases it into the fluid of cells for energy. In an interview Sinatra explained his awesome foursome metaphorically:

    D-ribose helps fill the body's gas tank while L-carnitine and CoQ10 help the body convert fuel to energy. Literally, D-ribose is a structural component of the ATP molecule, and L-carnitine and CoQ10 help recycle ATP by transporting fatty acids across mitochondrial membranes and shuttling electrons back and forth between enzymes, respectively. Co-Q10 then acts as an antioxidant to protect mitochondrial membranes from free-radical damage. Like a spark plug central to both processes, magnesium 'turns on' the enzymes that drive the entire metabolic reaction.

32. No adverse effects have been reported from CoQ10 at the doses Dr. Sinatra recommends. However he cautions that "if your heart is very starved for CoQ10, in other words, if the serum level is very low, then you want to start taking very low levels, like 10 mg once a day, or even twice a day, and just go very slowly. . . Alone, CoQ10 is great, but when we give CoQ10 in combination with the carnitine and magnesium and ribose, then you get the perfect combination for mitochondrial support. That's why people on metabolic cardiology approach absolutely thrive.

33. Research published in National Institute of Environmental Health Sciences reported that men carrying a cell phone in a hip pocket for an average of 15 hours daily over a period of six years had thinning of the pelvic bone corresponding to that hip pocket. Cell phone emissions have been linked to breast and brain cancers.

34. According to Dr. Mercola: A number of food ingredients can cause or aggravate depression, but the number one culprit is refined sugar and processed fructose, which feed pathogens in your gut, allowing them to overtake more beneficial bacteria. Sugar also suppresses the activity of a key growth hormone in your brain called brain-derived neurotrophic factor (BDNF). BDNF levels are critically low in both depression and schizophrenia. Diets high in sugar also triggers a cascade of chemical reactions in your body that promote chronic inflammation, which over the long term disrupts the normal functioning of your immune system and wreaks havoc on your brain.

35. **The EDF healthy fish list meets certain criteria for mercury contamination.**
   - Has low levels of mercury (below 216 parts per billion [ppb])
   - Provides at least 250 milligrams per day (mg/d) of omega-3s
   - Is classified as a Seafood Watch "Best Choice" (green)

   The list called Other Healthy "Best Choices"
   - Contain moderate amounts of mercury
   - Provide between 100 and 250 mg/d of omega-3s
   - Is classified as a Seafood Watch "Best Choice" (green)

36. Arjuna bark possesses glycosides, large quantities of flavonoids, tannins and minerals. Flavonoids have antioxidant, anti-inflammatory and lipid lowering effects while glycosides are cardiotonic. Experimental studies reveal its significant dose-related inotropic and hypotensive effect, increasing coronary artery flow and protecting myocardium against ischemic damage.

37. Arjuna [Terminalia arjuna] January 2005 in *Journal of Ethnopharmcology:* Oral administration of TA for 12 weeks in rabbits caused augmentation of myocardial antioxidants; superoxide dismutase (SOD), catalase (CAT) and glutathione (GSH) along with induction of heat shock protein72 (HSP72). In vivo ischemic-reperfusion injury induced oxidative stress, tissue injury of heart and hemodynamic effects were prevented in the

TA treated rabbit hearts. The study provides scientific basis for the putative therapeutic effect of TA in ischemic heart disease.

38. Western research on arjuna is limited, confused and bias. WebMD lists half a dozen herbs other than arjuna under the heading of Terminalia, For that reason Drugs.com reports these wide-ranging effects, "Terminalia has been evaluated to a limited extent for its cardiovascular properties as well as for its role in cancer therapy. Hepatoprotective, cholesterol-reducing, and antioxidant effects have been described. However, there is limited clinical information is too limited to recommend Terminalia for any use." Aside from incorrect grammar, this advice ignores the large body of world research and 3,000 years of use of the Terminalia category, which includes several different herbs such as haritaki and bibitaki as well as arjuna. No drug/herb interactions or contraindications are reported by WebMD. An interesting note is that Drugs.com contradicts itself and reports that 500 mg of arjuna herb every eight hours "can reduce angina or chest pain and increase exercise capacity in patients with cardiovascular diseases. In fact, it may be as effective isosorbide mononitrate, the most common drug used to treat angina."

39. The *Journal of Pharmacognosy and Phytochemistry* reported the study "Traditional Indian Herbs Punarnava and Its Medicinal Importance" done by researchers from Karpagam University, Coimbatore, Tamil Nadu, India. And R. K. Pharmacy College, Azamgarh, Uttar Pradesh, India. Their findings are "Being a diuretic and mild laxative, punarnava helps in detoxification and prevents fluid retention.

40. A triterpene called myrrhanol A was discovered in guggul that has potent anti-inflammatory effects. This would account for its use in arthritis and rheumatism. For that reason, guggul is an ingredient in Ayurvedic formulas used for reducing joint pain and swelling. Like myrrh guggul has antibacterial action and guggul's activity against acne has been compared to tetracycline. It decreases inflammation, reduces secretion of sebum and inhibits bacteria.

41. Heart drugs, blood thinners and guggul: Use caution and medical guidance when combining guggul with certain heart drugs such as calcium channel blockers Diltiazem (Cardizem, Dilacor, Tiazac) because taking guggul can decrease how much of the drug that the body absorbs and might decrease the drug's effectiveness.

Taking guggul along with some medications that are broken down by the liver can decrease their effectiveness. Before taking guggul talk to your healthcare provider if you are taking any medications that are changed by the liver such as lovastatin (Mevacor), atorvastatin (Lipitor), ketoconazole (Nizoral), itraconazole (Sporanox), fexofenadine (Allegra), triazolam (Halcion), and many others.

Taking guggul along with medications that also slow clotting might increase the chances of bruising and bleeding. Propranolol (Inderal) a beta-blocker heart drug interacts with guggul. Guggul might decrease how much propranolol (Inderal) the body absorbs and decrease the drug's effectiveness. Guggul might increase thyroid hormone in the body. Taking guggul along with thyroid hormone pills might increase the effects and side effects of thyroid hormones.

42. Modern research has discovered amla's wide spectrum of powerful anti-oxidants, polyphenols, tannic acids and bioflavonoids. Amla contains a high concentration of amino acids, trace minerals and other beneficial phytonutrients.

Raw Amla (Amalaki) contains the potent phenolic combination of ellagic acid, gallic acid and emblicanin A+B. Together these polyphenols are important for reducing cellular and oxidative stress, destroying immune damaging free radicals and supporting the overall detoxification of the body. The bioflavanoids, rutin and quercetin also contribute to the overall antioxidant, anti-inflammatory and youth promoting qualities of this remarkable fruit. Additionally, amla contains the potent antioxidant enzymes super oxide dismutase (SOD), glutathione peroxidase and catalase.

Online sources selling raw amla powder list these health benefits from regular daily use of cooling, detoxifying amla:

- Increasing blood flow & circulation even to the smallest capillaries

- Supporting healthy cholesterol levels
- Strong antioxidant properties
- Reducing clot-causing fibrin levels
- Acting as a body coolant
- Flushing out toxins
- Preventing oxidant-induced thickening of vessel walls
- Improving muscle tone
- Helping the urinary system
- Reducing total cholesterol & LDL in animal studies
- Improving heart health and blood vessel flexibility
- Supporting healthy cardiovascular system
- Increasing vitality
- Reducing blood sugar in diabetic laboratory animals
- Antibacterial
- Enhancing cellular regeneration
- Preventing inflammatory blood cells from sticking to endothelial linings
- Curbing free-radical oxidation of cholesterol in heart & arteries
- Reducing serum & tissue lipid levels in similar "statin" drugs—but without detectable adverse effects
- Lowering C-reactive protein
- Reducing both systolic & diastolic
- Protection against cardiovascular inflammation

43. "Total antioxidant activity of aqueous extract of amalaki, spirulina and wheat grass at 1mg/ml concentration were 7.78, 1.33 and 0.278 mmol/l respectively. At similar concentrations the total antioxidant activity of alcoholic extract of amalaki, spirulina and wheat grass was 6.67, 1.73 and 0.380 mmol/l respectively. Amalaki was also found to be rich source of phenolic compounds (241mg/g gallic acid equivalent)."

44. In a clinical study, healthy volunteers underwent two cold hands tests – one before amla supplementation, and one after. Volunteers were asked to put their hands in very cold water for a period of time which compromises endothelial function and raises blood pressure temporarily.

After the first test, the volunteers were supplemented with amla twice a day for fourteen days. All volunteers showed that same arterial stiffness and rise in blood pressure after the first cold pressure test. But after fourteen days of taking amla the second group using amla had a significant reduction of arterial stiffness (8%) as a measure of endothelial health and that showed amla supported healthy blood pressure.

45. In the *Journal of Ageing and Development*, scientists including Dr. Kalluri Subba Rao, a respected expert from Centre for Innovative Research, Nehru Technological University, Hyderabad, India, an article "Studies on the molecular correlates of genomic stability in rat brain cells following Amalakirasayana therapy" reported the successful use of amla to decrease DNA damage in brain cells caused by aging.

46. Evening primrose oil, According to University of Maryland: Along with omega-3 fatty acids, omega-6 fatty acids play a crucial role in brain function, as well as normal growth and development. Also known as polyunsaturated fatty acids they help stimulate skin and hair growth, maintain bone health, regulate metabolism, and maintain the reproductive system.

47. University of Maryland Medical Center reports, "There is some preliminary evidence that GLA may help reduce high blood pressure, either alone or in combination with the omega-3 fatty acids eicosapentaenoic acid (EPA) and docosahexaenoic acid (DHA), found in fish oil. In one study, men with borderline high blood pressure who took 6g of blackcurrant oil had a reduction in diastolic blood pressure compared to those who took placebo. Another study examined people with intermittent pain in the legs from reduced blood flow while walking which was caused by blockages in the blood vessels. Those who took GLA combined with EPA had a reduction in systolic blood pressure compared to those who took placebo."

48. If you are currently being treated with any of the following medications, you should not use omega-6 supplements without

first talking to your health care provider. They include blood thinning medications, Ceftazidime used to treat a variety of bacterial infections. Also avoid GLA with cancer chemotherapy and immunosuppressive drugs because GLA may increase their effects. People taking drugs called phenothiazines to treat schizophrenia should not take evening primrose oil or omega 6 supplements because they may increase the risk of seizures.

49. The peroxide that is 3.5% Pharmaceutical Grade which is the grade sold at your local drugstore or supermarket and contains an assortment of stabilizers which shouldn't be ingested. For example, acetanilide, phenol, sodium stanate and tertrasodium phosphate. Also 6% Beautician Grade is used in beauty shops to color hair and is not recommended for internal use.

Also 30% Reagent Grade used for various scientific experimentation also contains stabilizers. It is also not for internal use. Neither are 30% to 32% Electronic Grade which are used to clean electronic parts and 35% Technical Grade a more concentrated product than the Reagent Grade to help neutralize any chlorine from the water used to dilute it.

50. According to David G. Williams, "One of the most convenient methods of dispensing 35% H2O2 is from a small glass eye dropper bottle. These can be purchased at your local drugstore. Fill this with the 35% H2O2 and store the larger container in the freezer compartment of your refrigerator until more is needed. Store the eye dropper bottle in the refrigerator. The drops are mixed with either 6 to 8 ounces of distilled water, juice, milk or even aloe vera juice or gel. Don't use chlorinated tap water to dilute the peroxide!"

51. The May/June 2010 issue of *Nutrition Today* features the article, "Oregano: Overview of the Literature on Health Benefits" reporting that oregano has anticancer and liver protective properties. The large number of antioxidants found in oregano protect against age-related eye disease, muscle degeneration, and numerous nervous-system disorders including stress-related depression. It tastes spicy and invigorating.

52. A study published in *Cell Journal* reports carnosic acid found in rosemary "may protect against beta amyloid-induced neurodegeneration in the hippocampus." That acid has been found to be excessive in brains of people with dementia.

53. Ventricular tachycardia and ventricular fibrillation require immediate attention especially in people who have experienced heart failure or whose heart muscles are inflamed, dilated, and don't pump well, or when their left ventricle is dilated. One is ventricular tachycardia [AKA V-tach] an intense and prolonged racing of the heart. It becomes dangerous if it lasts for more than a few seconds. It can also turn into the second deadly arrhythmia ventricular fibrillation [V-fib] which occurs when chaotic electrical signals throw the ventricles off rhythm and they begin to quiver or vibrate. This is very dangerous because when the ventricles do not forcibly contract, the heart can not supply itself and the rest of the body with life-sustaining blood. V-fib may occur during a heart attack.

54. Scientific studies support the benefits of laughter in cardiac rehabilitation, pain perception, discomfort thresholds, coping with stress, and immune enhancement. One of Lee Berk's experiments involved 48 cardiac patients with diabetes who had suffered a heart attack and were receiving conventional rehabilitation care. He randomly assigned half the group to watch a 30-minute humorous video or sit-com of their choice on a daily basis. At the end of a year, the data showed that the comedy group had significantly lower blood pressure, needed fewer medications, registered healthier electrocardiograph readings. Most significantly only two of the comedy patients as compared to ten in the non-comedy group experienced new heart attacks.

55. According to University of Maryland Medical Center, laboratory studies report hawthorn contains antioxidants, including oligomeric procyandins (OPCs, also found in grapes) and quercetin. "Antioxidants found in hawthorn may help stop some of the damage from free radicals, especially when it comes to heart disease." Hawthorn's antioxidant flavonoids, including OPCs,

may help dilate blood vessels, improve blood flow, and protect the blood vessels from damage.

56. In one study participants took 1,200 mg hawthorn extract daily or placebo for 16 weeks. Those taking hawthorn had lower blood pressure than those taking the placebo. It is always best to monitor blood pressure and watch for other important signs such as sudden weight gain, swollen ankles or face that may indicate heart issues.

57. WebMD lists the following names for this respected Chinese medicinal herb: Ch'ih Shen, Chinese Red Sage, Chinese Salvia, Dan Shen, Dan-Shen, Huang Ken, Pin-Ma Ts'ao, Racine de Salvia, Radix Salviae Miltiorrhizae, Radix Salvie Miltiorrhiae, Red Rooted Sage, Red Sage, Sage Miltiorrhiza, Salvia bowelyana, Salvia miltiorrhiza, Salvia przewalskii, Salvia Przewalskii Mandarinorum, Salvia Root, Salvia yunnanensis, Salviae Miltiorrhizae, Sauge Rouge, Sauge Rouge Chinoise, Shu-Wei Ts'ao, Tan Seng, Tan-Shen, Tzu Tan-Ken. This long list of names indicates how wide-spread in the world the herb has been used to treat circulatory problems.

58. According to Chinese research reported at www.herbs2000.com: The herb [danshen] changes the rate at which the body absorbs and uses the mineral copper in metabolic processes; this has implications for blood clot formation in the human body and also has implications for chronic fatigue syndrome affected individuals. The active chemical compounds found in the danshen herb slow the production of a blood clotting protein called fibrin. . . enabling the maintenance of normal blood pressure in the circulatory system – this physiological action indirectly helps the brain to keep receiving enough oxygen necessary for normal functioning and overall fatigue in the system is beaten back.

59. Do not use danshen along with any of the following medicines because danshen can increase or replace their actions. Digoxin (Lanoxin) helps the heart beat more strongly. Some sources state that taking danshen along with digoxin may increase the effects of digoxin and increase the risk of side effects. However research

from May 2014 published in *Journal of Clinical Laboratory Analysis* reports that "LOCI digoxin assay is virtually free from interferences of Danshen and extract of bark of Arjuna tree."

Medications that slow blood clotting (anticoagulant /antiplatelet drugs) Danshen might slow blood clotting. Taking danshen might increase the chances of bruising and bleeding. For example do not use danshen along with aspirin, clopidogrel (Plavix), diclofenac (Voltaren, Cataflam, others), ibuprofen (Advil, Motrin, others), naproxen (Anaprox, Naprosyn, others), dalteparin (Fragmin), enoxaparin (Lovenox), heparin, warfarin (Coumadin), and others.

60. A 2010 controlled study published in *World Journal of Gastro-enterology* "Total salvianolic acid improves ischemia-reperfusion-induced microcirculatory disturbance in rat mesentery" investigates the effect of total salvianolic acid (TSA) on ischemia-reperfusion (I/R)-induced rat mesenteric microcirculatory dysfunctions. The danshen extract TSA was injected into veins of one of five control groups and the results concluded that the extract "protects from and ameliorates the microcirculation disturbance by inhibiting the production of oxygen-free radicals in the venular wall. When tissue is damaged and blood escapes the injury and the blood supply returns to that tissue following ischemia a lack of oxygen, the absence of oxygen and nutrients from blood during the ischemic period creates a condition in which the restoration of circulation results in inflammation and oxidative damage rather than restoration of normal function. That is called ischemia-reperfusion (I/R.) Danshen has been shown to reduce such damage to blood vessels and its use is wide-spread in China for treating stroke and related problems.

61. A 2008 study done by Department of Integration of Chinese and Western Medicine, Peking University, Beijing, China and published in *Pharmacology & Therapeutics* reports,

Ischemia and reperfusion (I/R) exerts multiple insults in microcirculation, frequently accompanied by endothelial cell injury, enhanced adhesion of leukocytes, macromolecular efflux, production of oxygen free radicals, and mast cell degranulation. Since the microcirculatory disturbance results in injury of organ involved, protection of organ after I/R is of great importance in clinic. Salvia miltiorrhiza root has long been used in Asian countries for clinical treatment of various microcirculatory disturbance-related diseases.

62. Arjuna's lipid lowering action stems from its inhibition of hepatic cholesterol biodynthesis, increased bile secretion, enhanced plasma lecithin, and stimulation of receptor mediated catabolism (reduction) of low density lipoprotein. Arjuna also inhibited development of atherosclerotic lesions despite a cholesterol rich diet (in rabbits.)

A significant study was carried out on angina heart patients for three months. There was a 50% reduction in angina (chest pain) episodes in stable angina patients, the time of the onset of angina and appearance of ST wave changes on stress tests after arjuna was significantly delayed. Unstable angina patients had no reduction in angina frequency. There was a reduction of systolic blood pressure, body mass index (which measures obesity) and marginal increase in HDL (healthy) cholesterol and some improvement in left ventricular ejection fraction in stable angina patients with no deleterious effects on liver or kidney function. With a dose of 500 mg every eight hour for one month, reduced ischemic mitral regurgitation and significantly improved diastolic dysfunction.

Another important issue is left ventricular hypertrophy – or a swollen left ventricle that is associated with a greater risk of heart failure, stroke, arrhythmias and sudden cardiac death. In the long term increasing left ventricle mass increases risk so that reduction of left ventricular hypertrophy LCH is associated with lower cardiovascular risk. In a study from 2008 published in *Food Chemistry Toxicology,* Arjuna was reported to reduce LVM along with improvement in LV ejection fraction in patients with angina. The ejection fraction is a result gained from the to-date most effective heart test, the echocardiogram, and the EF measures in effect the strength of the heart to push out blood to the rest of the body.

63. According to Carolinas Medical Center, danshen may prevent heart damage that leads to cardiomyopathy. According to Institute for Traditional Medicine in Portland, Oregon, "Salvia is reported to facilitate circulation by improving capillary bed circulation, dilating peripheral blood vessels, reducing excessive platelet aggregation (it's a blood thinner), inhibiting vascular smooth muscle cell proliferation, and having a positive iontropic effect."

64. HeartCare, by Himalaya herbal medicine company, has been clinically studied in human double-blind, placebo controlled trials to:

   • Support normal blood pressure and cholesterol levels both already within normal limits which are important measurements for overall cardiovascular wellness
   • It has mood supporting and relaxing herbs to support calmness and promote tranquility
   • Provides multifold beneficial support to the cardiovascular system, peripheral circulation, and support during physical exertion

HeartCare's ingredients combine a traditional formula called dashamula [AKA dahsmoola] with Himalaya's proprietary blend detailed below. Dashamula is a nourishing muscle tonic that strengthens the body and calms the nerves. Dashamula promotes healthy expectoration and respiration while supporting the proper function of the lungs and nervous system. The formula is very grounding and helps direct the flow of energy in the body downward. In India, a decoction of the whole herbs is used as an enema to eliminate natural toxins from the GI tract and to balance nervous irritation in the lower region of the body. According to Banyan Botanicals an online source of organic Ayurvedic herbs, "Dashamula literally means 'ten roots' referring to the traditional ingredients of the formula. Five of the plants are large trees and many of the roots are difficult to obtain sustainably. When necessary, other parts of the plants are used as effective substitutes to help ensure the protection of the species for future generations."

HeartCare ingredients:

The dashamula blend used in HeartCare is made of powdered bael tree (root), Malay bush beech (root), oroxylum (root), Clerodendrum phlomidis Linn. F. (root), fragrant padri tree (root), sarivan (root), (Uraria picta Desv. (root), solanum anguivi (root), yellow-fruit nightshade (root), tribulus (root).

Himalaya's proprietary herbal blend for HeartCare capsules is arjuna (bark), Indian catnip (whole plant), ashwagandha (root), shatavari (root), boerhavia (root), ajowan (seed), gotu kola (whole plant), Convolvulus pluricalis Choisy. (whole plant), eclipta (whole plant), amla (fruit), licorice (root), guggul (oleo-gum-resin), shilajeet (mineral pitch), holy basil (whole plant), long pepper (fruit), chebulic myrobalan (fruit rind), Indian tinospora (stem), ginger (rhizome), celastrus (fruit), cassia (bark), cyperus (tuber), cardamom (fruit), vidanga (fruit), fennel (seed), cabbage rose (flower), clove (flower bud), saffron (style & stigma).

Himalaya Herbal Healthcare company was founded in 1930. There have been over 1,200 human clinical trials on Himalaya herbal products and they are sold world wide in over seventy countries.

65. To date, over fifteen clinical trials involving 1776 people were reported for suxiao jiuxin wan at pubmed. http://www.ncbi.nlm. nih.gov/pubmed/18254051.

The conclusion of the trials was "Suxiao jiuxin wan appears to be effective in the treatment of angina pectoris and no serious side effects were identified." Another study cited at the website for University of Maryland Medical Center states: "suxiao jiuxin wan improved ECG measurements and reduced symptoms and frequency of acute angina attacks compared with nitroglycerin." The Chinese are slow to run strict clinical trials on herbs that have been in common use for hundreds of years. However, more research is being carried out on Asian herbs at NIH and at universities.

The small pill that tastes like medicinal camphor, its main ingredient, is commonly used for chest pain and prevention of blood vessel blockage. The camphor (AKA borneolum) dilates blood vessels.

The other ingredient chuanxiong (AKA *Ligusticum chuanxiong* Hort.; *L. wallichii* Franch.) stimulates heart action to sweep blood vessels clean. According to TCM the small pill that is dissolved slowly in the mouth or under the tongue, "Promotes qi and circulation. Relieves pain: like headaches, abdominal ache, chest pain, muscle pain, boils, difficulty in menses (painful period), amenorrhea (no period.) It corrects blood stasis." It feels cooling for your throat and sinus. It is relaxing and improves breathing. It may lower blood pressure and ease circulation in the head, neck and chest.

If you take this sort of natural nitroglycerine pill regularly, do not take it with food, but wait, if possible, to take it between meals. But it may be taken at any time for severe chest pain. The dose for prevention is 4 -6 small pills under the tongue three times daily. For acute heart attack 10 – 15 pills taken once or twice as needed. According to the manufacturer other uses for Suxiao jiuxin wan include:

- Dilates coronary arteries, improves blood flow to heart muscles, lowers oxygen consumption of heart muscles
- Improves blood flow to the brain and limbs, lowers resistance of the peripheral blood vessels
- Resists radiation
- Antibiotic effect
- Anti-coagulation of platelets
- Helps resist effects of lack of vitamin E

66. Bitter melon has been recommended to fight off tumors and malaria, and treat dyspepsia and constipation. In some parts of the world, bitter melon is used to treat chickenpox, measles, herpes simplex, dysentery, fever, painful menstruation, burns, scabies and other skin problems.

For every 100 grams, a boiled bitter melon contains carbohydrates (4.32 g), sugar (1.95 g), protein (0.84 g), water (93.95 g), calcium (1 mg), iron (0.38 mg), sodium (6 mg) and zinc (0.77 mg), as well as Vitamins A, B, C, E and K.

67. A study compared to the blood sugar spike of straight white rice, black beans and rice, and pinto beans and rice appeared to beat

out kidney beans and rice. Dr. Michael Greger tells us, "One of the reasons beans are so healthy is they contain compounds that partially block our starch digesting enzyme amylase which allows some starch to make it down to our colon to feed our good gut bacteria. And the inhibition of amylase by eating beans approximates that of a carb-blocking drug, acarbose, sold as Precose, a popular diabetes medication."

68. In one clinical trial, 22 people with type 2 diabetes who were taking oral diabetes drugs also took 400 mg of Gymnema sylvestre extract daily. Participants experienced significant reductions in blood sugar, hemoglobin A1c and glycosolated plasma protein levels. Significantly, at the end of the 18-month study, the participants were able to reduce their drug dosages, and five of the study subjects were able to effectively maintain normal blood sugar levels with the gymnema (GS4) alone. The researchers concluded, "the beta cells may be regenerated in type 2 diabetic patients on Gymnema sylvestre supplementation."

In other studies with type 1 (insulin-dependent) diabetes 400 mg of *Gymnema sylvestre* extract (GS4) daily a number of benefits I, including reductions in fasting blood sugar, hemoglobin A1c and glycosylated plasma protein levels. Insulin requirements were also reduced.

69. Dr. Fereydoon Batmanghelidj, M.D., who studied the effects of water in the human body for more than twenty-five years before his death in 2004, believed that chronic dehydration contributes to many of today's serious illnesses, such as heart disease, asthma, hypertension, lupus, arthritis, and multiple sclerosis. Another interesting fact is dehydration can influence cognition and even a mild level can disrupt mood, concentration, alertness, and short-term memory in children, young adults, and the elderly. Increased sweating during hot weather or after athletics is also dehydrating.

70. Reported benefits of apple cider vinegar:

- Improves insulin sensitivity during a high-carbohydrate meal by 19-34% and significantly lowers blood glucose and insulin responses
- Reduces blood sugar by 34% when eating 50 grams of white bread
- 2 tablespoons of apple cider vinegar before bedtime can reduce fasting blood sugars by 4%
- Numerous studies show that vinegar can increase insulin sensitivity and significantly lower blood sugar responses during meals
- Vinegar can be useful for people with diabetes, pre-diabetes, or those who want to keep their blood sugar levels low to normal for other reasons.

71. A 2012 study documents that Panax ginseng protects heart cells from oxygen-deprivation free radical damage and significantly reduces the amount of damage from experimentally induced heart attack. It improves the production of nitric oxide, in turn helping arteries relax and blood flow better. Another new study with spontaneously hypertensive rats found that Panax ginseng induced the release of friendly nitric oxide (eNOS), improved the health of arterial blood vessels, and eliminated their high blood pressure.

72. Scientific studies in June, 2006 Life Extension magazine support ashwagandha's ability to protect brain cells. For example, ashwagandha has been proven as effective as some tranquilizers and antidepressant drugs. Stress causes increased peroxidation of lipids, while decreasing levels of the antioxidant enzymes catalase and glutathione peroxidase. Ashwagandha extract normalizes these parameters of free radical damage in a dose-dependent manner. Premature aging and chronic nervous tension are abolished by antioxidants in ashwagandha extract. Another amazing study in Life Extension reports that 85% of the brain cells observed in animals exposed to chronic stress showed signs of degeneration and long-term cognitive difficulties. Ashwagandha

was administered daily and the number of degenerating brain cells was reduced by 80%.

Ashwagandha scavenges free radicals. Its steroidal alkaloids and steroidal lactones may account for its beneficial effects. To date, scientists have studied at least 12 alkaloids and 35 withanolides in ashwagandha, primarily withanolides, withaferin A and withanolide D.

73. Tibetan goji berry contains:

• Macronutrients:
~13% complete vegetarian protein with 18 amino acids, half of which are in free form (not bound up in proteins) ~8.2% essential fatty acids half of which are polyunsaturated fats ~67.7% carbohydrates with 10% being fiber, 36% being polysaccharides (very complex long chain sugars) and *only 21.7% being simple sugars* (making this a low-glycemic fruit)
• Vitamins:
~A ~B1, B2, B5 (in small amounts) and B6 ~C (although not in as high amounts as so many MLM companies claim) ~E (which is rarely found in fruits)
• Minerals:
~Calcium ~Copper ~Germanium ~Iron ~Magnesium ~Manganese ~Phosphorus ~Potassium ~Selenium ~Sodium ~Zinc ~and   many other trace minerals!
• Antioxidants (ORAC of 25,300):
~5 carotenoids (beta carotene, lutein, lycopene, cryptoxanthin and zeaxanthin) ~Riboflavin ~Ascorbic acid ~Cystine ~Copper ~Selenium ~Manganese
• Phytonutrients:
~5 *lycium barbarum* glycoconjugate polysaccharides (LbGp 1-5 are immuno-modulators, protect against DNA mutations and increase blood serum levels of superoxide dismutase) ~Betaine (protects DNA, increases choline production in the liver, calms the nervous system, enhances memory, promotes muscle growth, prevents fatty liver disease and detoxifies the liver) ~Physaline (anti-cancer, anti-leukemia, immune system booster and treats hepatitis B) ~Sesquiterpenoids (hgh

secretagogue, treats cervical cancer, treats menstrual discomfort and benefits the heart and blood pressure) ~Solavetivone (anti-fungal and anti-bacterial) ~Beta-sitosterol (anti-inflammatory, lowers cholesterol, treats sexual impotence and treats prostate enlargement.)

74. Rehmannia has been used for correcting the suppressive effects of corticosteroid (steroid) drugs. It improves anemia. It is used for mitigating certain side-effects of chemotherapeutic agents and HIV medications, curing eczema skin dryness, relieving pain from lung or bone cancer or disc protrusion, and helping ameliorate lupus nephritis (kidney inflammation) and type 2 diabetes with hyperlipidemia (high cholesterol).

Look for rehmannia [AKA di huang] in herbal formulas that combine it with digestive herbs because used along it is too gluey and sweet. Also using too strong a dose may have side-effects from one of its major components arginine which might bring out a herpes rash. Here are a couple of safe herbal blood tonics to give you an idea of how they can make life easier and more pleasant.

75. Red reishi mushroom (Ganoderma lucidum) from Japan or China has been shown to reduce DNA exposure to radiation damage. Researchers in the USA and Asia have long known that reishi is primarily composed of complex carbohydrates called water-soluble polysaccharides, triterpeniods, proteins and amino acids. Water-soluble polysaccharides are the most active element found in red reishi that have anti-tumor, immune modulating and blood pressure lowering effects.

Another major active ingredient found in red reishi are triterpenes, called ganoderic acids. Preliminary studies indicated that ganoderic acids help alleviate common allergies by inhibiting histamine release, improve oxygen utilization and improve liver functions. Triterpenes are bitter in taste and the level of the triterpene content contained in a product can be determined by the bitterness.

76. Astragalus research: A 2011 study published in *Nature* reported results from experiments done at Mayo Clinic. Researchers devised

a way to kill all senescent cells in genetically engineered mice. The animals aged far more quickly than normal, and when they were given a drug, the senescent cells would die. The researchers looked at three symptoms of old age: formation of cataracts in the eye; the wasting away of muscle tissue; and the loss of fat deposits under the skin, which keep it smooth. Researchers said the onset of these symptoms was "dramatically delayed" when the animals were treated with the drug. When it was given after the mice had been allowed to age, there was an improvement in muscle function.

The study raises the hopeful prospect of slowing the signs of ageing in humans. Senescent cells cannot be simply flushed out, however Dr Jan van Deursen, one of the principals in the study, told BBC news, "We were very surprised by the very profound effect. I really think this is very significant. . . I'm very optimistic that this could really have an impact. Nobody wants to live longer if the quality of life is poor." Young people can clear out their senescent cells. He said, "If you can prime the immune system, boost it a little bit, to make sure senescent cells are removed, that might be all it needs. "

How might we duplicate this cellular cleansing process naturally? By boosting our immune system. For example with tonics such as L. Carnitine and astragalus which spark cell rejuvenation.

77. Geriforte from India slows aging by regulating metabolism, improving digestion, reducing stress and fatigue and enhancing immunity. Geriforte promotes healthy cardiovascular and respiratory functions. Among its many vegetarian ingredients are Chyawanprash concentrate, turmeric, chicory, arjuna, asparagus, licorice, shilajeet, nutmeg, mace, saffron, clove, and iron (ferric oxide.)

Shilajeet [AKA shilajit, fulvic acid, mineral pitch] is worth volumes of information and praise as a rejuvenating adaptogen, and immune-enhancing stimulant. Shilajit's origin lies in the ancient, putrified organic plant material preserved by the darkness and pressure of the Himalayas. As the sun warms up the mountain, the snow melts and a soft, heavy shilajit resin seeps from rock crevices and is collected by local farmers. This thick resin is then dried and ground into a fine powder high in iron and important nutrients including fulvic acid, calcium, selenium and magnesium. Researched in India and Russia it is well known as a healer for broken bones and a weak constitution or slow recovery from illness. Shilajit gives our bones, muscles, and cells the strength of stone, the purity of diamonds in the rough. It smells like the inside of a damp cave. I do not recommend buying the expensive organic powder sold by health food stores because no matter how you try to cover the flavor by adding it to smoothies, it still tastes like melted rock or dung. I buy the capsules in East Indian health and food shops. The usual dosage is two capsules twice daily as a tonic. You can take it with an equal dose of ashwagandha to support muscles, bones, and blood. It is combined with many other beneficial herbs in Geriforte and Chyawanprash.

78. A study in the June 2011 issue of the *Journal of Ethnopharmacology* explored the anticancer activities of Eclipta alba on a line of liver cancer cells. The researchers noted that an alcoholic extraction of eclipta inhibited the growth of cancer cells and had cytotoxic effects (killing the cancer cells) by preventing proliferation of cancer cells through the disruption of the DNA molecules; thereby effectively inhibiting the spread of the disease. . . Eclipta alba has antimicrobial effects. An article appearing in the May 2011 issue of the *Annals of Clinical Microbiology and Antimicrobials* investigated the antimicrobial effects of Eclipta alba on secondary infections of patients undergoing anticancer treatment. At least nine different pathogenic bacterial species were identified, including Staphylococcus aureus causing staph infections, Escherichia coli, causing gastrointestinal problems, and Staphylococcus epidermis, a common cause of boils. Eclipta alba was an effective antimicrobial agent against all of the tested organisms,

79. Drug interactions: Serrapeptase might decrease blood clotting. Therefore, taking serrapeptase along with medications that also slow clotting might increase the chances of bruising and bleeding. Some medications that slow blood clotting include aspirin, clopidogrel (Plavix), diclofenac (Voltaren, Cataflam, others), ibuprofen (Advil, Motrin, others), naproxen (Anaprox, Naprosyn,

others), dalteparin (Fragmin), enoxaparin (Lovenox), heparin, warfarin (Coumadin), and others.

80. Cordyceps studies: See (Zhu, J.S., Halpern, G.M., and Jones, K. (1998): "The Scientific Rediscovery of a Precious Ancient Chinese Herbal Regimen: Cordyceps sinensis. Parts I and II." *Journal of Alternative and complementary Medicine*.) Another study was conducted on acute pulmonary edema (pneumonia) which causes systemic lack of oxygen, acidic body, and death. Research results show that animals taking cordyceps had a 400% improvement rate.

81. Aspiration pills by Health Concerns: The ingredients are Yuan Zhi (Polygala root) Herba Verbenae Officinalis (Vervain herb) Gou Teng (Uncaria stem) Zhi Zi (Gardenia Fruit) He Huan Hua (Albizzia flowers) Folium Turnerae aphrodisiacae (Damiana leaf) Bai Shao (White Peony root) Dang Gui (Tang Kuei root) Ban Xia (Pinellia rhizome) Fu Ling (Poria sclerotium) Chen Xiang (Aquilaria sinensis lignum.)

82. Bach Flower Remedies and what they treat:

Agrimony	You try to hide troubling thoughts and inner unrest behind cheerfulness and carelessness.
Aspen	You have unreasonable, vague trepidations, premonitions, secret fear of any threatening disaster.
Beech	You tend to be perfectionist, over-critical, arrogant, intolerant, lacking empathy.
Centaury	You over react to the wishes of others. You can't say "no".
Cerato	You lack confidence in your own intuition.
Cherry-Plum	You have fear of letting go, fear of losing your intellect and going crazy
Chestnut Bud	You make the same mistakes again and again because you don't process experiences and learn enough from it.

Chicory	You feel possessive, critical and expect everyone to be attentive and devoted to your will. You feel terrible if you don't get your way.
Clematis	You daydream, always somewhere else in thoughts, showing little attention to surroundings.
Crab Apple	You feel dirty inside and outside, impure or infected. "The cleansing blossom" for self-hatred.
Elm	You have the temporary feeling that your task or responsibility is too much for you to handle.
Gentian	You are discouraged, disappointed, doubting, pessimistic, easily dispiritedly.
Gorse	You are without hope, feel complete despair.
Heather	You like an audience. You have self concern like "the small needful child."
Holly	You feel strong hot emotions like jealousy, suspicion, hate and envy
Honeysuckle	You long for the past; feel sorry about things passed. You do not live in the present.
Hornbeam	You are tired, mentally exhausted at the thought of doing something.
Impatiens	You are impatient, easily irritably, over shooting reactions.
Larch	You expect to fail through lack of self-confidence, an inferiority complex.
Mimulus	You have specific fears that you can name; also timidity, fear of the world.
Mustard	You have periods of deep melancholy
Oak	You continue bravely and never gives up.
Olive	You feel total exhaustion, extreme fatigue of body and spirit.
Pine	You feel guilty, have self-reproach, discouragement.
Red Chestnut	You have over-concern, exaggerated worries about others.
Rock Rose	You have extremely acute anxiety, terror, panic feelings.
Rock Water	You have severe, rigid views and suppress your needs

Scleranthus	You can't decide what to do. Unbalanced your opinions and mood change from moment to moment
Star of Beth-lehem	You feel the after-effects of bodily, psychological or intellectual shocks no matter whether taking place long ago or recently. This remedy is "the soul comforter and pain calmer."
Sweet Chest-nut	You feel deepest despair, the end of your rope.
Vervain	You are zealous, feel righteous, irritable to fanatical. You can do no wrong
Vine	You like to feel dominating. You may be power-hungrily "The little tyrant."
Walnut	You seek protection from annihilation, you feel vulner-able, unsteady during decisive new beginning phases in the life. This is "the blossom that makes the break-through" possible.
Water Violet	You are at times stand-offish, proud and feel isolated superiority
White Chest-nut	You can't stop unwanted thoughts, inner self conversa-tions and dialogues again and again.
Wild Oat	You have frustrated ambitions, dissatisfaction because you don't find your direction in life.
Wild rose	You feel Indifference, apathy, resignation
Willow	You feel self-pity, hold a grudge, feel bitterness. You feel you are "the victim of destiny."

83. Python pills come with a manufacture's warning

NOT FOR USE BY INDIVIDUALS UNDER THE AGE OF 18 YEARS. Do not use if you are pregnant or nursing. Consult a physician or licensed qualified health care professional before using this product if you have, or have a family history of prostate cancer, prostate enlargement, heart disease, low "good cholesterol" (HDL), or if you are using any other dietary supplement, prescription drug, or over-the-counter drug. Do not exceed recommended serving. Exceeding recommended serving may cause serious adverse health effects. Possible side effects include acne, hair loss, hair growth on the face (in women), aggressiveness, irritability, and increase levels estrogen. Discontinue use and call a physician or licensed qualified health care professional immediately if you experience rapid heartbeat, dizziness, blurred vision, or other similar symptoms.

84. In a test of 75 healthy fertile men and 75 infertile men, in both cases, Ashwagandha increased sperm count, quality and motility and also increased serum testosterone and luteinizing hormone (LH), while reducing levels of follicle stimulating hormone (FSH) and prolactin. . . . Ashwagandha has been shown to increase the size and weight of testicles. . . increase the production of sperm, and the levels of lutenizing hormone which is responsible for the production of testosterone in the Leydig cells. Ashwagandha affects the gonadotropin releasing hormone (GnRH) neuronal activities and thus the release of LH and FSH in the Anterior pituitary by mediating the GABA(A) receptor. . . further testimony to the profound synergy we have with our herbal allies.

SELECT RESOURCE GUIDE

In my books, articles, and radio broadcasts I recommend many natural products for health, wellness and beauty. Product origin, quality control, and price are important factors. Here is a short list of recommended sources featuring products for heart care and related topics covered in this book. It is also updated in the "Product" section of www.asianhealthsecrets.com

Addictions:

Reduce nervous anxiety and stress, improve mood and reduce addictive behavior with a natural dietary salt of orotic acid and lithium in a capsule http://www.absorbyourhealth.com/product/lithium-orotate/?ref=4041

Energy/Immunity:

Liposomal Vitamin C absorbs 10 times more efficiently than traditional oral Vitamin C because it is broken down into nano-sized particles. http://www.absorbyourhealth.com/product/liposomal-vitamin-c-best-price-net-1-gram-vit-c-every-teaspoon/?ref=4041

Ashwagandha capsules an Ayurvedic tonic for energy, chronic pain, immunity and sexuality: http://www.absorbyourhealth.com/product/ashwagandha/?ref=4041

Chaga mushroom capsules a great tonic for energy and immunity, an anti-inflammatory painkiller and a powerful supplement for anti-aging. http://www.absorbyourhealth.com/product/chaga-mushroom-extract-30-polysaccharides-400mg-100-capsules/?ref=4041

Heart Health:

Pterostilobene similar to resveratrol, it reduces cholesterol, triglycerides, high blood sugar reducing hypertension and diabetes. http://www.absorbyourhealth.com/?ref=4041&s=pterostilbene

Magnesium Threonate improves memory and circulation, helps blood vessels stay healthy: http://www.absorbyourhealth.com/product/magnesium-threonate-500mg-100-capsules-nootropic-absorbable-mag3/?ref=4041

A combination of artemisinin, pterostilbene, and liposomal resveratrol. for heart protection and longevity. Artemisin is antiviral, pterostilbene and resveratrol fight cognitive decline and regulate cholesterol to protect the heart. http://www.absorbyourhealth.com/product/longevity-power-pack/?ref=4041

Medicinal mushroom capsules for antioxidants, immunity: http://www.absorbyourhealth.com/product/medicinal-mushroom-power-pack-2/?ref=4041

Pine Bark Extract: Anti-inflammatory, antioxidant, tonic: http://www.absorbyourhealth.com/product/pine-bark-extract-200mg-100-capsules-95-opc-flavanoids-powerful-antioxidant-free-radical-scavenger-dr-oz-recommended-skin/?ref=4041

Turmeric – liposomal curcumin
Curcumin the most absorbable form of turmeric extract, a powerful antioxidant: http://www.absorbyourhealth.com/product/liposomal-curcumin-best-price-net-95-curcuminoids-highest-dose/?ref=4041

Mental/Emotional Balance:

Brain Repair Power Pack improves memory and cognition, regulates cholesterol and blood sugar to protect immunity and correct brain deterioration. A combination of four capsules Acetyl L-Carnitine, Krill oil, Urdine, Choline Bitartrate: http://www.absorbyourhealth.com/product/brain-repair-power-pack/?ref=4041

Brain Repair Power Pack with auto-renewal: http://www.absorbyourhealth.com/product/brain-repair-power-pack-auto-renew/?ref=4041

Essential oil of grapefruit for depression, anxiety and vitality, for external use. http://www.absorbyourhealth.com/product/grape-fruit-essential-oil/?ref=4041

Lift Your Mood supplements: http://www.absorbyourhealth.com/product/mood-enhancer-power-pack/?ref=4041

Himalayan Bacopa [AKA brahmi] improves memory and understanding to improve sleep and refresh brain health. http://www.absorbyourhealth.com/product/bacopa-monniera-375mg-101-extract-100-capsules-memory-learning-supplement-himalaya-brahmi/?ref=4041

Sexuality:
PriMale sexual enhancement capsules that increase libido and male sexual potency with herbs to increase testosterone: http://www.absorbyourhealth.com/product/primale/?ref=4041

Weight Loss:
Garcinia, African mango and white kidney bean extract capsules enhance metabolism and improve heart health. http://www.absorbyourhealth.com/product/weight-loss-power-pack/?ref=4041

Ayurvedic herbs grown in the USA
Neem Tree Farms
Brandon, FL 33511
877-500-6336 www.neemtreefarms.com
Neem products for health and beauty

Ayurvedic Herbs, organic from India
Banyan Botanicals
Albuquerque, New Mexico
(800) 953-6424, www.banyanbotanicals.com
Organic health, beauty and wellness bulk herbs, powders, oils

Himalaya Herbal Healthcare
Sugar Land, Texas 77478
(800) 869-4640 **www.himalayausa.com**
Heart Care and Ayurvedic herbal capsules

Chinese Herbal Products
Health Concerns
Oakland, CA 94621
(800) 233 -9355 www.healthconcerns.com

Mayway Corporation
Oakland, CA 94607
(800 2MAYWAY **www.mayway.com**

Teas
Bird Pick Tea and Herbs
Pasadena, California
(888) 832-4372, http://www.birdpick.com/

Camellia Sinensis Tea Shop and Tea School
Montréal, QC H2X 1J2,
Canada
514.286.4002 http://camellia-sinensis.com

Colloidal silver, gold for energy and immunity
Colloids for Life LLC www.colloidsforlife.com

Information on protection against radiation and electromagnetic related illness
http://www.emfcenter.com/emffaqs.htm#B1.%20What%20
are%20Electromagnetic%20Fields%20%28EMFs%29

Information on health foods, non-antibiotic grown, free range eggs and meats etc.
from www.localharvest.org and www.eatwellguide.org

ABOUT THE AUTHORS

Letha Hadady, born into an old noble Hungarian family was raised in New Mexico, sang opera in Europe, has a Masters in psychology from the University of Paris and was nationally certified in acupuncture (NCCAOM) after studying at Tri-State Institute of Traditional Chinese Medicine, New York and the Institute of Acupuncture and Meridian in Shanghai. She studied Ayurveda in India and the U.S. with Dr. Vasant Lad and Tibetan wellness practices and philosophy with Drs. Yeshi Donden, Sogyal Rinpoche, and with HH the Dalai Lama.

Letha's books include
Asian Health Secrets (Random) Foreword by HH Dalai Lama
Personal Renewal (Crown/iUniverse) Foreword by Dr. Bernard Jensen
Healthy Beauty (Wiley/iUniverse) Foreword by Cliff deRaita
Feed Your Tiger (Rodale/iUniverse)
Naturally Pain Free (Sourcebooks)

The San Francisco Chronicle wrote, "Letha Hadady, one of the nation's leading experts on natural Chinese remedies, is leading a quiet lady-like revolution to bring herbal medicines from the Far East and elsewhere into everyday use in American homes." Since 2012 Letha has reached a world wide Internet radio audience along with host Marie Griffiths on "MG Live" at 105.1 mikefm.ca live from Montreal. Letha's natural health website is www.asianhealthsecrets. com Letha can be reached at Facebook and Twitter. https://www. facebook.com/letha.hadady.9

Michael Foster (1937-2016) was born in Coney Island, Brooklyn. His parents a loving happy couple, ran a lunch counter with a Murder Incorporated gambling operation in the back room. The tough kid on the block, Michael read the Russian classics by age ten, and was awarded a full scholarship to Cornell at sixteen and Harvard Law at twenty. A seeker of truth and adventure, he traveled to Haiti and North Africa and finally left Harvard to join Che's revolution in Cuba. He wrote historical novels, biographies, and erotic history. He was destined to create new ideas and relationships. His books have been translated into German, Spanish, Turkish, Slovenian and Korean.

Michael's books include
Freedom's Thunder (Avon Books)
The Serpent's Kiss (Kindle) (Amazon)
Forbidden Journey (Harper & Roe)
The Secret Lives of Alexandra David-Neel (Overlook)
Three in Love: Menages a Trois from Ancient to Modern Times (Harper Collins*)*
A Dangerous Woman: The Life, Loves and Scandals of Adah Isaacs Menken (Lyons Press)
As of 2016, Michael had written the sequel to *Three in Love* and a satirical graphic novel including stock market tips.

The New York Review of Books called his biography, *The Secret Lives of Alexandra David-Neel,* "one of the best books ever written" and *Entertainment Weekly* called *Three in Love* "racy and engaging." Michael's facebook page is https://www.facebook.com/mickey. stamler

70830984R00241

Made in the USA
Middletown, DE
21 April 2018